Hormones, Cognition and Dementia

State of the Art and Emergent
Therapeutic Strategies

Hormones, Cognition and Dementia

State of the Art and Emergent Therapeutic Strategies

Edited by

Eef Hogervorst PhD
Professor of Biological Psychology, Department of Human Sciences, Loughborough University, Loughborough, UK; Visiting Senior Research Fellow, Department of Public Health and Primary Care, University of Cambridge, UK; Visiting Professor, Department of Epidemiology and Public Health, University of Respati, Jakarta, Indonesia

Victor W. Henderson MD MS
Professor of Health Research and Policy (Epidemiology) and of Neurology and Neurological Sciences, Stanford University, CA, USA

Robert B. Gibbs PhD
Professor of Pharmaceutical Sciences, University of Pittsburgh, Pittsburgh, PA, USA

Roberta Diaz Brinton PhD
Professor of Molecular Pharmacology and Toxicology, Neuroscience and Biomedical Engineering, University of Southern California, Los Angeles, CA, USA

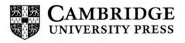

CAMBRIDGE
UNIVERSITY PRESS

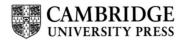

Shaftesbury Road, Cambridge CB2 8EA, United Kingdom

One Liberty Plaza, 20th Floor, New York, NY 10006, USA

477 Williamstown Road, Port Melbourne, VIC 3207, Australia

314–321, 3rd Floor, Plot 3, Splendor Forum, Jasola District Centre, New Delhi – 110025, India

103 Penang Road, #05–06/07, Visioncrest Commercial, Singapore 238467

Cambridge University Press is part of Cambridge University Press & Assessment, a department of the University of Cambridge.

We share the University's mission to contribute to society through the pursuit of education, learning and research at the highest international levels of excellence.

www.cambridge.org
Information on this title: www.cambridge.org/9780521899376

First published 2009

A catalogue record for this publication is available from the British Library

Library of Congress Cataloging-in-Publication data
Hormones, cognition, and dementia : state of the art and emergent therapeutic strategies / edited by Eef Hogervorst . . . [et al.].
     p. ; cm.
  Includes bibliographical references and index.
  ISBN 978-0-521-89937-6 (hardback)
1. Dementia–Prevention. 2. Estrogen–Therapeutic use.
I. Hogervorst, Eef.
  [DNLM: 1. Dementia–prevention & control. 2. Estrogen Replacement Therapy. 3. Cognition–drug effects. 4. Women's Health.
WP 522 H8135 2009]
  RC521.H68 2009
  616.8′3–dc22

                      2009024543

ISBN   978-0-521-89937-6   Hardback

....

Contents

Contents

Contributors

Farook Al-Azzawi MA PhD FRCOG
Gynaecology Research Unit,
University Hospitals of Leicester,
Leicester, UK

Wita Angrianni PhD
Faculty of Dentistry,
University of Trisaklti,
Jakarta, Indonesia

Sanjay Asthana MD FRCPC
Section of Geriatrics and Gerontology,
Department of Medicine,
University of Wisconsin School of Medicine and
Public Health,
Madison, WI;
Geriatric Research, Education and Clinical Center
(GRECC),
William S. Middleton Memorial Veterans Hospital,
Madison, WI, USA

Stephan Bandelow PhD
Department of Human Sciences,
Loughborough University,
Loughborough, UK

Kathryn J. Bryan PhD
Department of Pathology,
Case Western Reserve University,
Cleveland, OH, USA

Cynthia M. Carlsson MD MS
Section of Geriatrics and Gerontology,
Department of Medicine,
University of Wisconsin School of Medicine and
Public Health,
Madison, WI;
Geriatric Research, Education and Clinical Center
(GRECC),
William S. Middleton Memorial Veterans Hospital,
Madison, WI, USA

Jenna C. Carroll BA
Davis School of Gerontology and Neuroscience
Graduate Program,
University of Southern California,
Los Angeles, CA, USA

Gemma Casadesus PhD
Department of Neurosciences,
Case Western Reserve University,
Cleveland, OH, USA

Monique M. Cherrier PhD
Department of Psychiatry and Behavioral Sciences,
University of Washington School of Medicine;
Veterans Administration Puget Sound Health Care
System GRECC,
Seattle, WA, USA

Laura H. Coker PhD
Department of Public Health Sciences,
Wake Forest University School of Medicine,
Winston-Salem, NC, USA

María M. Corrada ScD
Institute for Brain Aging and Dementia,
Department of Neurology,
University of California, Irvine,
Irvine, CA, USA

Vita Priantina Dewi MHS
Center for Health Research,
University of Indonesia,
Jakarta, Indonesia

Roberta Diaz Brinton PhD
Department of Pharmacology and Pharmaceutical
Sciences,
University of Southern California School of
Pharmacy and Pharmaceutical Sciences Center,
Los Angeles, CA;
Program in Neuroscience,

University of Southern California,
Los Angeles, CA, USA

Mark A. Espeland PhD
Division of Public Health Sciences,
Wake Forest University School of Medicine,
Winston-Salem, NC, USA

Mirjam I. Geerlings PhD
Julius Center, University Medical Center Utrecht,
Utrecht, The Netherlands

Robert B. Gibbs PhD
University of Pittsburgh School of Pharmacy,
Pittsburgh, PA, USA

Carey E. Gleason PhD
Section of Geriatrics and Gerontology,
Department of Medicine,
University of Wisconsin School of Medicine and
Public Health,
Madison, WI;
Geriatric Research, Education and Clinical Center
(GRECC),
William S. Middleton Memorial Veterans Hospital,
Madison, WI, USA

Victor W. Henderson MD MS
Departments of Health Research and Policy
(Epidemiology) and Neurology and Neurological
Sciences, Stanford University,
Stanford, CA, USA

Patricia E. Hogan MS
Division of Public Health Sciences,
Wake Forest University School of Medicine,
Winston-Salem, NC, USA

Eef Hogervorst PhD
Department of Human Sciences,
Loughborough University,
Loughborough, UK

Claudia H. Kawas MD
Institute for Brain Aging and Dementia,
Departments of Neurology and Neurobiology and
Behavior, University of California, Irvine,
Irvine, CA, USA

Anna Khaylis MS
Department of Psychiatry and Behavioral Sciences,
Stanford University School of Medicine,
Stanford, CA, USA

Philip Kreager DPhil
Oxford Institute of Ageing, Oxford, UK

Linda Kushandy PhD
Faculty of Dentistry, University of Indonesia,
Jakarta, Indonesia

Donald Lehmann
University Department of Pharmacology,
Oxford, UK

Jin Li PhD
Gynaecology Research Unit,
University Hospitals of Leicester,
Leicester, UK

Mary E. McAsey PhD
Department of Obstetrics and Gynecology,
SIU School of Medicine,
Springfield, IL, USA

Pauline M. Maki MD
Center for Cognitive Medicine,
Neuropsychiatric Institute,
University of Illinois at Chicago,
Chicago, IL, USA

Ralph N. Martins PhD
School of Psychiatry and Clinical Neurosciences,
University of Western Australia,
Crawley, WA, Australia

Scott D. Moffat PhD
Institute of Gerontology and Department of
Psychology,
Wayne State University,
Detroit, MI, USA

Majon Muller MD PhD
Department of Geriatric Medicine,
University of Utrecht Medical Center,
Utrecht, The Netherlands

Theresia Ninuk PhD
University of Respati, Yogyakarta, Indonesia

Annlia Paganini-Hill PhD
Department of Preventative Medicine,
Keck School of Medicine,
University of Southern California;
Department of Neurology,
University of California,
Irvine, CA, USA

George Perry PhD
Department of Pathology,
Case Western Reserve University,
Cleveland, OH;
College of Sciences, University of Texas at San Antonio,
San Antonio, TX, USA

Christian J. Pike PhD
Davis School of Gerontology and Neuroscience
Graduate Program,
University of Southern California,
Los Angeles, CA, USA

Bevin N. Powers BA
Department of Psychiatry and Behavioral Sciences,
Stanford University School of Medicine,
Stanford, CA, USA

Tri Budi W. Rahardjo PhD
Center for Health Research, University of Indonesia,
Jakarta, Indonesia

Natalie L. Rasgon MD PhD
Department of Psychiatry and Behavioral Sciences,
Stanford University School of Medicine,
Stanford, CA, USA

Susan M. Resnick PhD
Laboratory of Personality and Cognition,
Intramural Research Program,
National Institute on Aging, NIH, Baltimore, MD, USA

Emily R. Rosario
Davis School of Gerontology,
University of Southern California,
Los Angeles, CA, USA

Sabarinah MD MSc
Center for Health Research,
University of Indonesia,
Jakarta, Indonesia

Tony Sadjimim MD PhD
University of Respati, Yogyakarta, Indonesia

Barbara B. Sherwin PhD
Department of Psychology, McGill University,
Montreal, Canada

Sally A. Shumaker PhD
Division of Public Health Sciences,
Wake Forest University School of Medicine,
Winston-Salem, NC, USA

Mark A. Smith PhD
Department of Pathology,
Case Western Reserve University,
Cleveland, OH, USA

Robert G. Struble PhD
Center for Alzheimer Disease and Related Disorders,
SIU School of Medicine,
Springfield, IL, USA

Chris Talbot PhD
Department of Genetics, Leicester University,
Leicester, UK

Wulf H. Utian MBBCh PhD DSc(Med)
North American Menopause Society,
Mayfield Heights, OH, USA

Giuseppe Verdile
Centre of Excellence for Alzheimer's Disease Research
and Care,
Sir James McCusker Alzheimer's Disease Research
Unit,
School of Exercise, Biomedical and Health Sciences,
Edith Cowan University,
Joondalup, WA, Australia

Robert B. Wallace MS MD
Department of Epidemiology,
The University of Iowa,
Iowa City, IA, USA

Whitney Wharton PhD
Section of Geriatrics and Gerontology,
Department of Medicine,
University of Wisconsin School of Medicine and
Public Health,
Madison, WI, USA

Katherine E. Williams MD
Department of Psychiatry and Behavioral Sciences,
Stanford University School of Medicine,
Stanford, CA, USA

Oliver T. Wolf PhD
Department of Cognitive Psychology,
Ruhr-University Bochum,
Bochum, Germany

Tonita E. Wroolie PhD
Department of Psychiatry and Behavioral Sciences,
Stanford University School of Medicine,
Stanford, CA, USA

Amina Yesufu BSc
Department of Human Sciences,
Loughborough University,
Loughborough, UK

Yudarini MPH
Center for Health Research,
University of Indonesia, Jakarta, Indonesia

Liqin Zhao PhD
Department of Pharmacology and Pharmaceutical
Sciences,
University of Southern California School
of Pharmacy and Pharmaceutical Sciences Center,
Los Angeles, CA, USA

Preface

In the 1980s and 1990s, laboratory and clinical research suggested that estrogens were promising candidates in women for the treatment of dementia due to Alzheimer's disease and for age-related cognitive decline. However, soon after the turn of the century, there was a remarkable change in attitude, which was almost comparable to a paradigm shift. As stated by Professor David Purdie (Edinburgh) in a 2003 BBC interview, "The only thing hormone replacement therapy has not yet been accused of is global warming and aggravating the national debt." To a major extent, this change was the result of the Women's Health Initiative, a large placebo-controlled clinical trial of conjugated equine estrogens with or without a progestogen, in which a number of health outcomes were examined. Beginning in 2002, Women's Health Initiative publications reported important adverse health effects of hormone treatment, including the heretofore unappreciated risk of coronary heart disease. An ancillary study of women aged 65 years and older, the Women's Health Initiative Memory Study (WHIMS), was an important milestone in scientific research on steroid hormones and cognition, and it is the logical starting point for work presented in this volume.

The WHIMS is the only clinical trial to have examined effects of estrogens on dementia risk, and it is one of the largest trials to have considered estrogenic effects on cognitive outcomes in older women without dementia. The primary finding of increased risk of dementia in women who were randomized to receive hormone therapy came at a time when several clinical trials failed to show clinical benefit of estrogens in women with Alzheimer's disease. Further, results from the WHIMS, as well as from other clinical trials in older postmenopausal women, were unable to document cognitive benefit of estrogens in women without dementia.

These largely unexpected findings constitute a clarion call to reassess where the field is today and to re-examine some of the basic and clinical underpinnings of our current knowledge in areas related to sex steroid hormones, cognitive aging, and dementia. This book brings together contributions from many of the most prominent researchers in areas of women's health, cognition, and steroid clinical endocrinology. These investigators have applied techniques from cell culture, animal models, human populations, clinical trials, and brain imaging in an attempt to understand effects of estrogens, androgens, progestogens, and the gonadotropins on human cognition and aging. Contributors to this volume summarize our current state of knowledge on selected topics and highlight areas where new research is needed. Through this means, we hope to promote collaborative, interdisciplinary research with translational goals: what can we learn from basic and clinical studies that we can apply to future therapies in older men and women?

This book is loosely divided into six sections. The first summarizes the most recent data from the WHIMS, including new brain imaging data, and it describes novel analytical techniques that attempt to find subgroups for whom cognitive outcomes might be improved by hormone therapy. Novel data from a study of nonogenarians and centurians substantiate increased risks for dementia among very old women using hormone treatment for long periods of time. One important question raised by the WHIMS is that of a critical window close to the time of natural menopause. During this so-called window, might estrogens reduce the risk of harmful outcomes, such as Alzheimer's disease, even if later therapy does not? If so, what factors might account for such a window of opportunity? The role of the basal forebrain cholinergic system could be of paramount importance. Another potential mechanism is described by the "healthy cell bias" theory.

In the laboratory, different estrogens can have different effects, depending on the model system under consideration. Are some estrogens, some hormonal formulations, or some routes of estrogenic administration more conducive to cognitive benefit? The second section of the book describes some of these options. Effects of transdermal estradiol on cognition in women with and without dementia are reviewed, and nasal administration of estradiol is discussed as an alternative to the oral administration. In this section also, effects of selective estrogen receptor modulators (SERM) on cognitive function are discussed. Phytoestrogens, whose impact can also be tissue selective, are considered as well.

It is difficult to consider estrogen actions in the brain without at the same time considering progestogen actions. The third section discusses potential modulators of estrogenic effects by progesterone, as well as other modifiers of estrogen actions, such as cortisol and folate. Some researchers suggest that estrogens can affect cognitive function indirectly, working to improve mood, sleep, or vasomotor symptoms. Estrogen effects on mood disorders are reviewed in this section. In Section 4, the focus is on genetic variation related to steroid hormone metabolism, Alzheimer's disease, and apolipoprotein E. This exciting research area may lead to new screening tools for assessment of risks and benefits of hormone treatment.

The relevance of testosterone to brain action in women and for men is being increasingly recognized. This steroid not only affects the nervous system directly, but it may also modulate brain effects of estradiol. Androgen research has received less attention than estrogen research, and substantial portions of Sections 5 and 6 are devoted to new insights on testosterone, cognition, and Alzheimer's disease. The role of gonadotropins is discussed here in relation to dementia, as is the role of sex hormone binding globulin, whose levels determine those of free sex hormones. Lowering levels of this globulin would increase free levels of both estradiol and testosterone, which could be of value in some clinical settings. Reducing gonadotropins will increase sex steroid levels, but in some models these peptides are also neurotoxic. Data from trials in women with Alzheimer's disease are presented, together with supportive results from animal and cell-culture experiments. The volume concludes with a perspective from Professor Wulf H. Utian, an expert in women's health and Executive Director of the North American Menopause Society.

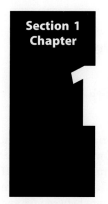

Estrogens and cognition: perspectives and opportunities
in the wake of the Women's Health Initiative Memory Study

Women's Health Initiative Memory Study (WHIMS) program: emerging findings

Mark A. Espeland, Sally A. Shumaker, Patricia E. Hogan, and Susan M. Resnick

Editors' introduction

The landmark Women's Health Initiative Memory Study (WHIMS) program has had an enormous impact on our understanding of how estrogens and estrogen-containing hormone therapy affect cognitive outcomes in postmenopausal women. It is the starting point and touchstone for any discussion on cognition and dementia in women. As reviewed in this chapter by principal WHIMS program investigators, the WHIMS comprised two large randomized placebo-controlled trials of conjugated equine estrogens with and without medroxyprogesterone acetate in women aged 65 years and older. In this study, the two hormone therapy formulations were associated with increased risk for probable dementia (hazard ratio 1.77, 95% confidence interval 1.22 to 2.58). They were also associated with a small adverse mean difference of 0.21 (0.06 to 0.37) points on the 100-point Modified Mini-Mental State examination. Adverse findings were similar for both hormone therapy formulations and for women with and without histories of prior hormone therapy use. The Women's Health Initiative Study of Cognitive Aging and the Women's Health Initiative Magnetic Resonance Imaging Study were conducted on subsets of WHIMS participants. The former found little evidence that conjugated equine estrogens with medroxyprogesterone acetate had a positive effect on cognitive aging. The latter found that the hormone therapy formulations were associated with decreased brain volumes, particularly among women with lower levels of cognitive function at baseline, but mean effects on ischemic lesions were not significant. No subgroups of WHIMS participants have been identified for which initiating hormone therapy appears to convey cognitive benefit.

Women's Health Initiative

Design of the Women's Health Initiative Hormone Therapy Clinical Trial

The Women's Health Initiative (WHI) trials of hormone therapy are landmarks in women's health research. These well conceived and well conducted randomized controlled clinical trials addressed whether the most prevalent form of postmenopausal hormone therapy in the USA should be prescribed to prevent cardiovascular disease, the leading cause of death in older women. Observational studies had supported this use in older women, who constituted a growing market share [1]. The WHI selected conjugated equine estrogens (CEE, 0.625 mg/day) as its estrogen therapy, because it had been extensively researched and was the most commonly prescribed postmenopausal estrogen therapy in the United States [2]. For women with a uterus, the WHI selected medroxyprogesterone acetate (MPA, 10 mg/day) to oppose CEE, because of its widespread use in the USA and because of prior research suggesting it conveyed similar cardiovascular risk profiles to other progestins [2, 3].

The stark finding of the WHI, that CEE therapy conveyed no cardiovascular benefits for older women, and indeed increased their overall risk of cardiovascular and cerebrovascular disease, has reverberated dramatically through the medical community and has led to a marked change in health care for women [4]. The findings are still widely studied and debated. While this chapter is focused on the impact of hormone therapy on cognition in older women, we first summarize the primary findings of the WHI on cardiovascular disease.

Hormones, Cognition and Dementia: State of the Art and Emergent Therapeutic Strategies, ed. Eef Hogervorst, Victor W. Henderson, Robert B. Gibbs, and Roberta Diaz Brinton. Published by Cambridge University Press.
© Cambridge University Press 2009.

Table 1.1 Hazard ratios and nominal 95% confidence intervals associated with assignment to hormone therapy reported by the Women's Health Initiative [6, 7].

Clinical event	CEE+MPA trial HR [95% CI]	CEE-alone trial HR [95% CI]
Stroke	1.41 [1.07, 1.85][a]	1.39 [1.10, 1.77][a]
Coronary heart disease	1.29 [1.07, 1.85][a]	0.91 [0.75, 1.12]
Pulmonary embolism	2.13 [1.39, 3.25][a]	1.34 [0.87, 2.06]
Death	0.98 [0.82, 1.18]	1.08 [0.88, 1.32]

Note: [a]95% Confidence interval excludes 1.0

Major findings of the Women's Health Initiative

The WHI trials of hormone therapy began in 1992 and were designed to continue until 2007 [2]. Following discovery of an unfavorable risk-to-benefit ratio of its non-cognitive endpoints, the CEE+MPA trial was discontinued in July, 2002 [5]. In March, 2004, the CEE-alone trial was also terminated earlier than planned due to an excess risk of stroke and the lack of a significant effect on other cardiovascular disease outcomes [6]. Table 1.1 summarizes the findings from these two trials for outcomes that may be most closely linked to mechanisms affecting cognitive function: stroke, coronary heart disease, pulmonary embolism, and all-cause death. Both trials found an increased risk for stroke associated with hormone therapy of about 40%. For CEE+MPA therapy, there was also an increased risk of coronary heart disease and pulmonary embolism. No significant interactions between treatment effect and age were found in either trial for these outcomes. When data are pooled across trials, a trend is evident for increased risks of these outcomes for women aged 60 and older compared to younger women; however, this finding is not as consistent within the individual trials [4].

The adverse risks for stroke within the CEE+MPA trial have been extensively studied [7]. Approximately 80% of the strokes were classified as ischemic. Increased rates of ischemic strokes accounted for the overall excess risk of stroke associated with CEE+MPA therapy.

Women's Health Initiative Memory Study

Design of the Women's Health Initiative Memory Study

The study design, eligibility criteria, and recruitment procedures of the WHIMS trials were described previously [8]. Participants were recruited from 39 WHI clinical sites; however, one was later dropped from the trial. To be eligible, women were between 65 and 79 years of age and free of dementia as ascertained by the WHIMS protocol (described below). Written informed consent was obtained; the National Institutes of Health and Institutional Review Boards for all participating institutions approved the protocols and consent forms.

Modified Mini-Mental State (3MS) examinations [9] were administered at baseline and annually thereafter by technicians who were trained and certified in their administration and masked to randomization assignment and reports of symptoms. Scores from the 3MS test may range from 0 to 100; a higher score reflects better cognitive functioning. The test includes items measuring temporal and spatial orientation, immediate and delayed recall, executive function, naming, verbal fluency, abstract reasoning, praxis, writing, and visuoconstructional abilities. Administration time averaged 10–12 minutes.

Women who scored below cutpoints based on education level proceeded to a second phase to classify their dementia status. At the start of the WHIMS, these cutpoints were ≤ 76 (for participants with nine or more years of education) and ≤ 72 (for participants with eight or fewer years of education). After 16 months the protocol was altered to increase the sensitivity of the 3MS by using cutpoints of ≤ 80 (for participants with eight or fewer years of education) and ≤ 88 (for participants with nine or more years of education). These second cutpoints were expected to provide a sensitivity of 80% and specificity of 85% based on earlier studies [8].

In the second phase of WHIMS screening, certified technicians administered a modified Consortium to Establish a Registry for Alzheimer's Disease neuropsychological battery [10]. This contained tests measuring verbal fluency, naming, verbal learning and memory, constructional praxis, and executive function. Technicians also administered standardized interviews to assess behavioral symptoms of generalized anxiety, major depression, and alcohol abuse [11] and the 15-item Geriatric Depression Scale [12]. Both the participant and her designated informant completed standardized interviews to identify acquired cognitive and behavioral deficits. An experienced local board-certified geriatrician, neurologist, or geriatric psychiatrist reviewed all data, completed a structured clinical evaluation, and classified women as having no dementia, mild cognitive impairment, or probable dementia, the latter based on standard DSM-IV criteria [13]. Clinicians were provided with reference scores for each test in the battery [14]. If the clinician suspected probable dementia, the participant was referred for a brain computerized tomography (CT) scan and laboratory blood tests to rule out possible reversible causes of cognitive decline and dementia and to classify subtypes of dementia.

A central expert panel adjudicated all probable dementia cases identified by the local clinicians, a random sample of 50% of mild cognitive impairment cases, and a random sample of 10% of no dementia cases. All information on participant's interviews and testing, except the field clinician's classification, was provided for initial classification by two independent adjudicators. The field clinician's diagnostic assessment was then shared with each adjudicator, who independently made a revised diagnosis. If the adjudicators agreed, this was considered the consensus diagnosis. If there was not agreement, discussions ensued among the entire adjudication committee until a consensus classification was made; however, agreement was generally high [15]. Regardless of their classification, all participants continued to be scheduled for annual 3MS tests.

The WHIMS has begun a Supplemental Case Ascertainment Protocol to identify additional classifications of probable dementia among women who had died or otherwise ceased full follow-up prior to a "determination" of cognitive status. The expectation has been that among these participants were women who would have been classified as having probable dementia had they completed the scheduled assessments. In order to capture these possible cases, the WHIMS, with the approval of the WHI, implemented a standardized telephone survey of proxies and/or family members of these women who provided consent. The survey consists of the Dementia Questionnaire [16], a standardized, validated instrument used to reliably diagnose dementia, and specifically Alzheimer's dementia, in deceased persons. It can be reliably administered

by telephone with good sensitivity and specificity [17], and includes items assessing memory and other cognitive functions, language, daily functioning, insight, and other medical and psychiatric difficulties. Data from these surveys are centrally adjudicated. Additional classifications of probable dementia are beginning to emerge from this protocol; however, these are not included in the results summarized below.

Major findings of the Women's Health Initiative Memory Study

The women who volunteered for and were enrolled in the WHIMS had mean ages of 69 years at enrollment. Approximately 40% of the 7,479 women had prior hysterectomy, and thus were drawn from the WHI CEE-alone trial (N = 2,947). The remainder, N = 4,532, were drawn from the CEE+MPA trial. Overall, about 30% reported use of hormone therapy at some time in the past, which, according to the WHI protocol, had been stopped at least three months prior to enrollment in the WHI. The early terminations of the WHI trials ended the WHIMS CEE + MPA and CEE-alone trials, with average follow-ups of 4.05 (SD = 1.19) and 5.21 (1.19) years, respectively [17].

At the time the primary publications from these trials were completed, central adjudication had yielded 108 cases of probable dementia and 310 cases of any cognitive impairment (i.e., probable dementia and/or mild cognitive impairment) [15, 17]. From these data, the hazard of probable dementia was increased by 76% among women assigned to hormone therapy compared to placebo (p = 0.005). The hazard of any cognitive impairment was increased by 41% (p = 0.003). The most common types of probable dementia were Alzheimer (52% overall), mixed (16%), and vascular (9%), with a trend towards greater numbers of each among women assigned to active therapy.

Adjudication of cases after the publication of these data has continued: 9 additional probable dementia cases and 17 additional cases of any impairment were identified as occurring during the follow-up periods of the trials. Figures 1.1 and 1.2 describe results of analyses of these completed data. The relative hazard of probable dementia associated with assignment to hormone therapy is now 1.77 [95% confidence interval: 1.22, 2.58]. For any impairment, the relative hazard is 1.36 [1.09, 1.69]. Treatment-related differences

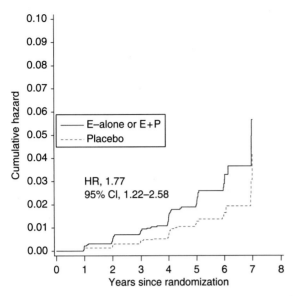

Fig. 1.1 Distribution of times until classification of probable dementia for women grouped by WHI treatment assignment.

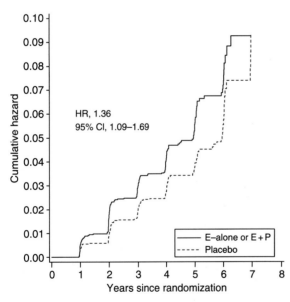

Fig. 1.2 Distribution of times until first classification of any impairment (probable dementia or mild cognitive impairment) for women grouped by WHI treatment assignment.

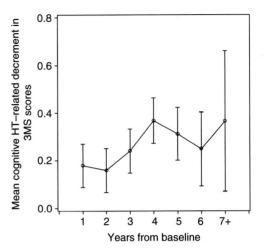

Fig. 1.3 Mean (± standard error) decrement in 3MS scores associated with assignment to hormone therapy, with adjustment for baseline 3MS score and age.

mean decrement in 3MS scores experienced by women assigned to hormone therapy relative to those assigned to placebo therapy. Covariate adjustment is made for baseline 3MS and age. Small relative decrements began to emerge within the first two years of therapy and continued throughout follow-up. The figure conveys no evidence that decrements diminish with time, even based on an intention-to-treat analysis in which non-adherence to medications was not factored. The average decrement in 3MS scores over time was 0.21 units (p = 0.006) on a scale ranging from 0–100 [19]. Such a deficit would clearly not be clinically detectable for an individual participant.

At the time of publication of the primary results of the trials, the hazard ratios of CEE-alone therapy versus its placebo and CEE+MPA therapy versus its placebo on the risk of probable dementia were 1.49 [0.83, 2.66] and 2.05 [1.21, 3.48], respectively [15, 17]. For any impairment, these were 1.38 [1.01, 1.89] and 1.37 [0.99, 1.89] [15, 17]. For the completed data described in this chapter, the hazard ratios of CEE-alone therapy versus CEE+MPA therapy on the risk of probable dementia were 1.55 [0.91, 2.65] and 2.05 [1.21, 3.47]; for any impairment, these were 1.34 [0.99, 1.80] and 1.39 [1.01, 1.92]. The mean relative deficits in on-trial 3MS scores were 0.26 [0.00, 0.52] and 0.18 [0.00, 0.37] [19]. Thus, the WHIMS found little evidence for a separate effect of MPA therapy when added to CEE therapy.

appear to emerge within the first two years of enrollment and extend throughout follow-up.

The WHIMS also found a small adverse effect of assignment to hormone therapy on global cognitive function, as measured by 3MS examinations [18, 19]. Figure 1.3 portrays, by year from randomization, the

The WHIMS has published the results of extensive subgroup analyses to examine the consistency of treatment-related effects on cognition among women grouped according to dementia risk factors and correlates of adherence to medications. These subgroups included age, prior use of hormone therapy, and history of cardiovascular disease. No factors have been found that appear to alter significantly the effect of CEE-based therapy, with or without MPA, on probable dementia or any impairment; however, power for these endpoints was low [17]. More definitive comparisons can be made for 3MS scores. Of the many factors examined, only one appears to identify women who are at greater potential risk for adverse effects [19, 20]. Women who scored relatively lower on the baseline measure of global cognitive function (3MS) on average had greater relative on-trial deficits in cognitive function ($p < 0.001$). The mean decrements in baseline cognitive function associated with hormone therapy were 0.10 [−0.07, 0.21] for women with scores of 95–100 at baseline, 0.38 [0.11, 0.65] for women with baseline scores above the screening cutpoint to 94, and 1.26 [0.75, 1.76] for women who scored at or below the screening cutpoint at baseline [19, 20]. These results suggest that the adverse impact of hormone therapy is most strongly expressed among women with underlying disease. It is important to note, however, that while subgroup differences were not statistically significant and the absolute risk was low, the relative hazard of probable dementia was greatest among women with baseline 3MS scores of 95–100: 2.82 [1.18, 6.70] [17]. Whether this results from the inability of 3MS tests to identify all women with underlying cognitive deficits, or for some other reason, is not known.

No subgroups emerged for which it appeared that hormone therapy had beneficial effects on cognition.

Women's Health Initiative Study of Cognitive Aging

Design of the Women's Health Initiative Study of Cognitive Aging

The Women's Health Initiative Study of Cognitive Aging (WHISCA) was designed to examine the impact of CEE-based therapy on longitudinal changes of cognitive tests targeting several different domains [21]. Participants were recruited from 14 of the 39 WHIMS sites. They were eligible for the WHISCA if they were English speaking, did not have probable dementia as determined by the WHIMS protocol, and provided written informed consent. The WHISCA was initiated after WHI randomization: its enrollees had been assigned to receive WHI treatment for 1.1–5.6 years (mean 3.0) prior to their initial WHISCA cognitive assessment.

The battery of cognitive measures used by WHISCA was designed to assess a broad range of cognitive functions (emphasizing tests that were expected to be sensitive to aging or the effects of hormones) and mood states. Included were assessments of verbal knowledge, phonemic and category fluency, short-term figural memory and visuo-construction, verbal learning and memory, attention and working memory, spatial rotational ability, fine motor speed, positive and negative mood states, and non-somatic features of depressed mood [21]. Test administrators were centrally trained using procedures consistent with those in the Baltimore Longitudinal Study of Aging [22]. Quality control was maintained through recertification of test administrators every six months for the first year and annually thereafter.

Major findings of the Women's Health Initiative Study of Cognitive Aging

The WHISCA enrolled 2,302 WHIMS participants [21]. In general, these women tended to be younger and healthier than the WHIMS women who chose not to enroll in WHISCA; however, there was good balance among treatment arms. To date, only WHISCA data from the CEE+MPA trial have been published [23]. When this trial was terminated in 2002, the 1,426 women enrolled in this trial had averaged 1.35 (SD = 0.61) years of WHISCA follow-up. Overall, none of the differences in this trial reached the protocol-specified criterion for statistical significance ($p < 0.01$). The largest difference between treatment groups was for verbal learning: women assigned to CEE+MPA therapy had slightly worse performance over time compared to women assigned to placebo. The primary conclusion from this analysis is that in these relatively healthy and cognitively intact women, there was little evidence that CEE+MPA therapy positively affected cognitive aging. The strongest signal was for a small adverse effect on changes in verbal learning over time.

Women's Health Initiative Memory Study of Magnetic Resonance Imaging

Design of the Women's Health Initiative Memory Study of Magnetic Resonance Imaging (WHIMS-MRI)

The WHIMS-MRI was designed to contrast neuro-radiologic outcomes among women who had been assigned to active versus placebo therapy during the WHIMS trials. It was conducted in 14 of the 39 WHIMS clinical sites, which were selected based on interest, experience in conducting multi-center MRI studies, participation in the WHISCA, and availability of necessary equipment. All participants in these centers were to be solicited for potential screening to join WHIMS-MRI, regardless of their prior adherence or cognitive function. Exclusion criteria included the presence of pacemakers, defibrillators, neurostimulators, prohibited medical implants, and foreign bodies that could pose a hazard to the participant during the MRI procedure. Other exclusion criteria included shortness of breath, inability to lie flat, and conditions that could be exacerbated by stress severe enough to preclude an MRI (e.g., anxiety panic disorders, claustrophobia, uncontrolled high blood pressure, and seizure disorders).

The standardized WHIMS-MRI scanning protocol was developed by investigators in its central reading center at the University of Pennsylvania. Included were oblique axial spin density/T2-weighted spin echo images from the vertex to skull base parallel to the anterior commissure–posterior commissure (AC–PC) plane; oblique axial FLAIR T2-weighted spin echo images matching these slice positions; and oblique axial 3D T1-weighted gradient echo images from the vertex to the skull base parallel to the AC–PC plane. The primary outcome measure for the WHIMS-MRI was total ischemic brain lesion volume from central readings. With this methodology, these volumes generally correspond to leukoaraiosis, ischemic white matter disease, and small vessel ischemia [24] and are generated by non-necrotic processes, i.e., ischemic effects on myelin that are secondary to the effects of aging, hypertension, and other small vessel pathologies of the brain [25, 26]. Ischemic lesion volumes within the basal ganglia may reflect lacunar infarcts.

Important secondary outcome measures for WHIMS-MRI were regional brain volumes [27]. To measure these, the T1-weighted volumetric MRI scans were first pre-processed according to a standardized protocol consisting of alignment to the AC–PC plane, removal of extra-cranial material, and segmentation of brain parenchyma into gray matter, white matter, and cerebrospinal fluid. Regional volumetric measurements were obtained with an automated computer-based template warping method based on a digital atlas labeled for brain lobes and individual structures [28].

Major findings of the Women's Health Initiative Magnetic Resonance Imaging Study

Enrollment in the WHIMS-MRI began in January, 2005, two-and-a-half years after the termination of the CEE+MPA trial and nearly a year after the completion of the CEE-alone trial. As in prior MRI studies that enrolled participants from existing cohorts, those willing and eligible to participate tended to be younger, healthier, and more cognitively intact than other members of the cohort [29]. Importantly, the enrollment rate of the WHIMS-MRI aligned with other major MRI studies, and there was no evidence that enrollment was differentially related to on-trial treatment assignment. Of the 1,426 women scanned, images on 1,403 (98%) met study quality control criteria for inclusion in primary data analyses. Of these, N = 530 (N = 257 HT; N = 273 placebo) had been enrolled in the CEE-alone trial and N = 883 (N = 436 HT; N = 447 placebo) had been enrolled in the CEE+MPA trial.

The WHIMS-MRI found that the random assignment to active therapy that occurred during the WHI trials did not have statistically significant associations with total ischemic lesion volumes and lesion volumes in the basal ganglia. Overall, women who had been assigned to active therapy during the WHI trials had only slightly (and non-significantly more) total ischemic lesion volume than those who had been assigned to placebo [26]. After adjustment for risk factors, women previously assigned to CEE+MPA therapy had mean (SE) ischemic lesion volumes of 5.10 (0.21) ml compared to 4.70 (0.20) ml for women previously assigned to its placebo (p = 0.25). Within the basal ganglia, these lesion volumes were 0.90 (1.19) ml versus 0.87 (1.08) ml respectively (p = 0.92). Among women previously assigned to CEE-alone therapy, mean ischemic lesion volumes were 5.41 (0.30) ml compared to 5.35 (0.29) ml among women previously assigned its placebo (p = 0.91). Within the basal ganglia, these lesion volumes were 0.91 (1.19) ml and 0.93 (1.23) ml respectively (p = 0.90). The hypothesis that the adverse effects of CEE-based therapy on cognition were primarily conveyed through increased lesion load and subclinical stroke is thus not supported by the WHIMS-MRI data. The slightly larger mean lesion volumes among women that had been assigned to CEE-based therapy were small and not statistically significant, despite the significantly increased incidence of ischemic strokes reported by the WHI [7].

The secondary outcomes of total and regional brain volumes, when adjusted for total intracranial volume, served as markers of brain atrophy. Women who had been assigned to CEE-based therapy during the WHI had smaller mean total, hippocampal, and frontal lobe brain volumes compared to those who had been assigned to placebo [27]. After adjustment for dementia risk factors, mean (SE) differences were 3.32 (1.84) ml for total brain (p = 0.07), 0.10 (0.05) ml for the hippocampus (p = 0.05), and 2.37 (0.004) ml for the frontal lobe (p = 0.004). When women were grouped according to their level of total ischemic lesion volume at the time of the MRI, no significant differences were found in the regional brain volumes between treatment groups among women in the lower quartile of lesion volumes (i.e., < 2 ml). However, differences were accentuated by about 40% among the three-quarters of women with ischemic lesion volumes ≥2: 4.67 (2.20) ml for total brain volume (p = 0.03), 0.16 (0.06) ml for hippocampal volume (p = 0.005), and 3.01 (0.98) ml for frontal lobe volume (p = 0.002).

The magnitudes of these differences were inversely related to the level of 3MS at enrollment into the WHIMS. Women whose baseline 3MS scores were less than 90 had mean HT-related decrements in adjusted brain volumes of 20.31 (8.14) ml, compared to 7.09 (4.57) for women with baseline scores of 90–94 and 0.43 (2.23) for women with baseline scores of 95 or greater. No other subgroupings were associated with differential treatment effects [27].

To date, the WHIMS-MRI has found little difference between the adverse effects of CEE-alone and CEE+MPA therapy on MRI outcomes.

Summary and conclusions

Taken together, findings from the WHI, WHIMS, WHISCA, and WHIMS-MRI provide a coherent set of evidence on the impact of CEE-based therapy on cognitive function in women aged 65 years or older. Four major conclusions can be drawn from the collective results, which we discuss in turn.

First, there is consistently no evidence that CEE-based hormone therapy has protective effects on cognition for women aged 65 years or older. Collectively, these studies have assessed cognitively related clinical events (dementia, mild cognitive impairment, and stroke), performance on a range of cognitive assessment tools, and MRI outcomes. For each of these, no overall benefits were found. Furthermore, across a range of clinical subgroups, none has been identified for which there is evidence of a material benefit on cognition. Nearly half the women in the CEE-alone trial and one-fifth the women in the CEE+MPA trial reported use of hormone therapy in the past, which by protocol had been terminated at least three months prior to enrollment. The on-trial resumption of CEE-based therapy was not beneficial to these women's cognitive health, regardless of the duration and timing of prior use [18]; however, the WHIMS program was not designed to assess whether hormone therapy may have some benefits on cognition when administered to women at the time of menopause.

Second, CEE-based therapy appears to be associated, on average, with a small adverse effect on cognition that is sustained over time. Overall, the risks of dementia, mild cognitive impairment, and stroke are significantly increased; there is a mean decrement in global cognitive function; and there is evidence that brain atrophy is accelerated. Less striking, and nonsignificant, may be decrements in other measures of cognitive function; however, the earlier termination of the WHISCA trial limited the ability to detect these. The WHISCA cohort consisted of women with relatively high levels of education, whose cognitive function may be more resilient in the face of underlying increases in neuropathology [30]. Also less striking and not statistically significant were associations with increased levels of ischemic lesion volumes. The decrements in global cognitive function were evident and unabated throughout the later spans of the WHIMS follow-up. The decrements in brain volumes were evident more than two years after the termination of the WHI assigned therapies.

The impact of CEE-based hormone therapy on cognition may be most strongly expressed among women with existing cognitive deficits. The only significant subgroup analyses across the range of outcomes has been that 3MS scores and brain volumes are more strongly adversely affected among women with lower cognitive function at baseline. Unfortunately, 3MS testing cannot be used as a means to identify accurately women without underlying cognitive deficits [20, 31], which may be why there remains an elevated risk for probable dementia among the relatively few high-scoring women who converted during follow-up.

Finally, it appears that the mechanism by which CEE-based therapy adversely affects cognition among older women is most likely complex and multifactorial. The WHI has clearly demonstrated that this therapy increases the risk of stroke, particularly ischemic stroke. While the absolute risk of clinical stroke is low, CEE-based therapy appears to increase this risk for women of all ages [7]. A second mechanism is expressed by an increased rate of brain atrophy, which appears to differentially affect women with evidence of existing disease. While the metabolic nature of this process has yet to be identified, it may not be strongly related to ischemic disease.

Observational data on US women can lead to spurious findings of health benefits of hormone therapy due to prescription practices [32, 33]. However, considerable evidence from well controlled basic science research remains that estrogens, and specifically components of CEE-based therapy, may have neuroprotective effects in vitro and in animal models [34]. These effects may be related to timing, dose, and duration of treatment [35]. The powerful evidence of the WHIMS program demonstrates that the beneficial effects of estrogens observed in basic science studies do not translate to cognitive benefits among older women, and signals that other overriding adverse consequences are in place to produce harm. Whether these are due to actions related to estradiol [36] or other components within CEE-based therapies [36, 37, 38], or differences among groups with respect to cognitive health and co-morbid conditions at the initiation of hormone therapy, requires further study.

Acknowledgments

The National Heart, Lung, and Blood Institute of the National Institutes of Health, US Department of Health and Human Services, Bethesda, Maryland, USA funded the Women's Health Initiative and the Women's Health Initiative Memory Study of Magnetic Resonance Imaging and co-funded the Women's Health Initiative Memory Study. Wyeth Pharmaceuticals, Inc., St. Davids, Pennsylvania, USA co-funded the Women's Health Initiative Memory Study and provided the medications and placebos used in the Women's Health Initiative. Wake Forest University Health Sciences, Winston-Salem, North Carolina, USA co-funded the Women's Health Initiative Memory Study. The Women's Health Initiative Study of Cognitive Aging was funded by the Department of Health and Human Services and the National Institute on Aging, NO1-AG-1–2106, National Institutes of Health, Bethesda, Maryland. Dr. Resnick is supported by the Intramural Research Program, National Institute on Aging, National Institutes of Health. Lists of participating centers and investigator groups appear in articles cited in this chapter.

References

1. Hersch AL, Stefanick ML, Stafford, RS. National use of postmenopausal hormone therapy: annual trends and response to recent evidence. *JAMA*. 2003;**291**:47–53.

2. The Women's Health Initiative Study Group. Design of the Women's Health Initiative clinical trial and observational study. *Control Clin Trials*. 1998; **19**:61–109.

3. The PEPI Investigators. Effects of estrogen or estrogen/progestin regimens on heart disease risk factors in postmenopausal women. The Postmenopausal Estrogen/Progestin Interventions (PEPI) Trial. *JAMA*. 1995;**273**:199–208.

4. Rossouw JE, Prentice RL, Manson KE, *et al.* Postmenopausal hormone therapy and risk of cardiovascular disease by age and years since menopause. *JAMA*. 2007;**297**:1465–77.

5. Writing Group for the Women's Health Initiative Investigators. Risks and benefits of estrogen plus progestin in healthy postmenopausal women: principal results from the Women's Health Initiative randomized controlled trial. *JAMA*. 2002;**288**:321–33.

6. The Women's Health Initiative Steering Committee. Effects of conjugated equine estrogens in postmenopausal women with hysterectomy: the Women's Health Initiative randomized controlled trial. *JAMA*. 2004;**291**:1701–12.

7. Wassertheil-Smoller S, Hendrix SL, Limacher M, *et al.* Effect of estrogen plus progestin on stroke in postmenopausal women. *JAMA*. 2003;**289**:2673–84.

8. Shumaker SA, Reboussin BA, Espeland MA, *et al.* The Women's Health Initiative Memory Study: a trial of the effect of estrogen therapy in preventing and slowing the progression of dementia. *Control Clin Trials.* 1998;**19**:604–21.

9. Teng EL, Chui HC. The Modified Mini-Mental State (3MS) examination. *J Clin Psychiatry.* 1987;**48**:314–18.

10. Morris JC, Heyman A, Mohs RC, *et al.* The Consortium to Establish a Registry for Alzheimer's Disease (CERAD). Part I. Clinical and neuropsychological assessment of Alzheimer disease. *Neurology.* 1989;**39**:1159–65.

11. Spitzer RL, Williams JB, Kroenke K, *et al.* Utility of a new procedure for diagnosing mental disorders in primary care. The PRIME-MD 1000 study. *JAMA.* 1994;**272**:1749–56.

12. Burke WJ, Roccaforte WH, Wengel SP. The short form of the Geriatric Depression Scale: a comparison with the 30-item form. *J Geriatr Psychiatry Neurol.* 1991;**4**:173–8.

13. American Psychiatric Association. *Diagnostic and Statistical Manual of Mental Disorders*, 4th edn. Washington, DC: American Psychiatric Association, 1994.

14. Welsh KA, Butters N, Mohs RC, *et al.* The Consortium to Establish a Registry for Alzheimer's Disease (CERAD). Part V. A normative study of the neuropsychological battery. *Neurology.* 1994;**44**:609–14.

15. Shumaker S, Legault C, Rapp S, *et al.* The effects of estrogen plus progestin on the incidence of dementia and mild cognitive impairment in postmenopausal women: The Women's Health Initiative Memory Study. *JAMA.* 2003;**289**:2651–62.

16. Ellis RJ, Jan K, Kawas C, *et al.* Diagnostic validity of the dementia questionnaire for Alzheimer disease. *Arch Neurol.* 1998;**55**:360–5.

17. Shumaker SA, Legault C, Kuller L, *et al.* Conjugated equine estrogens and incidence of probable dementia and mild cognitive impairment in postmenopausal women: the Women's Health Initiative Memory Study. *JAMA.* 2004;**291**:2947–58.

18. Rapp SR, Espeland MA, Shumaker SA, *et al.* Effect of estrogen plus progestin on global cognitive function in postmenopausal women: Women's Health Initiative Memory Study: a randomized controlled trial. *JAMA.* 2003;**20**:2663–72.

19. Espeland MA, Rapp SR, Shumaker SA, *et al.* Conjugated equine estrogens and global cognitive function in postmenopausal women: the Women's Health Initiative Memory Study. *JAMA.* 2004;**291**:2959–68.

20. Espeland MA, Robertson J, Albert M, *et al.* Benchmarks for designing two-stage studies using

modified mini-mental state examinations: experience from the Women's Health Initiative Memory Study (WHIMS). *Clin Trials.* 2006;**3**:99–106.

21. Resnick SM, Coker LH, Maki PM, *et al.* The Women's Health Initiative Study of Cognitive Aging (WHISCA): a randomized clinical trial of the effects of hormone therapy on age-associated cognitive decline. *Clin Trials.* 2004;**1**:440–50.

22. Shock NW, Greulich RC, Andres R, *et al.* Normal human aging: the Baltimore Longitudinal Study of Aging. Washington, DC: US Government Printing Office, 1984.

23. Resnick SM, Maki PM, Rapp SR, *et al.* Effects of combination estrogen plus progestin hormone treatment on cognition and affect: the Women's Health Initiative Study of Cognitive Aging (WHISCA). *J Clin Endocrinol Metabol.* 2006;**91**:1802–11.

24. Pantoni L, Garcia JH. Pathogenesis of leukoaraiosis: a review. *Stroke.* 1997;**28**:652–9.

25. Moody DM, Bell MA, Challa VR. Features of the cerebral vascular pattern that predict vulnerability to perfusion or oxygenation deficiency: an anatomic study. *AJNR Am J Neuroradiol.* 1990;**11**:431–9.

26. Coker LH, Hogan PE, Bryan NR, *et al.* Postmenopausal hormone therapy and subclinical cerebrovascular disease: the WHIMS-MRI study. *Neurology.* 2009;**72**:125–34.

27. Resnick SM, Espeland MA, Jaramillo SA, *et al.* Effects of postmenopausal hormone therapy on regional brain volumes in older women: the Women's Health Initiative Magnetic Resonance Imaging Study (WHIMS-MRI). *Neurology.* 2009;**72**:135–42.

28. Shen D, Davatzikos C. HAMMER: hierarchical attribute matching mechanism for elastic registration. *IEEE Trans Med Imaging.* 2002;**21**:1421–39.

29. Jaramillo SA, Felton D, Andrews LA, *et al.* Enrollment in a brain magnetic resonance study: results from the Women's Health Initiative Memory Study Magnetic Resonance Imaging Study (WHIMS-MRI). *Acad Radiol.* 2007;**14**:603–12.

30. Elkins JS, Longstreth WT, Manolio TA, *et al.* Education and the cognitive decline associated with MRI-defined brain infarct. *Neurology.* 2006;**67**:435–40.

31. Bland RC, Newman SC. Mild dementia or cognitive impairment: the Modified Mini-Mental State examination (3MS) as a screen for dementia. *Can J Psychiatry.* 2001;**46**:506–10.

32. Prentice RL, Langer R, Stefanick ML, *et al.* Combined postmenopausal hormone therapy and cardiovascular disease: toward resolving the discrepancy between observational studies and the Women's Health

Initiative clinical trial. *Am J Epidemiol.* 2005;**162**: 404–14.

33. Prentice RL, Langer RD, Stefanick MR, *et al.* Combined analysis of Women's Health Initiative observational and clinical trial data on postmenopausal hormone treatment and cardiovascular disease. *Am J Epidemiol.* 2006;**163**:589–99.

34. Zhao L, Brinton RD. Select estrogens within the complex formulation of conjugated equine estrogens (Premarin) are protective against neurodegenerative insults: implications for a composition of estrogen therapy to promote neuronal function and prevent Alzheimer's disease. *BMC Neurosciences.* 2006;7:24.

35. Chen S, Nilsen J, Brinton RD. Dose and temporal pattern of estrogen exposure determines neuroprotective outcome in hippocampal neurons: therapeutic implications. *Endocrinology.* 2006;**147**: 5303–13.

36. Ravaglia G, Forti P, Maioli F, *et al.* Endogenous sex hormones as risk factors for dementia in elderly men and women. *J Gerontol.* 2007;**62A**:1035–41.

37. Dhandapani KM, Wade FM, Mahesh VB, Brann DW. Astrocyte-derived transforming growth factor-β mediates the neuroprotective effects of 17β-estradiol: involvement of nonclassical genomic signaling pathways. *Endocrinology.* 2005;**146**:2749–59.

38. Rozovsky I, Hoving S, Anderson SP, O'Callaghan J, Finch CE. Equine estrogens induce apolipoprotein E and glial fibrillary acidic protein in mixtures of glial cultures. *Neurosci Lett.* 2002;**323**(3):191–4.

Identifying risk factors for cognitive change in the Women's Health Initiative: a neural networks approach

Stephan Bandelow, Mark A. Espeland, Victor W. Henderson, Susan M. Resnick, Robert B. Wallace, Laura H. Coker, and Eef Hogervorst

Editors' introduction

The Women's Health Initiative Memory Study (WHIMS) has been much criticized and it has been suggested that subgroups of women exist for whom hormone therapy (HT) might improve or impair cognitive function. Possible modifying variables could be age, smoking, body mass index, and menopausal symptoms. These were included in artificial neural networks (ANN) analyses, which allow testing of complex non-linear higher order interactions of variables to predict outcomes. Artificial neural networks analyses without hidden units could predict responders and non-responders to treatment as well as logistic regression models that included only main effects, which indicated that higher order interactions were not necessary and did not add to the value of the models. There seemed to be no subgroups (e.g., older women who smoke and have a high body mass) for whom HT has a worse or better effect on cognitive function over time. This study also showed that cross-validation is essential in building robust models with many independent variables and should be applied as a standard technique in complex multivariate analyses.

Introduction
Hormone therapy and cognitive function

Results of recent large randomized controlled trials of elderly healthy women [1, 2, 3, 4] and women with Alzheimer's disease (AD) [5, 6, 7] indicated that HT increased the risk for AD and could not prevent cognitive decline. Many women have stopped taking HT because of these and other associated risks of HT use, such as breast cancer, stroke, and thromboembolism

[1, 8]. However, it remains unclear whether subgroups of women are at additional risks for cognitive impairment when using HT, or whether subgroups of elderly postmenopausal women exist for whom HT may still be indicated.

The impact of the largest trial to date, the Women's Health Initiative Memory Study (WHIMS) [1, 2, 3, 4], has been extensive. The main explanations for the unexpected negative effects have focused on the older age of women, the under-representation of women with severe menopausal symptoms, the long duration and/or the type of treatment [9, 10, 11, 12, 13, 14]. The WHIMS study using combined HT (conjugated equine estrogens (CEE) and medroxy-progesterone acetate (MPA)) had included over 4,000 women aged 65 years and older. These women did not have diagnoses of dementia at baseline and were followed up for four years on average. Results suggested that prescribing HT could result in an additional 23 cases of dementia per 10,000 women per year, a two-fold increase in risk [3]. The risk for ischemic stroke was also 1.5 times higher in women with combined HT and it was suggested that silent infarcts may have mediated the increased risk for dementia [3]. Risk factors for (cerebro)vascular disease are often the same as those for AD and cognitive decline, and less AD pathology is needed to induce cognitive deficits when cerebrovascular disease is also present [15]. The WHIMS estrogen-only trial (CEE) [1] showed a similar trend for an increased dementia risk and there was a significant increased risk for stroke, with an absolute excess risk of 12 additional strokes per 10,000 person-years.

The findings of the WHIMS contrasted with the biological plausibility of protective effects of HT on brain function as evidenced by animal and cell-culture studies; small positive early treatment studies; and most observational studies, which showed associations between HT use and decreased risk for dementia [16]. Importantly, cross-sectional observational studies have a high likelihood of bias because women with AD (by the nature of their disease) systematically have lower recall of their actual HT use than controls [17]. In addition, prospective observational studies may be biased because HT users are often better educated women of high socioeconomic status (SES) with healthy profiles (low blood pressure, body weight, cholesterol) that could protect them against AD [18, 13].

Surprisingly, in our earlier review [16] we found that those cohort studies of women without dementia that had included women with a lower SES and education [19] actually reported greater advantages of HT use on cognitive function. This finding could indicate that HT effects are more profound in women with less education, which was substantiated in another observational study [20]. Women who have received less education may have fewer resources to cope with cognitive decline and are at higher risk for AD [21]. Hormony therapy could potentially enhance residual resources, e.g., through its effect on cholinergic function, nerve growth factors, and dendritic sprouting [22, 23], and be particularly useful for this vulnerable group. Analyses stratified for education in the WHIMS study, however, did not indicate that treatment would have been beneficial for women with low levels of education [3].

It is unclear whether lifelong estrogen exposure, determined by a younger age at menarche and later age at menopause, affects the risk for AD and whether this interacts with HT effects after menopause. One study reported a decreased risk for AD with a younger age at menarche [24], but several others did not [25, 26, 27]. Some studies found that a later age at menopause [25, 28] was protective for AD, but others did not replicate this finding [24, 26, 27]. One observational study actually found the opposite [29]. In this cohort, a longer reproductive period increased the risk for AD, but only in those women genetically at risk for AD (APOE ε4 carriers). Socioeconomic status of women may also affect lifelong exposure to estrogen levels as women of higher SES were found to have an earlier age at menarche [30].

To further complicate matters, lifestyle factors, such as smoking, may also interact with lifelong estrogen exposure and HT use. Smokers have an earlier menopause than non-smokers [31] and are more likely to develop AD [32]. Smoking induces hepatic enzymes that metabolize estrogen [33], which would lower estrogen levels and also render HT less effective. One study that controlled for smoking found no protective effect of HT against AD [34]. In contrast, another study reported a possible synergistic effect of smoking and HT in risk reduction [35]. Smoking, of course, is also a known risk factor for cerebro- and cardiovascular disease and AD [15].

In addition, detailed analyses of results from our meta-analyses of women without dementia indicated that significant effects of HT seemed to be limited to women who had undergone surgical menopause [36]. It is unclear whether having undergone surgical menopause would affect HT use at a later age. Surgical menopause may be an initial risk factor for accelerated cognitive impairment and observational and experimental studies suggested that giving these women HT would reduce that risk [37, 38, 39]. However, long-term use of HT for this group could have negative effects on cognitive function [40, 41]. Another theory is that cognitive function was only improved in earlier HT studies because of alleviation of severe menopausal symptoms [42, 43], which are common in surgically menopausal women.

These findings suggest complicated interactions between age, education, smoking, duration and type of treatment, type of menopause, prior exposure to estrogens, and whether women were/are symptomatic (which could reflect heightened sensitivity to estrogen withdrawal, possibly influencing effects of treatment at a later age). Consequently, it could be the case that only higher order interactions identify those cases who are at an additional risk for dementia and cognitive impairment when using HT. For instance, such interactions might identify a high-risk group as those with high levels of education and who are prone to silent infarcts (e.g., those who smoke and have high blood pressure) and underwent surgical menopause at an early age without treatment at the time.

In sum, complex patterns of demographic and lifestyle factors may modify effects of HT, and interactions may occur on different levels. In the present study we used artificial neural networks (ANN) to model complex higher order interactions. Neural networks that account for higher order interactions may perform better than logistic regression models in assessing risks and benefits for the individual if the independent variables contain complex patterns. We assessed the performance of these networks in predicting cognitive outcomes, and estimated whether these multiple interactions can improve predictive accuracy and assist in identifying women who are more or less vulnerable to HT effects.

Neural network models as statistical classification devices

Binary outcomes such as improvements versus decline in cognitive function are often analyzed via logistic regression models. In the simplest and generally most robust case, such a model focuses on the main effects of the independent variables. The resulting model provides a linear scaling factor for each of those variables, and the sum of all scaled inputs yields the prediction of the outcome value. Such a linear discriminant approach is also the basis of classifications by ANN without hidden units. Each independent variable is assigned to an input node, and each of these input nodes has one link to the output node. The strength of this link is adapted during training to provide the best approximation of the required output values, and the resulting model uses the link weights to produce an outcome estimate in a manner that is equivalent to the scaling factors of the logistic regression. The main difference is that link weights in the ANN are adapted during training (i.e., the model-building stage) via a heuristic method. In the present work we used backpropagation of error [44]. An optimal model is not guaranteed in the ANN case, but simple networks in particular tend to arrive at the best solution.

The added advantage of ANN models rests in their ability to provide non-linear transformations of the input data via the inclusion of hidden units. Hidden units receive the input data, transform it in a manner similar to what is provided by two-way or many-way interactions in a regression model, and then add these transformed data to the output node. The discrimination ability of neural networks can be superior to that of linear discriminant analysis because of the highly non-linear transformation that ANN can apply to the data, and the use of multiple higher order interactions to achieve the best fit [45]. For a large and complex dataset like that of the WHIMS, which contains many independent variables, neural networks with hidden units may be able to provide much better models than logistic regression, because of their

ability to automatically include simple and complex interactions. This possibility was empirically tested in the present work.

In the case of neural networks with hidden units, the interactions are derived in an unsupervised manner by the backpropagation algorithm – they do not need to be specified before training the models. As a result, connectionist neural networks can readily achieve very high classification accuracy on many types of data, but the solution they find may include spurious interactions that result in poor performance on novel data from the same or different datasets. In general, more hidden units introduce more mathematical complexity into the neural network models, usually leading to better fits for the training data, but often sacrificing generality so that novel data are actually processed less accurately. Such problems with the generality of models are also a problematic issue for complex regression models that include interactions between the independent variables. In the present work, we employ cross-validation, where the models are trained on a part of the available data and then tested on the trained data and the remaining novel data, to deal with this problem and derive scores specifically for the classification of trained and novel data.

Objectives

The main aim of this study was to determine if increasingly complex statistical models can account better for cognitive outcomes (mild cognitive impairment (MCI), probable dementia, and a global cognitive measure using the 3MS examination score) in the WHIMS data. The independent variables included risk and protective factors that had been obtained in the entire study sample, such as age, education, socioeconomic status, region of the USA, ethnicity, physical activity, body mass index, smoking, alcohol use, prior cardiovascular disease, hypertension, diabetes mellitus, vasomotor symptoms, prior HT use, age at hysterectomy, and bilateral oophorectomy (for the CEE-alone trial). The most basic models only accounted for main effects, while more complex neural network models made use of increasing numbers of hidden units to account for higher order interactions, which are derived heuristically during model training. Cross-validation then allowed us to assess the impact of model complexity separately for trained and novel data, which provides reliable estimates of the robustness and generality of the model architectures tested here. Consequently, the current study could provide ways that predict whether either form of HT might be beneficial or additionally risk inducing for women with specific combinations of characteristics (e.g., those who had a stroke, those who are older, those who underwent a surgical menopause, those with low levels of education, and those who are smokers), as was suggested by our earlier review [16].

Methods

The Women's Health Initiative Memory Study (WHIMS)

The WHIMS [46] is an ancillary study to the Women's Health Initiative (WHI) Trials of Hormone Therapy [47, 48], two large, randomized, double-blind, placebo-controlled, clinical trials examining hormone-related outcomes. The WHIMS was conducted to assess the relative effect of estrogen alone (CEE-alone) or in combination with a progestin (CEE+MPA) on the incidence of dementia and global cognitive functioning in postmenopausal women. Following discovery of an unfavorable risk-to-benefit ratio of its non-cognitive endpoints, administration of study drug in the WHI CEE+MPA trial was discontinued (July, 2002) [49]. The WHI CEE-alone was discontinued later due to an adverse risk profile with respect to stroke, and a lack of benefit for cardiovascular disease (Feb, 2004) [50]. These decisions also ended the CEE+MPA and CEE-alone trials of WHIMS, which subsequently reported that both regimens had adverse affects on dementia and global cognitive function [3, 1, 4, 2].

The study design, eligibility criteria, and recruitment procedures of the WHI Hormone Trials have been described elsewhere [46, 51, 52]. Women aged 50–79 years were enrolled if they were postmenopausal. Major exclusion criteria were a history of breast cancer or any cancer within the previous ten years except non-melanoma skin cancer; acute myocardial infarction, stroke, or transient ischemic attack in the previous six months; known chronic active hepatitis or severe cirrhosis; and current use of corticosteroids, anticoagulants, tamoxifen, or other selective estrogen receptor modifiers. A history of venous thromboembolism was added as an exclusion criterion in 1997. A three-month washout period was required for women who were current hormone users at the initial screening visit. Women with a uterus at baseline were randomized with equal probability to take one daily tablet that contained either 0.625 mg of CEE with 2.5 mg MPA (PremPro™, Wyeth Pharmaceuticals, Inc., St. David's, PA) or a matching placebo. Women without a uterus at baseline were randomized with equal probability to take one daily tablet that contained either 0.625 mg of CEE (Premarin™, Wyeth Pharmaceuticals, Inc., St. David's, PA) or a matching placebo.

Participants in the WHIMS trials were recruited between May, 1996 and December, 1999 from women in the WHI trials who were at least 65 years of age and free of dementia as ascertained by the WHIMS protocol [46]. Written informed consent was obtained. The National Institutes of Health (NIH) and institutional review boards approved the protocol and consent forms.

Global cognitive function was measured with the Modified Mini-Mental State (3MS) examination [53] at baseline and annually for up to eight years. The 3MS examination consists of 15 items that sum to 0–100; higher scores reflect better cognitive functioning. Test items measure temporal and spatial orientation, immediate and delayed recall, executive function, naming, verbal fluency, abstract reasoning, praxis, writing, and visuo-constructional abilities. The 3MS test has good reliability, sensitivity, and specificity for detecting cognitive impairment and dementia [54, 55].

Modified Mini-Mental State examinations were administered by trained and certified technicians who were masked to other outcomes. Participants who scored below pre-established cut points were scheduled for a more extensive neurocognitive assessment and neuropsychiatric examination to determine the presence or absence of probable dementia and mild cognitive impairment, which was centrally adjudicated [46]. Regardless of adjudicated dementia status, women continued to be scheduled for their annual 3MS assessments.

Baseline demographic data and medical histories were collected via self-report and standardized assessments. Hypertension was defined as present when indicated by self-reported current drug therapy for hypertension or clinical measurement of BP > 140/90 mmHg at enrollment. Cardiovascular disease (CVD) history was coded as positive if the participant had reported a history of myocardial infarction, stroke, angina, coronary bypass surgery, or angioplasty of coronary arteries at their baseline visit. Factors included in our analyses were those found to be significantly related to 3MS test scores [4, 2] and/or which we hypothesized may identify important patient subgroups.

Dataset description

The variables listed in Table 2.1 were used as independent variables for the neural net and logistic regression models. As women included for the CEE alone and CEE combination therapy were different between studies (age and a history of oophorectomy and/or hysterectomy), which may have affected the outcome, analyses were split for type of treatment. A total of 3,014 and 3,092 participants with valid 3MS examination data for year 0 and year 4 were present in the CEE-alone trial and the CEE+MPA trial datasets, respectively. After excluding all rows with missing data for any variable, 2,448 and 2,527 participants (including those assigned to active treatment and placebo) remained available in the CEE-alone and CEE+MPA trial datasets, respectively.

The ANN models used in this work require input values with the range {0,1}. Hence, only binary variables, which are listed with "binary" in the transformation column in Table 2.1, could be used directly without any transformation. All continuous variables were transformed by subtracting the minimum value and dividing by the range. This procedure did not cause any information loss because all new values were stored with sufficient numeric precision. The label "range" in the transformation column of Table 2.1 indicates these continuous variables. Finally, categorical variables were transformed into a "localist" code, where every possible value of the variable (i.e., each category) is encoded by a dedicated binary variable.

Outcome variables

We chose to use changes in 3MS scores and clinical dementia/mild cognitive impairment diagnoses as the outcome variables for this study, because our aim was to predict changes in cognitive function and cognitive impairment. Due to the early termination of the WHI trials, only four years of planned follow-up were available for the majority of women, so we focus on changes over the four-year study period. The WHIMS analyses support the utility of examining changes of at least

four units on the 3MS examination (approximately one standard deviation) [4, 2].

We thus examined models that contrasted women whose four-year 3MS examination showed >3 units improvement or worsening from baseline. Due to its maximum score at 100, a baseline 3MS examination of >96 precluded women from being classified as improving under this approach. The number of participants with changes of >3 units were 1,788 (CEE-alone) and 1,882 (CEE+MPA). The binary outcome measure 'd3MS' was calculated in the following way:

$$d3MS = \left\{ \begin{array}{l} 1 \ if \ 3MS_{year4} - 3MS_{year0} > 3 \\ 0 \ if \ 3MS_{year4} - 3MS_{year0} < -3 \end{array} \right\}$$

We also analyzed the predictability of clinical diagnoses related to dementia. Two diagnostic categories for cognitive impairment were present in the data: mild cognitive impairment (MCI) and probable dementia (PD). However, the numbers of PD diagnoses at year 4 were very small, with only 41 and 26 cases present in the CEE-alone and CEE+MPA datasets. Excluding rows with missing data would have reduced these numbers further, making it very difficult to derive any reliable prediction of PD diagnosis alone. Since an MCI diagnosis confers an increased risk of converting to Alzheimer's disease [56], we grouped MCI and PD diagnoses together, which created a larger group of participants with a "cognitively impaired" or "dementia-related" diagnosis. Diagnosis during the previous study period was not considered in this outcome measure. All participants whose 3MS examination scores remained stable or improved between year 0 and year 4 were grouped into the opposite outcome. The clinical diagnosis outcome "diagnosis" was defined as follows:

$$diagnosis = \left\{ \begin{array}{l} 1 \ if \ CDIAG_{year4} = MCIorPD \\ 0 \ if \ 3MS_{year4} - 3MS_{year0} \geq 0 \end{array} \right\}$$

Statistical models

We chose to evaluate and compare the performance of logistic regression models and ANN. Logistic regression modeling and other statistical analyses were carried out using R (www.r-project.org). All independent variables that were available to the ANN simulations were also included in the regression models. Despite the fact that many of these variables did not reach significance, reducing the logistic regressions to

Table 2.1 Predictor variables and how they were transformed into inputs for the neural network models.

Variable	Description	Source	Transformation
BMI	body mass index	c1	range
SCRNAGE	age at enrollment	c1	range
EDU	education (1–11 levels)	c1	range
BASE3MS	3MS score at enrollment (0–100)	c1	range
HT	HT/placebo	c1	binary
MI	myocardial infarct history	c1	binary
CABG	coronary artery bypass	c1	binary
PTCA	PTCA, ever	c1	binary
ANGINA	history of angina (0 = no, 1 = yes)	c1	binary
ASPIRIN	use of aspirin at baseline	c1	binary
HYPT	previous or current hypertension	c1	binary
DIAB	diabetes mellitus, ever	c1	binary
TOTH	history of HT use (0 = no, 1 = yes)	c1	binary
TOTESTAT	past/currrent unopposed estrogen use	c1	binary
TOTPSTAT	past/current combination HT use	c1	binary
SMOKING	never/previous or current smoking	c1	localist
RACE	racial/ethnic backgroup (1–8)	c1	localist
INCOME	income group (4 levels)	d1	range
NIGHTSWT	presence of night sweats	d1	range
HOTFLASH	presence of hot flashes	d1	range
SYST	systolic blood pressure (continuous)	d1	range
DIAS	diastolic blood pressure	d1	range
LMSEPI	moderate to limited activity	d1	range
ALCSWK	alcohol units/week	d1	range
MENOPSEA	age at last regular menstrual period	d1	range
ANYMENSA	age at last bleeding	d1	range
HTGRP	HT use and duration, 4 levels	d1	range
STARTHT	HT onset wrt last period, 4 levels	d1	range
HYST	having undergone hysterectomy	d1	binary
STROKE	having had a stroke	d1	binary
CVD	cardio/cerebrovascular disease	d1	binary
BASESTAT	baseline statin use	d1	binary
STATIN	statin use while participating in study	d1	binary
OOPHGRP	oopherectomy (no/single/both)	d1	binary

include only significant independent variables resulted in lower area under the curve (AUC) scores. Hence, we decided to retain all independent variables for the logistic regressions in order to make the results of the logistic regression directly comparable to the ANN simulations.

Neural network simulations were built with the "lens" neural network simulator (http://tedlab.mit.edu/~dr/Lens) and contained 46 input units and 1 output unit. Hidden unit numbers included 0 (i.e., only direct connections from the input to the output layer were present), 1, 2, . . . , 10, 15 and 20 in order to allow estimates of the effect of hidden unit numbers, a measure of model complexity, on the predictive quality of the ANN. The direct input–output connections were left in place in all networks that included hidden units. Networks without hidden units were trained for 5,000 epochs and evaluated every 1,000 epochs. Networks with hidden units were trained for 10,000 epochs and evaluated every 2,000 epochs. To calculate true and false positive and negative rates, neural network outputs were evaluated with a cut-off of 0.5, i.e., any output below 0.5 was counted as 0 (negative) and any output above 0.5 was classified as 1 (positive).

Cross-validation

Connectionist networks can readily achieve very high classification accuracy on many types of data, but the solution they find may not always generalize very well to novel data from the same or different datasets. To guard against overfitted models, which may give undue weight to outliers or unusual patterns in the dataset, we used cross-validation to ensure robust generalization of the results. With this method, only a subset of the data, in our case 90% of the available participants, was used to train each given ANN model, whose performance was then tested on the remaining (and to the model previously unseen) 10% of the data. This was repeated ten times for each dataset, so that in the end each model had been tested on 100% (10×10%) of the data without having used any of the testing data for model building. Via this method, all models were assessed for their predictive performance for each participant in the dataset without ever having been exposed to the data from that participant previously. The performance scores derived in this manner can thus provide a fair estimate of how well the models could predict the cognitive function for entirely new patients.

Results

Changes of more than three points in 3MS examination scores

The CEE-alone and CEE+MPA trial datasets contained 660 and 645 participants, with positive outcome (>3 units improvement on the 3MS) prevalences of 72% and 67%, respectively. The neural networks were trained on the task of predicting the outcome from the baseline data, and their performances were evaluated on the training data and on the novel testing data. Figure 2.1 shows the accuracy of these models in terms of the percentage of correct classifications.

A linear regression model of the percentage of correct classifications by the ANN models showed a significant interaction between testing on trained versus novel data and hidden unit numbers in the CEE trial ($t = 20.3$, $p < 0.0001$). The interaction is a result of the beneficial effect of increasing hidden unit number on model performance on trained data ($\beta = 0.8$, $t = 23.9$, $p < 0.0001$), as opposed to decreased model performance with more hidden units for novel data ($\beta = -0.2$, $t = -5.9$, $p < 0.0001$). The same significant interaction between hidden unit number and testing on trained versus novel data was found in the CEE+MPA trial ($t = 14.4$, $p < 0.0001$), where more hidden units provided better performance on trained data ($\beta = 0.7$, $t = 23.7$, $p < 0.0001$) while leading to decreased performance on novel data ($\beta = -0.4$, $t = -3.1$, $p < 0.003$ after removing the significant non-linear component).

Artificial neural network models without hidden units yielded 77% and 80% correct predictions for novel data in the CEE-alone and CEE+MPA trials, respectively. This performance is considerably better than chance when considering that the positive outcome prevalences were 72% and 67% for the CEE-alone and CEE+MPA trials. Focusing exclusively on participants with 3MS changes of four points or more made it possible to build quite robust models that were able to generalize to novel data with a good degree of accuracy.

We also included a comparison of ANN classifier performance to a logistic regression model, which contained the main effects of all the variables available to the ANN models and was built and tested on the entire dataset for each treatment trial (Fig. 2.2).

The neural networks without hidden units performed similarly to the logistic regression model.

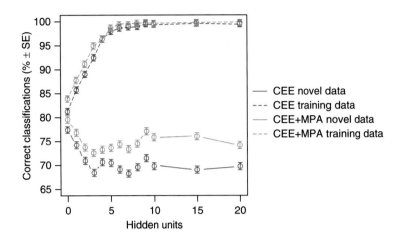

Fig. 2.1 Artificial neural network model accuracy (percent correct classifications ± SE) on training and novel data for the CEE-alone and CEE+MPA trials for 3MS examination changes of four points or more as a function of hidden unit number. (See color plate section.)

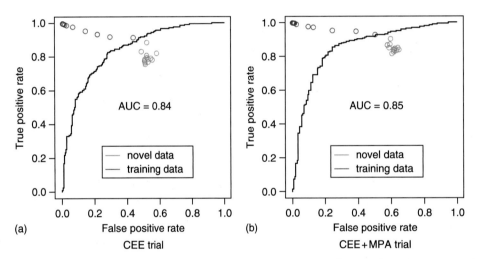

(a) CEE trial

(b) CEE+MPA trial

Fig. 2.2 The full logistic regression model ROC compared to ANN model performance for 3MS examination changes of four points or more. (See color plate section.)

Those with more hidden unit resources achieved better scores on the training data (red circles), but again this performance gain did not translate into improved performance on novel data (green circles). Hence, although changes in 3MS score of four points or more appeared to be more reliably predictable than the smaller changes analyzed above, cross-validation suggests that the simpler models provided a more robust and general description of the data in both treatment trials.

Clinical diagnosis

After removing all entries with missing data, the CEE-alone trial contained 1,756 participants with a positive diagnosis prevalence of 3.2% (56 cases) and the CEE+MPA trial included 1,863 participants with a positive diagnosis prevalence of 1.8 % (34 cases). The neural networks were trained to predict this outcome, and their performance on trained and novel data as a function of hidden unit number is shown in Fig. 2.3.

A regression model with the percentage of correct classifications as outcome and hidden unit number and trained versus novel data as input variables indicated a significant interaction between hidden unit number and the type of testing data in the CEE-alone trial ($t = 8.9$, $p < 0.0001$). This interaction results from the positive effect of increasing hidden unit number on model performance on trained data ($\beta = 0.1$, $t = 20.6$, $p < 0.0001$), as opposed to decreased

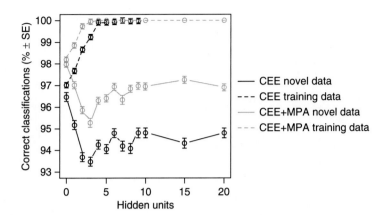

Fig. 2.3 Artificial neural network model accuracy (percent correct classifications ± SE) on training and novel data for the CEE-alone and CEE+MPA trials for the clinical diagnosis outcome as a function of hidden unit number. (See color plate section.)

model performance with more hidden units for novel data ($\beta = -0.2$, $t = -4.4$, $p < 0.0001$ after removing the significant non-linear component). The results for the CEE+MPA trial were similar when a non-linear component was included to account for the initial drop in correct classifications on novel data with very few hidden units only (see Fig. 2.3). There was a significant interaction between hidden unit number and testing on trained versus novel data ($t = 3.0$, $p < 0.004$). More hidden units provided better performance on trained data ($\beta = 0.2$, $t = 22.0$, $p < 0.0001$ after removing the non-linear component), and produced a trend for worse performance on novel data ($t = -0.2$, $p = 0.06$ after removing the non-linear component).

Compared to the previous results, the absence of a significant correlation between increasing model complexity and the predictive accuracy for novel data in the CEE+MPA trial leaves open the possibility that more complex models might work well for the CEE+MPA trial with the diagnosis outcome. However, the positive outcome prevalence of only 1.8% in this trial provides an alternative explanation: most models scored between 97% and 98% correct predictions, which was roughly at chance level. The low sensitivity scores for novel data (0–20%) indicate that this is driven by erring on the side of caution, i.e. mostly predicting outcomes of 0, for novel data. Hence, absence of a significant correlation between more hidden units and accuracy of outcome predictions for the CEE+MPA trial may have been driven by a ceiling effect that resulted from the very low prevalence of positive outcomes in this dataset. In the CEE+MPA trial, where the prevalence was slightly less skewed at 3.2%, ANN models without hidden units

were able to make 97% correct classifications on novel data, thus also not performing better than chance.

Artificial neural network classifier performance was also compared to a logistic regression model that contained the main effects of all the variables available to the ANN models and was built and tested on the entire dataset for each treatment trial (Fig. 2.4).

Neural networks without hidden units performed similarly to the logistic regression model on trained data. Those with more hidden unit resources achieved better scores on the training data (red circles), but again this performance gain did not translate into improved performance on novel data (green circles). Overall, cross-validation suggests that the simpler models provided a more robust and general description of the diagnosis outcome in both treatment trials.

Discussion

We used neural network models to try to predict cognitive test score changes and clinical diagnoses of cognitive impairment (mild cognitive impairment and probable dementia combined) in an HT treatment study. The study contained two treatment trials, one for estrogen alone (CEE-alone) and one with combination therapy (CEE+MPA), which were analyzed separately. We also compared the performance of the neural network models to that of logistic regression models, but performed no cross-validation on the latter because one would expect their performance to be similar to that of the neural networks without hidden units. Indeed, we found that the regression models performed just as well as the neural networks without hidden units on the data that had been used for model building, for all outcome

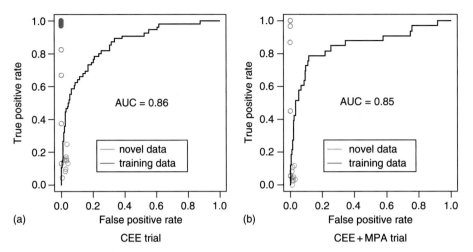

Fig. 2.4 The full logistic regression model ROC compared to ANN model performance on the clinical diagnosis outcome. (See color plate section.)

measures that were evaluated. Furthermore, we never observed a case where more complex models provided better fits for novel data. Instead, we found consistent and statistically significant decreases in predictive accuracy for novel data with more complex models. These findings are important as they show that the inclusion of higher order interactions does not result in more robust models that give a better fit for the data. Hence, our analysis of the WHIMS data does not support the idea that some women with specific profiles of the independent variables would benefit from HT while others might be at additional risk.

Using ANN yielded poor accuracy in predicting subtle changes in cognitive test scores (no change and/or decreased 3MS scores vs. improved scores over a period of four years, analyses not shown), indicating that the information contained in the independent variables was insufficient for a reliable model of overall treatment outcome. Similar effects were found for the clinically diagnosed cognitively impaired group. This fact may tie in with the earlier WHIMS papers showing no effect of HT on MCI prevalence [4, 2]. However, using a less noisy and more clinically relevant four-point change in 3MS scores as outcome appeared to be predictable with much higher accuracy. Even the ANN models with just a few hidden units could achieve 100% correct classifications on the training data. However, increasing hidden unit numbers actually decreased classification accuracy on novel data significantly. The same effect was found

for the other outcome measures that were evaluated. Hence, the inclusion of higher order interactions increased the explanatory value of the ANN model for trained data, but produced poorer classifications for novel data.

One possibly problematic aspect of the model building approach taken here is that the neural networks were supplied with a large number of independent variables, many of which had no significant correlation with the outcome. This might have been a driving factor in the sometimes low generalization of model accuracy to novel data, especially for networks with many hidden units, as they would have been likely to make use of spurious interactions in order to achieve better fits for the training data. Indeed, it is possible that ANN with fewer inputs could actually provide more accurate classifications when tested on novel data. However, all included independent variables were chosen because prior research has indicated that they may modify the effect of HT on cognitive function.

Independent variables that do not contribute to model accuracy are commonly eliminated via logistic regression with stepwise backward removal of individual variables. However, this is very problematic because relevant independent variables are often excluded if they are partially correlated with other variables. Indeed, we found that minimal models constructed in this way produced significantly poorer fits also for novel data than the models that included the main effects of all variables listed in Table 2.1.

Determining the most relevant independent variables and interactions that should be included to predict cognitive outcomes was beyond the scope of this research and remains an important question for future research. The current work only allows the conclusion that a full model of all available independent variables and their interactions is not the best way to predict cognitive outcomes in this body of data. Furthermore, we can conclude that any complex models should be evaluated for their generality via cross-validation, since only testing on novel data can reveal overfitted models.

A further possibly problematic aspect of our modeling approach is the use of compound scores (e.g., CVD) as well as the single factors related to those compound scores within the same model. In a logistic regression model, intercorrelations can confound main effects of either or both variables (e.g., where both variables sometimes no longer significantly contribute to the variance explained in the model because of inter-relatedness). However, this would not have caused analogous problems for the ANN as these models do not rely on testing the amount of variance explained. Instead, neural networks will treat correlated inputs with similar weights, or ignore the less relevant inputs.

The use of a combined MCI/PD group is by no means uncontroversial. Mild cognitive impairment in WHIMS was defined differently than by Petersen (1999) [56], and WHIMS-MCI has not been validated as a sensitive predictor of AD. However, considering the low numbers of cases with PD, it would have been very difficult to build cross-validated models for the probable dementia alone. In fact, the combined MCI and PD group amounted to only 2–3% of the entire WHIMS group. The small size of the cognitively impaired group may have caused ceiling effects, because there was a corresponding 97% chance level for guessing the outcome by predicting non-case membership.

Our findings suggest that variables predicting treatment outcome were heterogeneous and were not limited to one or more small group(s) with a certain pattern of predictors. We were unable to predict reliably subgroups of women who would benefit and/or not benefit from HT. Effects did not seem to be modified by other risk and protective factors in elderly women. Previous work suggests that HT may have some benefit for women who have recently undergone menopause [12]. However, the WHIMS

data do not address this possibility because women were aged 65 years and older. Moreover, the hypothesis that more recently postmenopausal women would show cognitive benefit from HT has not been tested with an appropriately sized, randomized controlled clinical trial. The hypothesis is supported by animal research indicating a "window of opportunity," where effects of estrogens were only beneficial for a limited period of time after onset of (surgically induced) menopause [23, 22]. This could perhaps relate to desensitization or down-regulation of receptors or other hormone-sensitive systems necessary for optimal brain function. Women in WHIMS were on average more than 15 years past their menopause, which may have been too late for estrogens to exert putative positive effects.

Finally, there may be an interaction of HT with genetic factors and HT could be more or less effective in women with particular polymorphisms. For instance, some polymorphisms associated with estrogen biosynthesis and metabolism can result in high levels of estrogens and the formation of toxic metabolites, which, when not inactivated, could potentially lead to DNA damage and subsequently AD pathology [13]. In addition, having at least one APOE ε4 allele is approximately two to three times more common in cases with AD [15]. While some observational studies found that cognitive decline was only prevented in women who were negative for the ε4 allele [57, 58], several reported that having the ε4 allele made no difference in risk reduction or that associations were not significant [59, 60, 61, 62, 63]. Discrepancies between studies could potentially be explained by complex interactions with the APOE genotype and differences in age of participants combined with the onset of treatment and/or duration of HT use. However, in the present analyses, genotyping was not available for cases and these variables could not be included.

The present study showed that neural networks that had many independent variables and their interactions available to predict cognitive outcomes led to suboptimal models of cognitive function outcomes when tested on novel data. The simplest models, comparable to logistic regression models limited to main effects, were most robust when assessed with cross-validation. More complex models that included non-linear interactions could fit the training data with 100% accuracy, but did not achieve better predictive accuracy on novel data. This indicates the presence of unusual patterns of interactions that are inconsistent across the dataset, and suggests that the most parsimonious statistical models, e.g., regression models limited to main effects, possibly including plausible interactions, may offer the most robust description of the WHIMS cohort. Our results also suggest that it is important to assess the quality of any complex regression models with cross-validation. Of all the outcome measures we evaluated, clinically significant changes in 3MS examinations of more than three points were most reliably predictable.

References

1. Shumaker SA, Legault C, Kuller L, *et al.* Conjugated equine estrogens and incidence of probable dementia and mild cognitive impairment in postmenopausal women: Women's Health Initiative Memory Study. *JAMA.* 2004;**291**(24):2947–58.

2. Espeland MA, Rapp SR, Shumaker SA, *et al.* Conjugated equine estrogens and global cognitive function in postmenopausal women: Women's Health Initiative Memory Study. *JAMA.* 2004; **291**(24):2959–68.

3. Shumaker SA, Legault C, Rapp SR, *et al.* Estrogen plus progestin and the incidence of dementia and mild cognitive impairment in postmenopausal women: the Women's Health Initiative Memory Study: a randomized controlled trial. *JAMA.* 2003;**289** (20):2651–62.

4. Rapp SR, Espeland MA, Shumaker SA, *et al.* Effect of estrogen plus progestin on global cognitive function in postmenopausal women: the Women's Health Initiative Memory Study: a randomized controlled trial. *JAMA.* 2003;**289**(20):2663–72.

5. Henderson VW, Paganini-Hill A, Miller BL, *et al.* Estrogen for Alzheimer's disease in women. *Neurology.* 2000;**54**:295–301.

6. Mulnard RA, Cotman CW, Kawas C, *et al.* Estrogen replacement therapy for treatment of mild to moderate Alzheimer's disease. *JAMA.* 2000;**283**:1007–15.

7. Wang PN, Liao SQ, Liu RS, *et al.* Effects of estrogen on cognition, mood, and cerebral blood flow in AD. *Neurology.* 2000;**54**:2061–6.

8. Barrett-Connor E, Grady D, Stefanick ML. The rise and fall of menopausal hormone therapy. *Annu Rev Public Health.* 2005;**26**:115–40.

9. Brinton RD. Impact of estrogen therapy on Alzheimer's disease: a fork in the road? *CNS Drugs.* 2004;**18**(7):405–22.

10. Sherwin BB. Estrogen and memory in women: how can we reconcile the findings? *Horm Behav.* 2005; **47**(3):371–5.

11. Maki PM. Hormone therapy and risk for dementia: where do we go from here? *Gynecol Endocrinol.* 2004;**19**(6):354–9.

12. Resnick SM, Henderson VW. Hormone therapy and risk of Alzheimer disease: a critical time. *JAMA.* 2002;**288**(17):2170–2.

13. Hogervorst E. The short-lived effect of hormone therapy on cognitive function. In Rasgon NL, ed. *The Effects of Estrogen on Brain Function.* Baltimore, MD: John Hopkins Press, 2006, pp. 46–78.

14. Pinkerton JV, Henderson VW. Estrogen and cognition, with a focus on Alzheimer's disease. *Semin Reprod Med.* 2005;**23**(2):172–9.

15. Hogervorst E, Mendes-Ribeiro H, Molyneux A, Budge M, Smith AD. Serum homocysteine, cerebrovascular risk factors and white matter low attenuation on CT scans in patients with post-mortem confirmed Alzheimer's disease. *Arch Neurology.* 2002;**59**:787–93.

16. Hogervorst E, Williams J, Budge M, Riedel W, Jolles J. The nature of the effect of female gonadal hormone replacement therapy on cognitive function in postmenopausal women: a meta-analysis. *Neuroscience.* 2000;**101**:485–512.

17. Petitti DB, Buckwalter JG, Crooks VC, Chiu V. Prevalence of dementia in users of hormone replacement therapy as defined by prescription data. *J Gerontol A Biol Sci Med Sci.* 2002;**57**:M532–8.

18. Matthews KA, Kuller LH, Wing RR, Meilahn EN, Plantinga P. Prior to use of estrogen replacement therapy: are users healthier than nonusers? *Am J Epidemiol.* 1996;**143**(10):971–8.

19. Jacobs DM, Tang M-X, Stern Y, *et al.* Cognitive function in non-demented older women who took estrogen after menopause. *Neurology.* 1998;**50**(2):368–73.

20. Matthews K, Cauley J, Yaffe K, Zmuda J. Estrogen replacement therapy and cognitive decline in older community women. *JAGS.* 1999;**47**:518–23.

21. Launer LJ, Andersen K, Dewy ME, *et al.* Rates and risk factors for dementia and Alzheimer's disease. *Neurology.* 1999;**1**(52):78–84.

22. Henderson VW. Hormone therapy and Alzheimer's disease: benefit or harm? *Expert Opin Pharmacother.* 2004;**5**(2):389–406.

23. Gibbs R. Preclinical data relating to estrogen's effects on cognitive performance. In Rasgon NL, ed. *The Effects of Estrogen on Brain Function.* Baltimore, MD: John Hopkins Press, 2006, pp. 9–45.

24. Paganini-Hill A, Henderson VW. Estrogen deficiency and risk of Alzheimer's disease in women. *Am J Epidemiol.* 1994;**140**:256–61.

25. Balderischi M, DiCarlo A, Lepore V, *et al.* Estrogen-replacement therapy and Alzheimer's disease in the

Italian longitudinal study on aging. *Neurology.* 1998; **50**:996–1002.

26. Kawas C, Resnick S, Morrison A, *et al.* A prospective study of estrogen replacement therapy and the risk of developing Alzheimer's disease. *Neurology.* 1996;**48**:1517–21.

27. Waring SC, Rocca WA, Peteresen RC, *et al.* Postmenopausal estrogen replacement therapy and risk of AD. *Neurology.* 1999;**52**(2):965–70.

28. McLay RN, Maki PM, Lyketsos CG. Nulliparity and late menopause are associated with decreased cognitive decline. *J Neuropsychiatry Clin Neurosci.* 2003;**15**(2):161–7.

29. Geerlings MI, Ruitenberg A, Witteman JC, *et al.* Reproductive period and risk of dementia in postmenopausal women. *JAMA.* 2001;**285**(11):1475–81.

30. Ayatollahi SM, Dowlatabadi E, Ayatollahi SA. Age at menarche in Iran. *Ann Hum Biol.* 2002;**29**(4):355–62.

31. Kato I, Toniolo P, Akhmedkhanov A, *et al.* Prospective study of factors influencing the onset of natural menopause. *J Clin Epidemiol.* 1998;**51**(12):1271–6.

32. Merchant C, Tang M-X, Albert S, *et al.* The influence of smoking on the risk of Alzheimer's disease. *Neurology.* 1999;**52**(7):1408–12.

33. Meek MD, Finch GL. Diluted mainstream cigarette smoke condensates activate estogen receptor and aryl hydrocarbon receptor-mediated gene transcription. *Environ Res.* 1999;**80**(1):9–17.

34. Brenner DE, Kukull WA, Stergachis A, *et al.* Postmenopausal estrogen replacement therapy and the risk of Alzheimer's disease: a population based case-control study. *Am J Epidemiol.* 1994;**140**:262–7.

35. Lerner A, Koss E, Debanne S, *et al.* Smoking and oestrogen replacement therapy as protective factors against AD. *Lancet.* 1997;**349**(Feb 8):403–4.

36. Hogervorst E, Smith AD. The interaction of serum folate and estradiol levels in Alzheimer's disease. *Neuroendocrinol Lett.* 2002;**23**:155–60.

37. Verghese J, Kuslansky G, Katz M, *et al.* Surgically menopausal women on estrogen have better cognitive performance. *Neurology.* 2000;**54**(Suppl 3):A210–A211.

38. Sherwin BB. Cognitive assessment for postmenopausal women and general assessment of their mental health. *Psychopharmacol Bull.* 1998;**34**(3):323–6.

39. Nappi RE, Sinforiani E, Mauri M, *et al.* Memory functioning at menopause: impact of age in ovariectomized women. *Gynecol Obstet Invest.* 1999;**47**:29–36.

40. File SE, Heard JE, Rymer J. Trough oestradiol levels associated with cognitive impairment in post-menopausal women after 10 years of oestradiol implants. *Psychopharmacology (Berl).* 2002; **161**(1):107–12.

41. Szklo M, Cerhan J, Diez-Roux AV, *et al.* Estrogen replacement therapy and cognitive functioning in the Artherosclerotic Risk In Communities (ARIC) study. *Am J Epidemiol.* 1996;**144**:1048–57.

42. Yaffe K, Sawaya G, Lieberburg I, Grady D. Estrogen therapy in postmenopausal women. *JAMA.* 1998; **279**(9):688–95.

43. LeBlanc ES, Janowsky J, Chan BK, Nelson HD. Hormone replacement therapy and cognition: systematic review and meta-analysis. *JAMA.* 2001; **285**(11):1489–99.

44. Rumelhart DE, Hinton G, Williams R. Learning internal representations by error propagation. In McClelland JL, Rumelhart DE and the PDP research group, ed. *Parallel Distributed Processes: Explorations in the Microstructure of Cognition. Volume 2: Foundations.* Cambridge, MA: Bradford Books/MIT Press, 1986.

45. French BM, Dawson MR, Dobbs AR. Classification and staging of dementia of the Alzheimer type: a comparison between neural networks and linear discriminant analysis. *Arch Neurol.* 1997;**54**:1001–9.

46. Shumaker SA, Reboussin BA, Espeland MA, *et al.* The Women's Health Initiative Memory Study (WHIMS): a trial of the effect of estrogen therapy in preventing and slowing the progression of dementia. *Control Clin Trials.* 1998;**19**(6):604–21.

47. Women's Health Initiative Study Group. Design of the Women's Health Initiative clinical trial and observational study. *Control Clin Trials.* 1998;**19**:61–109.

48. Stefanick ML, Cochrane BB, Hsia J, *et al.* The Women's Health Initiative postmenopausal hormone trials: overview and baseline characteristics of participants. *Ann Epidemiol.* 2003;**13**(9 suppl):578–86.

49. Writing Group for the Women's Health Initiative Investigators. Risk and benefits of estrogen plus progestin in healthy postmenopausal women: principal results from the Women's Health Initiative randomized controlled trial. *JAMA.* 2002;**288**:321–33.

50. The Women's Health Initiative Steering Committee. Effects of conjugated equine estrogen in postmenopausal women with hysterectomy: the Women's Health Initiative randomized controlled trial. *JAMA.* 2004;**291**:1701–12.

51. Anderson GL, Manson J, Wallace R, *et al.* Implementation of the Women's Health Initiative study design. *Ann Epidemiol.* 2003;**13**:S5–17.

52. Hayes J, Hunt JR, Hubbell FA, *et al.* The Women's Health Initiative recruitment methods and results. *Ann Epidemiol.* 2003;**13**:S18–77.

53. Teng EL, Chui H. The Modified Mini-Mental State (3MS) examination. *J Clin Psychiatry*. 1987;**48**:314–18.

54. McDowell I, Kristjansson B, Hill GB, Herbert R. Community screening for dementia: the Mini Mental State Examination (MMSE) and Modified Mini Mental State Examination (3MS) compared. *J Clin Epidemiol*. 1997;**50**:377–83.

55. Bravo G, Herbert R. Age- and education-specific reference values for the Mini-Mental and Modified Mini-Mental State Examinations derived from a non-demented elderly population. *Int J Geriatr Psychiatry*. 1997;**12**:1008–18.

56. Petersen RC, Smith GE, Waring SG, *et al.* Mild cognitive impairment: clinical characterization and outcome. *Arch Neurol*. 1999;**56**(3):303–8.

57. Yaffe K, Haan M, Byers A, Tangen C, Kuller L. Estrogen use, APOE, and cognitive decline. *Neurology*. 2000;**54**:1949–53.

58. Burkhardt MS, Foster JK, Laws SM, *et al.* Oestrogen replacement therapy may improve memory functioning in the absence of APOE epsilon4. *J Alzheimer's Dis*. 2004;**6**(3):221–8.

59. Tang MX, Jacobs D, Stern Y, *et al.* Effect of estrogen during the menopause on risk and age of onset of Alzheimer's disease. *Lancet*. 1996;**348**:429–32.

60. Steffens DC, Noron MC, Plassman BL, *et al.* Enhanced cognitive performance with estrogen use in nondemented community dwelling older women. *JAGS*. 1999;**47**:1171–5.

61. Slooter AJC, Bronzova J, Witteman JCM, van Broekhoven C, van Duijn C. Estrogen use and early onset Alzheimer's disease: a population based study. *J Neurol Neurosurg Psychiatry*. 1999;**67**(6):779–81.

62. Zandi PP, Carlson MC, Plassman BL, *et al.* Hormone replacement therapy and incidence of Alzheimer disease in older women: the Cache County study. *JAMA*. 2002;**288**(17):2123–9.

63. Henderson VW, Benke KS, Green RC, Cupples LA, Farrer LA. Postmenopausal hormone therapy and Alzheimer's disease risk: interaction with age. *J Neurol Neurosurg Psychiatry*. 2005;**76**:103–5.

Chapter 3

Estrogen therapy – relationship to longevity and prevalent dementia in the oldest-old: the Leisure World Cohort Study and the 90+ Study

Claudia H. Kawas, María M. Corrada, and Annlia Paganini-Hill

Editors' introduction

To our knowledge, the study by Kawas et al. is the first observational study to describe a significant increase of dementia risk in older women who had been using hormones for five to nine years. The Leisure World Cohort Study was initiated in 1981 and consisted of women residing in a California retirement community (N = 8,801) who had completed a postal survey including details of estrogen therapy [ET]. After 22 years of follow-up, ET users (ever) had a 10% lower age-adjusted mortality than lifetime non-users. This risk was further decreased with increasing duration, but was not related to dose (0.625 mg vs. 1.25 mg). The relationship did not significantly change when adjusted for potential confounders, including exercise, body mass index, smoking, and medical histories related to mortality. The 90+ Study was initiated to directly examine surviving members of the cohort to determine clinical and functional status. Research participants who were alive and aged 90 and older on January 1, 2003 were invited to participate (N = 706 women, 90–106 years old). Prevalence of all-cause dementia was 45% in these women, but was not lower in ever-users of estrogen. Somewhat surprisingly, women who had used estrogen for five to nine years appeared to have an increased prevalence of dementia (odds ratio (OR) = 2.02, 95% CI 1.17–3.45), but longer or shorter duration of use was not associated with increased or decreased risk. This chapter discusses these results with regards to timing of exposure and age.

Introduction

In recent years, randomized clinical trials with post-menopausal estrogen therapy (ET) found increased risks of dementia, coronary heart disease, stroke, and venous thromboembolic disease among women assigned to conjugated equine estrogens alone or in combination with medroxy-progesterone acetate compared with placebo [1–5]. These results contradict the numerous observational studies that suggested that use of estrogens is associated with lower risk of dementia, cognitive decline, other conditions, and mortality. The randomized trials minimized confounding, an important consideration since women who take estrogens undoubtedly differ from those who do not in many lifestyle factors, use of health services, and other ways. However, the randomized studies were of relatively short duration and could not address issues regarding long-term use or the long-term effects of more limited perimenopausal use. For practical considerations, it is unlikely that randomized trials involving large numbers of women with follow-up of 15 years or more will be conducted. In this chapter, we describe results from a 22-year observational study of ET, mortality, and dementia. Long-term observational studies such as the Leisure World Cohort Study and the 90+ Study will continue to contribute valuable data that will complement those from clinical trials.

Study cohorts

In the early 1980s, investigators from the University of Southern California established a prospective cohort study of 8,877 postmenopausal women with the goal of studying the risks and benefits of ET [6]. After 7.5 years of follow-up, women who had used estrogens had 20% lower risk of death compared to women who had not used estrogens. This cohort provides the foundation for our investigations of the relationships between estrogen use and longevity and dementia in older women. With follow-up extended to 22 years, we investigated estrogen use and menstrual factors in relation to long-term mortality in the Leisure World Cohort Study. With additional neurological and neuropsychological examinations for dementia as part of the 90+ Study [7, 8] we also investigated estrogen use in relation to prevalent dementia in these women aged 90 years and older.

Estrogen therapy and longevity: the Leisure World Cohort Study

For the Leisure World Cohort Study, a health survey was mailed to all residents who owned homes in Leisure World Laguna Hills, a California retirement community, on June 1, 1981; June 1, 1982; June 1, 1983; and October 1, 1985. Of the 13,978 residents who returned the questionnaire and constitute the Leisure World Cohort, 8,877 are women. Reflecting the local community, they are predominantly white, well-educated, and upper middle class. The health survey asked demographic information, brief medical history, personal lifestyle habits, and use of medications, including postmenopausal ET, and other menstrual factors. The women were classified as "ever" or "never" users of ET. Duration of ET is the total number of years during which any ET was taken. Dose of ET is the dose of the oral conjugated estrogens taken for the longest period.

These female cohort members, the subjects for our study of estrogens and longevity, were followed to June 1, 2003, by periodic resurvey, review of hospital discharge records, and search of death indexes. Age-adjusted risk ratios (RRs) for death were obtained using proportional hazard regression analysis and controlling for potential confounding baseline factors (age, smoking, exercise, body mass index, and histories of hypertension, angina, heart attack, stroke, diabetes, rheumatoid arthritis, and cancer). After excluding 27 women who did not report their use of ET and 49 women with missing information on the potential confounding variables, data of 8,801 women were analyzed.

We found no association between death and most menstrual-related variables. Mortality was unrelated to age at menarche, age at first child, and type of menopause (natural vs. artificial). In addition, neither practice of breast self-examination nor having had a mammogram reduced risk of death.

However, as shown in Fig. 3.1, ET users had a 10% lower mortality rate compared to non-users [9]. Consistent with the time period, the majority of ET in these women was in the form of oral conjugated equine estrogens (CEE) without opposing progestin. Lower dose (0.625 mg) CEE users had a slightly better (but not statistically significant) survival than higher dose (>1.25 mg) users. Users of ET experienced a decreasing mortality rate with increasing duration of use. In summary, after adjustment for multiple factors, women who used ET initiated in the perimenopausal period lived longer with the longest-lived being in the group who used estrogens the longest.

Estrogen therapy and longevity: previous studies

Although observational studies have consistently shown a 20–50% reduction in mortality among users of estrogens [10–15], the randomized clinical trials of short-term ET found no decrease in mortality among estrogen users in both primary and secondary prevention trials. In the secondary prevention trials, the risk of death was increased by 8–20%, although these associations were also not statistically significant. In these trials, the RRs were 1.08 (95% CI = 0.84–1.38) during 4.1 years of follow-up in the Heart and Estrogen/Progestin Replacement Study (HERS) [5], 1.10 (95% CI = 0.91–1.31) during 6.8 years of observations in HERS and HERS II [16], and 1.2 (95% CI = 0.8–1.8) in the Women's Estrogen for Stroke Trial (WEST) [17]. In the primary prevention trials of the Women's Health Initiative (WHI), estrogens and placebo groups also did not differ in short-term mortality for combined estrogens–progestin during five years of follow-up (RR = 0.98, 95% CI = 0.82–1.18) [3] or for the estrogens-alone therapy with an average of 6.8 years of follow-up (RR = 1.04, 95% CI = 0.88–1.22) [4].

In these clinical trials, ET was initiated in women well past menopause (average age in HERS was 67 years; WEST, 71 years; WHI, 71 years). Interestingly, HERS data suggested that ET and risk of coronary heart disease (CHD) might change over time. Coronary heart disease events (non-fatal myocardial infarctions and CHD deaths) were increased in ET users in year 1 after randomization (RR = 1.52, 95% CI = 1.01–2.29). Over time, however, CHD risk became similar in both groups, and in years 4 and 5 a non-significant

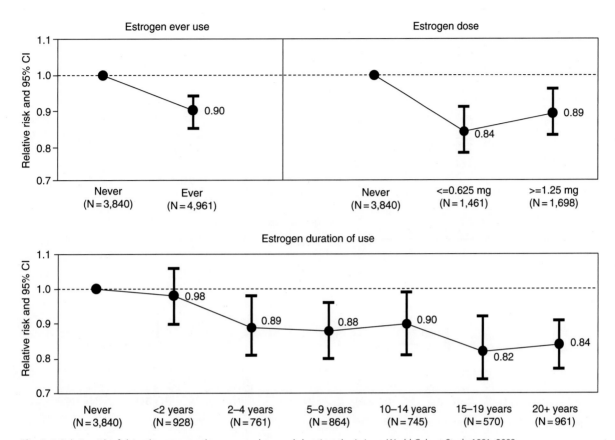

Fig. 3.1 Relative risk of dying by estrogen therapy use, dose, and duration: the Leisure World Cohort Study 1981–2003.

protective trend was seen for those randomized to ET (RR = 0.67, 95% CI = 0.43–1.04). In fact, a similar trend of protection over time was observed for all events of interest, except venous thrombotic events, which remained elevated in ET users.

Estrogens and dementia: the 90+ Study

Participants in the Leisure World Cohort who were alive and 90 years or older on January 1, 2003 comprise the subjects of the 90+ Study (N = 1150, 77% women). As of July 1, 2006, 941 participants had been recruited into the study. These participants are followed longitudinally every six months with in-person neuropsychological evaluations and neurological examinations, telephone interviews, and informant questionnaires. We investigated the relationship between prevalent dementia in the oldest-old and use of estrogens reported 21 years earlier in the 706 women of the 90+ Study. Estrogen use was

reported on their baseline Leisure World Cohort health survey in the early 1980s. A determination of dementia was done using in-person examinations as well as telephone and informant questionnaires and applying *Diagnostic and Statistical Manual of Mental Disorders*, 4th Edition (DSM-IV) criteria for dementia or age- and education-specific cutpoints on screening tests [18]. Adjusted odds ratios (ORs) for dementia were obtained using logistic regression analysis and controlling for potential confounding factors (age, education, and smoking) measured at the baseline evaluation of the 90+ Study.

The average time between the baseline Leisure World Cohort health survey and the baseline evaluation of the 90+ Study was 21 years (range: 15–22 years). The average age of these women at the 90+ Study baseline evaluation was 93 years (range: 90–105 years). Of the 706 women in the study, 317 (45%) were determined to have dementia at their 90+ Study baseline evaluation. Estrogen therapy showed little, if any, relationship with dementia prevalence

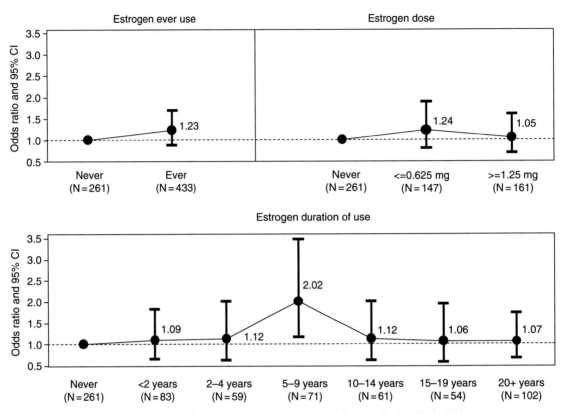

Fig. 3.2 Odds ratio of prevalent dementia by estrogen therapy use, dose, and duration: the 90+ Study 2003.

at the baseline visit (Fig. 3.2). After adjustment for age, education, and smoking, neither ever use of ET nor dose of ET was associated with prevalent dementia. Duration of ET was also generally unrelated to prevalent dementia. Only women who had used ET for 5–9 years had increased odds of dementia (OR = 2.02, 95% CI = 1.17–3.45). Interestingly, as discussed below, this is somewhat similar to the duration of use in the WHIMS randomized trial of dementia prevention, which showed a paradoxical increased risk for dementia after a mean exposure of 4.5 years.

Estrogens and dementia: previous studies

Although not all studies agree, most published observational studies on the effects of ET on dementia have reported a decreased risk of dementia and Alzheimer's disease (AD) among users of estrogens compared to non-users. Initial results regarding ET and AD were from case-control or cross-sectional studies and were somewhat inconclusive, with some studies

finding a significant decrease in risk with ET [19–21], and others finding no association [22–27]. The first prospective study of estrogens and AD was published in 1994 and reported results from the Leisure World Cohort Study [28]. In this report, AD and related dementias occurred less often in women using ET compared to non-users. Furthermore, this study showed a significant dose and duration effect, with AD risk decreasing with increasing dose and duration. Subsequently, other prospective studies also found a lower risk of AD and dementia among ET users [29–32] with many finding greater effects with longer durations of use [29, 31]. A 1998 meta-analysis of ET and AD did not find a significant risk reduction when combining data from case-control studies but did find a 52% reduction in risk of AD among ET users when combining the results of two prospective cohort studies [33]. A more recent meta-analysis of 12 case-control and cohort studies also found a reduction in the risk of dementia among ET users compared to non-users when combining the results of 12 case-control and cohort studies [34].

Results from randomized clinical trials described above are in sharp contrast with results from the observational studies. In 2003, the Women's Health Initiative Memory Study (WHIMS) reported results from over 7,000 women aged 65–79 who were randomized to conjugated equine estrogens (CEE) alone, conjugated equine estrogens plus medroxy-progesterone acetate (MPA), or placebo and who were followed for the development of dementia and memory loss. Women in the CEE+MPA group had twice the risk of developing dementia when compared to the placebo group (hazard ratio [HR] = 2.05, 95% CI = 1.21–3.48) [1]. Although the risk of dementia among the CEE-alone group was not significantly increased compared to placebo (HR = 1.49, 95% CI = 0.83–2.66), when the data from the two CEE arms were pooled, the risk of dementia was significantly increased (HR = 1.76, 95% CI = 1.19–2.60) [2]. The average time between randomization and last examination was 5.2 years in the CEE-alone trial, 4.1 years in the CEE+MPA trial, and 4.5 years in the pooled data. These women were followed up to about 8 years, and a few were followed beyond 8 years. Considering the results of observational and randomized studies, the possibility is suggested that ET and the risk of dementia may vary by timing of initiation and duration of therapy.

In the 90+ Study, the OR of prevalent dementia for women who used ET for 5–9 years differed significantly from that of non-users, but it is difficult to explain biologically such a duration-specific result. Moreover, studies of prevalent cases may detect factors relevant to the duration of disease rather than risk. Finally, there is always the concern of finding a spurious significant result when doing multiple comparisons. We are in the process of prospectively examining estrogen use and risk of developing dementia in the 90+ Study (incident cases), which will hopefully provide additional insight into the issues of timing and duration.

Conclusion

In the Leisure World Cohort Study, we found use of ET by women was associated with longer life. Our results are consistent with numerous other observational studies that have suggested mortality benefits for women who start estrogen therapy in the perimenopausal period. Moreover, most observational studies have also shown estrogen-related benefits in regards to dementia. In contrast, randomized trials, with ET generally initiated later in life, have shown no benefits in regards to mortality and dementia and have even suggested an increase in risk of dementia and AD. The effects of timing (duration of use and initiation of exposure) require further investigation because it is possible that the benefits and risks of ET exposure change with time. Exposure to ET in the perimenopausal period is likely to have different effects than novel exposure later in a woman's life, as was studied in the large randomized clinical trials that showed increased risks for dementia. Long-term randomized clinical trials would be ideal to explore the issues of timing further, but these studies are unlikely to be conducted for practical and ethical reasons. It is always a concern in observational studies that factors other than estrogens may be responsible for the observed benefit (confounding). Although observational studies have shown beneficial associations for women with exposure to estrogens, the available evidence at present does not support a role for the clinical use of estrogens in the prevention of dementia. It is likely that the risks and benefits of ET change in women over time and at different ages, formulations, doses, and durations of ET. More research in the clinic and laboratory is necessary to understand more fully the effects of hormonal factors, including the putative role of estrogens in longevity and the prevention of dementia and other age-related conditions.

References

1. Shumaker SA, Legault C, Thal L, *et al.* Estrogen plus progestin and the incidence of dementia and mild cognitive impairment in postmenopausal women: the Women's Health Initiative Memory Study: a randomized controlled trial. *JAMA.* 2003;**289**:2651–62.

2. Shumaker SA, Legault C, Kuller L, *et al.* Conjugated equine estrogens and incidence of probable dementia and mild cognitive impairment in postmenopausal women: the Women's Health Initiative Memory Study. *JAMA.* 2004;**291**:2947–58.

3. Rossouw JE, Anderson GL, Prentice RL, *et al.* Risks and benefits of estrogen plus progestin in healthy postmenopausal women: principal results from the Women's Health Initiative randomized controlled trial. *JAMA.* 2002;**288**:321–33.

4. Anderson GL, Limacher M, Assaf AR, *et al.* Effects of conjugated equine estrogen in postmenopausal women with hysterectomy: the Women's Health Initiative randomized controlled trial. *JAMA.* 2004;**291**:1701–12.

5. Hulley S, Grady D, Bush T, *et al.* Randomized trial of estrogen plus progestin for secondary prevention of coronary heart disease in postmenopausal women. Heart and Estrogen/Progestin Replacement Study (HERS) Research Group. *JAMA.* 1998;**280**: 605–13.

6. Henderson BE, Paganini-Hill A, Ross RK. Decreased mortality in users of estrogen replacement therapy. *Arch Intern Med.* 1991;**151**:75–78.

7. Whittle C, Corrada MM, Dick M, *et al.* Neuropsychological data in non-demented oldest-old: the 90+ Study. *J Clin Exp Neuropsychol.* 2006;**29**:290–9.

8. Kahle-Wrobleski K, Corrada MM, Li B, Kawas C. Sensitivity and specificity of the mini-mental state examination for identifying dementia in the oldest-old: the 90+ Study. *J Am Geriatr Soc.* 2007;**55**:284–9.

9. Paganini-Hill A, Corrada MM, Kawas CH. Increased longevity in older users of postmenopausal estrogen therapy: the Leisure World Cohort Study. *Menopause.* 2006;**13**:12–18.

10. Bush TL, Barrett-Connor E, Cowan LD, *et al.* Cardiovascular mortality and noncontraceptive use of estrogen in women: results from the Lipid Research Clinics Program Follow-up Study. *Circulation.* 1987;**75**:1102–9.

11. Criqui MH, Suarez L, Barrett-Connor E, *et al.* Postmenopausal estrogen use and mortality. Results from a prospective study in a defined, homogeneous community. *Am J Epidemiol.* 1988;**128**:606–14.

12. Hunt K, Vessey M, McPherson K. Mortality in a cohort of long-term users of hormone replacement therapy: an updated analysis. *Br J Obstet Gynaecol.* 1990;**97**:1080–6.

13. Sturgeon SR, Schairer C, Brinton LA, Pearson T, Hoover RN. Evidence of a healthy estrogen user survivor effect. *Epidemiology.* 1995;**6**:227–31.

14. Ettinger B, Friedman GD, Bush T, Quesenberry CP, Jr. Reduced mortality associated with long-term postmenopausal estrogen therapy. *Obstet Gynecol.* 1996;**87**:6–12.

15. Rodriguez C, Calle EE, Patel AV, *et al.* Effect of body mass on the association between estrogen replacement therapy and mortality among elderly US women. *Am J Epidemiol.* 2001;**153**:145–52.

16. Hulley S, Furberg C, Barrett-Connor E, *et al.* Noncardiovascular disease outcomes during 6.8 years of hormone therapy: Heart and Estrogen/Progestin Replacement Study follow-up (HERS II). *JAMA.* 2002;**288**:58–66.

17. Viscoli CM, Brass LM, Kernan WN, *et al.* A clinical trial of estrogen-replacement therapy after ischemic stroke. *N Engl J Med.* 2001;**345**:1243–9.

18. Corrada M, Brookmeyer R, Berlau D, Paganini-Hill A, Kawas C. Prevalence of dementia after age 90: results from the 90+ Study. *Neurology.* 2008;**71** (5):337–43.

19. Henderson VW, Paganini-Hill A, Emanuel CK, Dunn ME, Buckwalter JG. Estrogen replacement therapy in older women. Comparisons between Alzheimer's disease cases and nondemented control subjects. *Arch Neurol.* 1994;**51**:896–900.

20. Lerner A, Koss E, Debanne S, *et al.* Smoking and oestrogen-replacement therapy as protective factors for Alzheimer's disease. *Lancet.* 1997;**349**:403–4.

21. Baldereschi M, Di Carlo A, Lepore V, *et al.* Estrogen-replacement therapy and Alzheimer's disease in the Italian Longitudinal Study on Aging. *Neurology.* 1998;**50**:996–1002.

22. Broe GA, Henderson AS, Creasey H, *et al.* A case-control study of Alzheimer's disease in Australia. *Neurology.* 1990;**40**:1698–707.

23. Mortel KF, Meyer JS. Lack of postmenopausal estrogen replacement therapy and the risk of dementia. *J Neuropsychiatry Clin Neurosci.* 1995;**7**:334–7.

24. Graves AB, White E, Koepsell TD, *et al.* A case-control study of Alzheimer's disease. *Ann Neurol.* 1990; **28**:766–74.

25. Brenner DE, Kukull WA, Stergachis A, *et al.* Postmenopausal estrogen replacement therapy and the risk of Alzheimer's disease: a population-based case-control study. *Am J Epidemiol.* 1994;**140**:262–7.

26. Heyman A, Wilkinson W, Stafford J, *et al.* Alzheimer's disease: a study of epidemiological aspects. *Ann Neurol.* 1984;**15**:335–41.

27. Amaducci L, Fratiglioni L, Rocca WA, *et al.* Risk factors for clinically diagnosed Alzheimer's disease: a case-control study of an Italian population. *Neurology.* 1986;**36**:922–31.

28. Paganini-Hill A, Henderson VW. Estrogen deficiency and risk of Alzheimer's disease in women. *Am J Epidemiol.* 1994;**140**:256–61.

29. Tang MX, Jacobs D, Stern Y, *et al.* Effect of oestrogen during menopause on risk and age at onset of Alzheimer's disease. *Lancet.* 1996;**348**:429–32.

30. Kawas C, Resnick S, Morrison A, *et al.* A prospective study of estrogen replacement therapy and the risk of developing Alzheimer's disease: the Baltimore Longitudinal Study of Aging. *Neurology.* 1997;**48**: 1517–21.

31. Waring SC, Rocca WA, Petersen RC, *et al.* Postmenopausal estrogen replacement therapy and risk of AD: a population-based study. *Neurology.* 1999;**52**:965–70.

32. Zandi PP, Carlson MC, Plassman BL, *et al.* Hormone replacement therapy and incidence of Alzheimer disease in older women: the Cache County study. *JAMA.* 2002;**288**:2123–9.

33. Yaffe K, Sawaya G, Lieberburg I, Grady D. Estrogen therapy in postmenopausal women: effects on cognitive function and dementia. *JAMA.* 1998;**279**:688–95.

34. Nelson HD, Humphrey LL, Nygren P, Teutsch SM, Allan JD. Postmenopausal hormone replacement therapy: scientific review. *JAMA.* 2002;**288**:872–81.

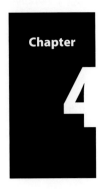

Chapter 4

The critical window hypothesis: hormone exposures and cognitive outcomes after menopause

Victor W. Henderson

Editors' introduction

Critical windows are a common phenomenon in biological systems. An exposure or experience at one point in time may elicit a different response, or even no response, at another time. In this chapter, Henderson considers several versions of the so-called critical window hypothesis as it relates to a woman's estrogenic exposures during middle age or during a later period of her life. These versions are based on timing of exposure, type of cognitive outcome, and timing of cognitive outcome assessment. At present, long-term cognitive effects of estrogenic exposures around the time of natural menopause are essentially unknown. As Henderson points out, some important but controversial clinical issues will be extraordinarily difficult to resolve. Partial answers may come from the ongoing Early versus Late Intervention Trial and the Kronos Early Estrogen Prevention Study. Truly convincing evidence regarding the critical window hypothesis can come only from randomized controlled trials in midlife women with follow-up extending into old age. Surrogate biomarkers may make some trial designs more feasible, and animal models and well designed observational studies can continue to provide valuable data. In the future, a variety of selective estrogen receptor modulators alone or in combination with an estrogen are certain to come to market, and similar issues may arise as more women are exposed to these compounds.

Prologue: effects of estrogens on brain processes implicated in memory and Alzheimer 's disease

Episodic memory refers to the conscious recollection of information linked to specific events or episodes. It is usually assessed by presenting something new, such as a list of words, and then asking for recall of these words after some interval. Integrity of the hippocampus and other medial temporal lobe structures is required for episodic memory formation. Some decline in memory performance is common as part of the aging process, and later in life impaired episodic memory can be an ominous sign of impending Alzheimer's disease (AD) or some less common form of dementia [1]. In AD, cognitive decline begins insidiously and progresses gradually over a period of years. An early and consistent feature is impairment in episodic memory. Key histopathological features of AD are extracellular neuritic plaques and neurofibrillary tangles. Key biochemical abnormalities are β-amyloid, a polypeptide proteolytically derived from its precursor protein, and a hyperphosphorylated form of tau, a microtubule-associated protein.

A surprising number of estrogen actions seem relevant to episodic memory, other cognitive functions, and AD [2], and the postmenopause would thus appear to be a time of cognitive vulnerability. The production of estrogens by ovarian follicles – primarily estradiol and estrone – begins to decline about two years before a woman's final menstrual period, and circulating concentrations reach a stable nadir about four years later [3]. The brain is an important target organ for estrogens, and the two estrogen receptor types – alpha and beta – are expressed by neurons within specific brain regions. Other estrogen receptors located in the cell membrane help regulate intracellular signaling cascades and mediate rapid effects that do not require genomic activation [4]. Some estrogen actions, for example antioxidant effects, may occur independently of binding to the estrogen receptor [5]. In addition to these direct neural effects, estrogens can influence brain function indirectly through effects on blood flow, glucose transport, coagulation cascades, the cerebral and systemic vasculature, and the immune system [2].

Estrogens promote neurite extension, hippocampal synaptic plasticity, long-term potentiation in the hippocampus, and hippocampal neurogenesis. Estrogens also protect against apoptosis and neural toxicity, including experimental injury by ischemia, β-amyloid, excitatory neurotransmitters, and oxidative stress [2]. Among neurotransmitter systems, effects on acetylcholine seem most relevant. Cholinergic neurons located in the basal forebrain express estrogen receptors [6] and project widely to hippocampus and neocortex. Estradiol preserves neuronal function after injury to the cholinergic system [7]. Over time, use of postmenopausal hormone therapy is associated with increased cerebral blood flow in medial temporal lobe structures implicated in memory [8], and estrogens modulate neural activity during performance of some cognitive tasks [9, 10].

With respect to AD, estradiol reduces the formation of β-amyloid in the brain [11, 12] and diminishes tau phosphorylation [13]. In a rodent model of AD, estradiol reduces β-amyloid accumulation after ovariectomy [14]. Different genetic and non-genetic factors contribute to the characteristic clinical and pathological features of AD. Risk is influenced by polymorphic variations in the gene that encodes apolipoprotein E. Apolipoprotein E is a lipid transport protein, and estradiol increases the expression of apolipoprotein E in the brain [15]. Elevated Alzheimer risk is associated with the ε4 allele, and this polymorphism increases risk more for women than for men [16].

Critical window: a look back

Critical windows are a common phenomenon in physiology and psychology. Konrad Lorenz famously showed that goslings would imprint a moving stimulus – be it a mother goose or a human – as an object to be followed about, but only during a critical period within the first days after hatching. Cataracts, strabismus, or refractive errors in infancy lead to largely irreversible changes in visual cortex organization and permanently impair visual acuity, even if the underlying ocular problem is later corrected. Similar eye problems later do not have the same deleterious

consequences for vision. In many mammalian species, male castration in utero affects brain organization and sexually dimorphic adult behaviors far more profoundly than castration at later developmental stages.

Interest in the so-called critical window of opportunity in relation to adult estrogen exposures and human cognition has emerged only during the past decade. In 2000, Gibbs at the University of Pittsburgh described hormonal influences on a form of spatial memory in female Sprague-Dawley rats whose ovaries had been removed [17]. After ovariectomy at 13 months of age, these middle-aged animals were randomly assigned to receive different regimens of ovarian hormones (parenteral estradiol with or without progesterone). Animals were allocated to one of five treatment groups, with treatment initiated at varying intervals after ovariectomy. About a year later, these now old animals were trained on a delayed matching-to-position task. At first, one arm of the T-maze was blocked, allowing the rat to enter the open arm for a food reward. On the next trial, both arms were open, but the animal was rewarded only if it visited the same arm as before. Thus, for the second reward it had to recall which arm of the maze had previously contained the reward. Delays between first and second trials ranged from 10 to 60 seconds. Gibbs analyzed several aspects of learning and memory. Among his findings, animals for which hormone replacement began immediately after surgery learned the delayed matching-to-position task better than animals who never received hormones. Animals whose treatment began three months after ovariectomy learned as well as animals treated immediately. However, animals for which treatment was delayed for ten months performed like animals that had never been treated. Gibbs interpreted differences between the three month and ten month regimens as "suggesting a window of opportunity after the loss of ovarian function during which hormone replacement can effectively prevent the effects of aging and hormone deprivation on cognitive function" (p. 107) [17].

Two years later, Zandi and colleagues reported a prospective study of incident AD among 1,889 women residing in Cache County, Utah [18]. Current and former use of hormone therapy (HT) was ascertained at baseline, when participants were at least 65 years of age (mean 74.5 years). When women were reassessed three years later, 88 now had AD. Women who had reported hormone use had a 41% reduction

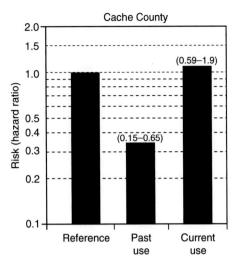

Fig. 4.1 Risk (hazard ratio) of Alzheimer's disease in the Cache County cohort study among older women reporting no hormone therapy use (reference), past use, or current use. 95% confidence intervals are given in parentheses. Data are from Zandi *et al.* [18].

in the risk of developing AD during the follow-up period (hazard ratio [HR] = 0.59, 95% confidence interval [CI] = 0.17–0.86). By itself, this finding was not new; similar protective associations had been reported previously for HT and AD [19, 20]. Among Cache County women, no effect was observed for multivitamin or calcium use, which like HT is generally linked to a healthy lifestyle, suggesting that the association was specific for HT. Importantly, when hormone exposure in Cache County was broken down into past use and current use, the associated reduction in AD incidence was confined to former hormone users (HR = 0.33, 95% CI = 0.15–0.65) (Fig. 4.1). This association with past use raised the question of "an apparent limited window of time during which sustained [HT] exposure seems to reduce the risk of [AD]" (p. 2128) [18].

An editorial that accompanied the report of Zandi *et al.* further discussed implications of a possible critical window with respect to estrogens and AD [21], under the assumption that most prior hormone use in Cache County occurred during midlife. It was pointed out that primary prevention trials of HT then in progress, which included the Women's Health Initiative Memory Study (WHIMS) and two other trials that eventually failed to come to completion, would provide useful information on women's health. However, it was important to recognize that

these trials were not designed to assess effects of estrogen exposures during a midlife window on later dementia risk.

Critical issues and some supporting evidence

The critical window hypothesis or, alternatively, the window of opportunity hypothesis, implies that estrogen-containing HT has health-related consequences that vary according to age at initiation or use, or in relation to some other lifespan marker, such as menopause. As commonly applied to cognitive outcomes, HT might benefit aspects of cognition if used during midlife or used at a time close to menopause but might have no effect or a deleterious effect if used at an older age or at a time more remote from menopause. Although this concept is fairly simple, assessing its validity is far from straightforward.

Is the putative critical window based on a woman's absolute age or on some temporal relation with menopause? The two – i.e., age and timing – are closely correlated, but they are not identical. If age but *not* timing is critical, is the usual wear-and-tear of age per se the key variable, or is it some specific age-associated pathological process, say, atherosclerosis? Atherosclerosis is more prevalent and more severe with increasing age, even though some women remain substantially free of atherosclerosis even in late old age. If timing but *not* age is critical, is the window related to down-regulation of the estrogen receptor or receptor insensitivity to its ligand, or to some other mechanism, and is the relevant tissue the brain itself or another organ or tissue that impacts brain indirectly? More generally, it has been argued that "healthy" neurons can respond more favorably to estrogens, at least in vitro [22].

In the laboratory, both animal age and the timing of a hormonal intervention can influence physiological and behavioral responses observed after ovariectomy. Old rats are more refractory than young animals to estradiol treatment with respect to expression of brain-derived neurotrophic factor and neurotrophin receptors [23]. In primates, estradiol injections begun 10 days after ovariectomy, but not 30 days after ovariectomy, restore the density of dopamine-containing neurons in the substantia nigra [24]. For synaptic density in rat hippocampus, the window of opportunity is apparently quite short, with increased density after initiation of conjugated estrogens at 4 days after ovariectomy but not at 12 days [25]. In an animal model of ischemic stroke, estradiol given immediately after ovariectomy attenuates production of proinflammatory cytokines but has no effect if administration is delayed by ten weeks [26]. Certain cognitive effects of estradiol implants after ovariectomy are preserved in middle-aged rats but not in old rats [27], or are preserved when estradiol is initiated immediately after ovariectomy but not when initiated five months later [28].

Particularly for the vascular system, accumulating evidence tends to support the critical window concept. This research is relevant to cognitive outcomes because cerebral vascular disease is associated with cognitive impairment and may predispose to AD [29], and because vascular pathology appears to work synergistically with Alzheimer pathology in producing symptoms of dementia [30]. Favorable estrogenic effects on endothelial-mediated blood flow [31] and atherosclerosis [32, 33] may be confined to younger postmenopausal women. Monkey studies indicate that an estrogen given immediately after ovariectomy reduces coronary artery atherosclerosis, but this benefit is lost if hormonal treatment is delayed [34]. Several mechanisms may be important. Estrogen actions on inducible nitric oxide synthase and endothelial nitric oxide synthase may be blocked in the presence of atherosclerosis [35]. Nitric oxide has important effects on vascular endothelium and smooth muscle. A cholesterol metabolite found in atherosclerotic plaques, 27-hydroxycholesterol, acts as a selective estrogen receptor modulator to antagonize these vascular effects of estradiol [35]. Another effect of estrogens could be to increase production of the matrix metalloproteinases, which can destabilize a complicated atheromatous plaque and lead to plaque rupture and thrombus formation [34]. Obviously, this particular adverse action depends on pre-existing atherosclerosis. Consistent with these laboratory findings, women in the Women's Health Initiative clinical trials who were randomized to hormone therapy closer to the time of menopause had a somewhat lower risk of developing coronary heart disease than women randomized later [36].

What are the critical cognitive outcomes?

"Usual" aging is associated with cognitive decline. Fortunately, such cognitive decrements are typically modest in severity, and some cognitive domains (e.g., semantic memory) are less affected during aging than others (e.g., episodic memory).

Should critical cognitive outcomes focus on usual age-associated decline? Or should the concern be for specific illnesses such as AD, which are defined in part by characteristic neuropathological features and which do not affect everyone during the aging process? For age-associated cognitive change, is one concerned with all cognitive domains (measured by, for example, a global cognitive assessment tool), with domains particularly impacted by age (e.g., episodic memory or executive functions), or with domains putatively influenced by hormonal status (e.g., verbal episodic memory or perhaps working memory)? The fact that the issue is complicated is no indication that the issue is unimportant or that answers cannot be achieved. However, it does mean that unambiguous, clinically relevant answers may be hard to come by.

The following discussion examines evidence on whether there is a critical midlife window during which estrogen exposures – and especially exposure to estrogen-containing HT – affect cognition or affect the risk of developing AD later in life. For cognition, the emphasis is on episodic memory. There are four reasons for this focus. Episodic memory is affected by usual aging; it is assessed more often in aging studies than other domains, so more data are available; in some settings verbal [37] and perhaps non-verbal [38] forms of episodic memory are affected by estrogen status; and finally, it is a domain affected early in the course of AD. The discussion includes an indirect comparison of late-life hormone exposures and midlife hormone exposures. As will be shown, current evidence supporting the critical window hypothesis is better developed for AD than for cognitive outcomes in the absence of dementia.

Estrogen exposures and Alzheimer's disease later in life

Many observational studies have addressed the association between HT use by healthy women and AD risk, but the relation with dementia has been examined experimentally only in the WHIMS trials. Most but not all of these observational studies report protective associations. Meta-analyses suggest reductions in Alzheimer risk of about one-third to two-fifths [39, 40]. In some of these studies, long-term hormone use is associated with greater risk reductions than short-term use [18–20]. The association with treatment duration is germane because there is an inverse relation between the duration of hormone use and the age at hormone initiation [41].

The interpretation of these associations is called into question by relatively small clinical trials in which women with AD failed to benefit from an estrogen [42, 43], although not all findings are congruent [44]. A more serious challenge comes from results of the WHIMS trials, where hormone therapy failed to reduce dementia risk [45]. The WHIMS participants were community-dwelling women, 65 to 79 years of age at the time they entered the study. The trials were reported as primary prevention trials because women were without recognized dementia at the time of treatment randomization, but simultaneous recruitment into other WHIMS studies led to a study population in which some women were probably less healthy than the general population (e.g., there was a high prevalence of obesity).

Active treatment in the WHIMS was with conjugated equine estrogens (CEE, 0.625 mg/day) with or without a progestogen (medroxy-progesterone acetate, MPA, 2.5 mg/day), depending on the presence or absence of a uterus [46, 47]. The parent trials were halted prematurely because of adverse health outcomes among women with a uterus (the CEE+MPA) and because of no overall health benefit among women who had undergone hysterectomy (the CEE–alone trial). During the course of the WHIMS trials, 108 women developed dementia during mean follow-up intervals of about five years. Because the WHIMS trials were stopped early, the number of incident cases of dementia was less than anticipated, and separate outcomes were not reported for specific types of dementia.

In the CEE+MPA trial, the risk of dementia among women in the active treatment group (40 cases) was doubled compared to women in the placebo group (21 cases) (HR = 2.01, 95% CI = 1.21–3.48). In the CEE–alone trial, the risk was increased by about half (28 vs. 19 cases; HR = 1.49, 95% CI = 0.83–2.66). The increased risk in these studies represents about two additional cases of dementia per 1,000 women per year of hormone use. Alzheimer's disease was the most common cause of dementia in each group.

Women with lower baseline cognitive scores and older women were much more likely to develop dementia during the course of the WHIMS trials. Most other examined factors did not appear to

modify the risk of developing dementia during the trials. However, as in other observational reports, WHIMS participants who had used HT prior to the trial were less likely to develop dementia during the trial, regardless of treatment arm; effects of on-trial therapy were not modified by prior use [45, 48]. The increase in dementia risk appeared soon after treatment began [45]. Histopathological features of AD are believed to begin years before the onset of overt appearance of dementia, and the WHIMS investigators speculated that vascular effects of estrogens on the cerebral vasculature may have led to the relatively quick appearance of dementia symptoms among women randomized to hormone therapy. Other possibilities, in addition to direct neural effects, include adverse estrogen actions on the coagulation cascade or on inflammatory processes [49].

The apparent discrepancy between the WHIMS findings (increased dementia incidence) and observational findings (decreased Alzheimer risk) undoubtedly involves various factors [50]. Two are especially relevant. The first concerns bias. Women who use HT are generally better educated and are believed to enjoy better health and to engage in healthier lifestyle practices than women who do not use hormones [51]. Such differences are important and could account for protective associations seen in most observational studies [50]. In some observational studies, differential recall of prior hormone usage (recall bias) might also underestimate cognitive risks of HT, contributing to positive findings in these analyses.

The second factor relates to the critical window hypothesis. As recognized even before completion of the WHIMS trials [21], on-trial hormone use in the WHIMS would come at an older age remote from the time of menopause, in contrast to the timing of hormone use by most women in most observational studies. Hormone therapy is most often prescribed for vasomotor symptoms around the time of menopause, taken for several years, and then discontinued [41]. Thus, most hormone use in observational studies probably occurred at a relatively young age, close to the time of menopause, and was discontinued before the age at which women would have become eligible for WHIMS enrollment. All on-trial hormone use during the WHIMS trials occurred after age 64, years or even decades after women had experienced natural or surgical menopause.

Do other human data support the interpretation that the WHIMS results, although vitally important

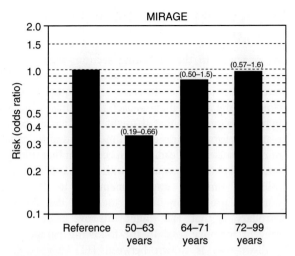

Fig. 4.2 Risk (odds ratio) of Alzheimer's disease based on hormone therapy exposure among postmenopausal women in the Multi-Institutional Research in Alzheimer Genetic Epidemiology (MIRAGE) case-control study. There was a significant interaction by age (p = 0.03), and results for hormone use are shown as age tertiles. The reference is no hormone therapy use; 95% confidence intervals are given in parentheses. Data are from Henderson *et al.* [52].

for older women, might not generalize to younger women, closer to the age of menopause? Evidence that putative estrogen effects on Alzheimer risk are modified by age of hormone use or by use during a critical window close to the time of menopause is indirect and not yet robust. However, some of the observational findings are suggestive.

As already described, Alzheimer risk reduction in Cache County was limited to former users of HT (HR = 0.33, 95% CI = 0.15–0.65). For current users the hazard ratio was 1.1 (95% CI = 0.59–1.9) [18] (Fig. 4.1). One of several plausible interpretations is that only early estrogen exposure was protective. In the Multi-Institutional Research in Alzheimer Genetic Epidemiology case-control study, investigators compared HT among postmenopausal women: 426 with AD and 545 relatives without dementia [52]. Here again, HT was associated with reduced Alzheimer risk (odds ratio [OR] = 0.70, 95% CI = 0.51–0.95), but this association was significantly modified by age. In stratified analyses, the protective association was evident only in the youngest age tertile (50–63 years), where the OR was 0.35 (95% CI = 0.19–0.66) [52] (Fig. 4.2). These results could be interpreted as suggesting that hormone use protects younger women from AD or that hormone use only during the menopause transition or early postmenopause reduces Alzheimer risk.

Case-control studies from Seattle [53] and the United Kingdom [54] had unbiased and relatively precise measures of hormone exposure. Using computerized pharmacy databases, neither study showed protective associations between hormone prescriptions and Alzheimer risk. However, in both instances, the databases extended back only about a decade, meaning that early hormone use would have been systematically missed. Speculatively, the absence of a protective association in these two studies could have been due to the absence of data on early hormone exposures.

Estrogen exposures and cognition later in life

Results of observational research involving older women are not fully congruent in delineating putative cognitive effects of HT in the late postmenopause. In the Nurses' Health Study [55], comparisons between current hormone users and never-users suggested only a few differences, but long-term users were at increased risk of cognitive decline, particularly when HT was initiated at older ages. In contrast, Cache County women who reported hormone use showed slower rates of cognitive decline [56].

Results from large randomized clinical trials of older postmenopausal women provide a more consistent picture for the cognitive effects of late-life HT [57]. Most studies have examined episodic memory, usually using verbal materials, so inferences are most secure for this particular cognitive domain.

The WHIMS trials involved postmenopausal women who were 65 years of age or older at the time of randomization. During follow-up that averaged about five years, hormone initiation in the WHIMS did not substantially affect global cognition measured by the Modified Mini-Mental State examination; small differences tended to favor women in the placebo groups [46, 47]. More detailed neuropsychological assessment was conducted in a subset of WHIMS participants (the Women's Health Initiative Study of Cognitive Aging, WHISCA) [58]. Here, analyses among women with a uterus showed no differences or only small differences on a variety of cognitive tasks, including memory tasks. For measures of verbal episodic memory, small differences favored placebo (total word-list recall score, short and long free delayed word-list recall scores); for a measure of non-verbal episodic memory (visual retention), the trend favored HT [58]. The magnitude of these differences was small, and no differences were found on other tests.

Several other large randomized clinical trials have assessed the impact of late-life hormone therapy initiation on episodic memory and on other aspects of cognition [57]. As described in the following paragraph, these include secondary prevention trials of women with pre-existing coronary heart disease [59] and cerebrovascular disease [60], and primary prevention trials in generally healthy women [61, 62].

Over a four-year period, the Heart and Estrogen/ Progestin Replacement Study treated 1,063 women with coronary heart disease (mean age 71) with CEE combined with MPA, or placebo [59]. Verbal episodic memory was assessed with word-list learning and delayed recall. The two treatment groups did not differ on these outcomes; significant differences on one of four non-memory tasks (verbal fluency) favored placebo. The Women's Estrogen for Stroke Trial studied effects of oral estradiol versus placebo in postmenopausal women (mean age 70) with recent stroke or transient ischemic attack [60]. Among 461 women without stroke three years later, episodic memory (incidental recall of words from a naming test) was similar in both groups, and estradiol had no effect on other cognitive tasks. However, in post hoc analyses confined to women who scored normally at baseline on a global cognitive measure, there was less global decline among women in the estradiol group compared to the placebo group [60]. In a 20-week trial of 115 Australian women without a uterus (mean age 74), oral estradiol showed no benefit over placebo on verbal episodic memory (word-list learning and delayed recall) or on other cognitive tasks [61]. Finally, 417 women without osteoporosis (mean age 67) were followed for two years after randomization to very low-dose transdermal estradiol or a placebo patch [62]. There were no effects of treatment on tasks of memory (paragraph learning and delayed recall; word-list learning and delayed recall; memory for complex visual patterns) or other domains.

The conclusion from this consistent series of randomized clinical trials is that hormone initiation in older postmenopausal women does not have a substantial effect on episodic memory and probably not on other domains either, at least over the intermediate term. Some caveats, however, regarding this conclusion are mentioned below.

Estrogen exposures and cognition in midlife

As reviewed in the preceding section, starting HT after about age 60 does not benefit episodic memory, but is the outcome different if initiation occurs closer to the age of menopause? The critical window hypothesis suggests that it might be. After all, complaints of forgetfulness are common around the time of menopause [63], leading to speculation that midlife hormonal changes associated with the loss of ovarian follicular function impair memory. If declining hormone production impairs memory, the obvious corollary is that HT might improve memory or prevent memory loss. In the following paragraphs, a distinction is drawn between HT after natural menopause and after surgical menopause.

Circulating levels of estradiol are unrelated to objective measures of memory performance in middle-aged women [64–66]. This finding could mean that estradiol levels are unimportant to memory in this age group, but it is also possible that estrogen exposures in the brain, i.e., what neurons actually encounter, are not closely related to peripheral concentrations. However, reports from several cohorts indicate that natural menopause per se does not appear to have important effects on episodic memory. This conclusion is inferred from cross-sectional and longitudinal analyses in population-based cohorts of middle-age women in Melbourne [64], Taiwan [67], the UK [68], Sweden [65], and the USA [66]. For example, for women 52–63 years of age in the Melbourne Women's Midlife Health Project, which excluded women with surgical menopause, word-list learning and recall were unrelated to reproductive stage (among 250 non-users of hormones), years from final menstrual period or years of reproductive life (among 139 never-users of hormones who had experienced a final menstrual period), or HT use (among 299 women in late menopausal transition or early postmenopause) [64]. In a unique cohort of 1,261 British women born in 1946, reproductive stage at age 53 had no effect on word-list learning, nor did HT use [68]. These findings on natural menopause are necessarily observational, of course.

For midlife women, only a few clinical trials have examined cognitive outcomes after therapy with an estrogen or with an estrogen and a progestogen. Most trials in this age range have not reported significant effects on an objective measure of episodic memory

[57]. An important caveat is that clinical trial data on HT in this age group are still fairly limited. The largest randomized trial lasted four months and involved 180 healthy postmenopausal women aged 45 to 55 [69]. There were no significant between-group differences on episodic memory measures in this trial, and one verbal memory task showed a non-significant trend in favor of placebo therapy [69].

How can one reconcile the frequency of subjective complaints and the paucity of objective deficits? An important consideration is that a woman's perception of stress, mood changes, and physical health may contribute to memory symptoms [70] even in the absence of demonstrable memory loss. In the Melbourne study, for example, nearly two-fifths of women aged 55 to 66 years self-reported "particular trouble remembering recent events" during the preceding month, yet objective measures of episodic memory did not distinguish these women from those without similar symptoms (Szoeke *et al.*, unpublished data). It remains possible that midlife memory symptoms might reflect deficits in cognitive domains other than episodic memory. A three-week clinical trial among midlife women (mean age 51 years), for example, showed improvements in oral reading skills among women randomized to receive CEE [71]. However, clinical trial evidence thus far has not substantiated large effects of HT in most aspects of cognitive function (e.g., Maki *et al.* [69]). Still, experimental evidence is less substantial than for late-life HT initiation [57].

Thus, there is currently no strong evidence to indicate that natural menopause or use of hormone therapy in the early postmenopause after natural menopause has much effect on episodic memory. The situation may differ, however, when the hormonal milieu changes precipitously. Some data – albeit limited – support the view that abrupt hormonal withdrawal (surgical menopause or pharmacological suppression of ovarian function) may adversely affect verbal episodic memory. Small clinical trials by Sherwin and colleagues in Montreal suggest that prompt administration of an estrogen may be beneficial in this setting, at least over the short term [37, 72]. Consistent with this perspective, a recent case-control study from the Mayo Clinic found unilateral or bilateral oophorectomy associated with increased risk of cognitive decline or dementia, with greatest risk occurring in women undergoing oophorectomy at younger ages [73]. Even if the critical window hypothesis

with respect to cognitive aging has thus far not proven especially germane for middle-aged women who have experienced natural menopause (and evidence here is far from definitive), the issue is almost totally unsettled for large numbers of women with menopause induced by oophorectomy before the age of natural menopause.

Midlife estrogen exposures and cognition later in life

Midlife cognitive consequences of estrogenic exposures are beginning to be understood, but very little research addresses long-term cognitive consequences of these midlife exposures. There are no clinical trials with adequate long-term follow-up, and extant observational findings at best serve only to suggest the need for further research. One such observational study involved a random selection of households in Adelaide, Australia [74]. Four hundred twenty-eight women older than 60 were administered a series of cognitive tasks. Differences were small, but comparisons in this cohort generally suggested that women who initiated HT before age 56 or within 5 years of surgical menopause tended to perform better than women who initiated HT at a later age [74].

In a provocative follow-up of clinical trial enrollees, Danish investigators assessed women who had participated in trials of HT for osteoporosis prevention [75]. Women were postmenopausal at the time of initial randomization to hormone therapy or placebo, with a mean age of 54 years. The on-study treatment duration was 2 or 3 years, and 5 to 15 years later the authors attempted to track down women who had completed their trial. Women who were thus identified were then administered a short cognitive screening test. Women initially randomized to active therapy had reduced risk of scoring below a cutoff score for cognitive impairment, compared to women randomized to placebo (OR = 0.33, 95% CI = 0.13–0.84); these analyses were confined to women who had not used HT after the trial [75].

Critical window: a look ahead

Loose formulations of the critical window hypothesis may provide a shifting target that is difficult to substantiate or refute. This chapter has considered several versions based on timing of exposure, timing of outcomes, and type of cognitive outcome. Some possible underlying mechanisms have been mentioned (e.g., those based on nervous system effects and those based on vascular system effects), and others are also feasible.

In recent years, considerable progress has been made in understanding cognitive effects of estrogens after menopause. Evidence from randomized clinical trials seems to show that beginning an estrogen or an estrogen plus a progestogen in the late postmenopause – after about age 60 or 65 – probably does not improve episodic memory and probably does increase dementia risk. These two conclusions might be stated more firmly if it is assumed that commonly used estrogen formulations and doses have similar effects on cognitive outcomes, and if it is assumed that estrogenic effects are not substantially modified by a concomitant progestogen. Until stronger, clinically relevant evidence is on hand, these assumptions are probably reasonable as a first approximation. However, in some circumstances the type of estrogen or the type of progestogen clearly does make a difference. Dosage and route of administration (e.g., oral versus transdermal or parenteral) are also important variables. Even the convenience of continuous estrogen therapy could have unintended adverse consequences on neural responsiveness [76]. Further, our simple models may inadequately capture what is actually happening. As an example, secondary analyses from a randomized clinical trial of estradiol suggest that hormonal effects on subclinical atherosclerosis are mediated not only by resultant levels of estrogens and sex hormone binding globulin, but by testosterone as well [77].

Natural menopause probably has no substantial effect on cognition, and weaker evidence indicates that beginning hormone therapy before age 60, even if initiated close to the time of natural menopause, probably has no important effect on memory during midlife. Thus, there may be no critical window with respect to midlife memory, although this inference is based only on limited short-term (weeks to months) outcomes in younger naturally menopausal women. Two on-going placebo-controlled trials will test this inference more carefully, the Kronos Early Estrogen Prevention Study (ClinicalTrials.gov identifier NCT00154180) and the Early versus Late Intervention Trial with Estrogen (NCT00114517). The former proposes to enroll 720 women within three years of natural menopause, and the latter proposes to study 650 postmenopausal women divided into an early group within six years of menopause and a late group

more than ten years beyond menopause. Estrogen interventions differ slightly in the two trials, but each incorporates robust cognitive outcome measures.

Evidence that is even more limited suggests that surgical menopause – which by definition occurs before the age of natural menopause – may adversely affect short-term [72] and perhaps long-term cognitive outcomes [73] (but see [78]). Here, a still sparse animal literature supports the contention that there may be a critical window soon after ovariectomy during which an estrogen may preserve or enhance cognitive task performance [17, 27, 28], although the duration of the window is unknown. It may be quite short for some brain effects but longer for others.

The greatest challenge lies in the fact that long-term cognitive effects of estrogenic exposures around the time of natural menopause are essentially unknown. If the outcome of interest is AD and not memory preservation in the absence of dementia, observational evidence suggests there might indeed be an opportunity for estrogen-containing hormone therapy to reduce risk if – and this *if* is crucial – reported associations are not adequately accounted for by bias. There is no way of being certain, but many investigators believe that bias is an incomplete explanation. The finding that all-cause dementia risk was increased by HT in the WHIMS trials implies that this theoretical window is closed by age 65. As with long-term cognitive outcomes apart from dementia, the issue will be extraordinarily difficult to resolve. Neither the Kronos Early Estrogen Prevention Study nor the Early versus Late Intervention Trial were designed to answer this question, but their results could provide useful illumination.

Convincing data can come only from randomized controlled trials in midlife women with follow-up that extends into old age. Surrogate biomarkers (for example, brain imaging based on β-amyloid load) may make some trial designs more feasible. In the years to come, exogenous hormone exposures are likely to shift as new drugs come to market, and the impetus for such trials may diminish. A variety of selective estrogen receptor modulators alone or in combination with an estrogen are certain to claim increasing market shares for several health concerns. However, animal models and well designed observational studies can continue to provide valuable evidence that will inform scientists, clinicians, and patients in deciding whether the estrogen critical window hypothesis is valid for these very important long-term cognitive outcomes.

Acknowledgments

Supported in part by AG023038 and AG024154. There is no approved indication for sex steroid hormones or selective estrogen receptor modulators for the prevention or treatment of cognitive impairment or dementia.

References

1. Petersen RC, Doody R, Kurz A, et al. Current concepts in mild cognitive impairment. *Arch Neurol.* 2001; **58**:1985–92.

2. Henderson VW. *Hormone Therapy and the Brain: a Clinical Perspective on the Role of Estrogen.* New York: Parthenon Publishing, 2000.

3. Burger HG. The endocrinology of the menopause. *Maturitas.* 1996;**23**:129–36.

4. Edwards DP. Regulation of signal transduction pathways by estrogen and progesterone. *Annu Rev Physiol.* 2005;**67**:335–76.

5. Behl C, Skutella T, Lezoualch F, et al. Neuroprotection against oxidative stress by estrogens: structure–activity relationship. *Mol Pharmacol.* 1997;**51**:535–41.

6. Shughrue PJ, Scrimo PJ, Merchenthaler I. Estrogen binding and estrogen receptor characterization (ERα and ERβ) in the cholinergic neurons of the rat basal forebrain. *Neuroscience.* 2000;**96**: 41–9.

7. Luine V. Estradiol increases choline acetyltransferase activity in specific basal forebrain nuclei and projection areas of female rats. *Exp Neurol.* 1985; **89**:484–90.

8. Maki PM, Resnick SM. Longitudinal effects of estrogen replacement therapy on PET cerebral blood flow and cognition. *Neurobiol Aging.* 2000;**21**:373–83.

9. Shaywitz SE, Shaywitz BA, Pugh KR, et al. Effect of estrogen on brain activation patterns in postmenopausal women during working memory tasks. *JAMA.* 1999;**281**:1197–202.

10. Joffe H, Hall JE, Gruber S, et al. Estrogen therapy selectively enhances prefrontal cognitive processes: a randomized, double-blind, placebo-controlled study with functional magnetic resonance imaging in perimenopausal and recently postmenopausal women. *Menopause.* 2006; **13**:411–22.

11. Petanceska SS, Nagy G, Frail D, Gandy S. Ovariectomy and 17β-estradiol modulate the levels of Alzheimer's amyloid β peptides in brain. *Neurology.* 2000;**54**: 2212–17.

12. Zheng H, Xu H, Uljon SN, et al. Modulation of Aβ peptides by estrogen in mouse models. *J Neurochem.* 2002;**80**:191–6.

13. Alvarez-De-La-Rosa M, Silva I, Nilsen J, et al. Estradiol prevents neural tau hyperphosphorylation characteristic of Alzheimer's disease. *Ann N Y Acad Sci.* 2005;**1052**:210–24.

14. Carroll JC, Rosario ER, Chang L, et al. Progesterone and estrogen regulate Alzheimer-like neuropathology in female 3xTg-AD mice. *J Neurosci.* 2007;**27**: 13357–65.

15. Stone DJ, Rozovsky I, Morgan TE, et al. Astrocytes and microglia respond to estrogen with increased apoE mRNA *in vivo* and *in vitro. Exp Neurol.* 1997;**143**:313–18.

16. Farrer LA, Cupples LA, Haines JL, et al. Effects of age, sex, and ethnicity on the association between apolipoprotein E genotype and Alzheimer disease. *JAMA.* 1997;**278**:1349–56.

17. Gibbs RB. Long-term treatment with estrogen and progesterone enhances acquisition of a spatial memory task by ovariectomized aged rats. *Neurobiol Aging.* 2000;**21**:107–16.

18. Zandi PP, Carlson MC, Plassman BL, et al. Hormone replacement therapy and incidence of Alzheimer's disease on older women: the Cache County study. *JAMA.* 2002;**288**:2123–9.

19. Paganini-Hill A, Henderson VW. Estrogen replacement therapy and risk of Alzheimer's disease. *Arch Intern Med.* 1996;**156**:2213–17.

20. Tang M-X, Jacobs D, Stern Y, et al. Effect of oestrogen during menopause on risk and age at onset of Alzheimer's disease. *Lancet.* 1996;**348**: 429–32.

21. Resnick SM, Henderson VW. Hormone therapy and risk of Alzheimer disease: a critical time. *JAMA.* 2002;**288**:2170–2.

22. Brinton RD. Investigative models for determining hormone therapy-induced outcomes in brain: evidence in support of a healthy cell bias of estrogen action. *Ann N Y Acad Sci.* 2005;**1052**:57–74.

23. Jezierski MK, Sohrabji F. Neurotrophin expression in the reproductively senescent forebrain is refractory to estrogen stimulation. *Neurobiol Aging.* 2001;**22**:309–19.

24. Leranth C, Roth RH, Elswoth JD, et al. Estrogen is essential for maintaining nigrostriatal dopamine neurons in primates: implications for Parkinson's disease and memory. *J Neurosci.* 2000;**20**:8604–9.

25. Silva I, Mello LEAM, Freymüller E, Haidar MA, Baracat EC. Onset of estrogen replacement has a critical effect on synaptic density of CA1 hippocampus in ovariectomized adult rats. *Menopause.* 2003;**10**:406–11.

26. Suzuki S, Brown CM, Dela Cruz CD, *et al.* Timing of estrogen therapy after ovariectomy dictates the efficacy of its neuroprotective and antiinflammatory actions. *Proc Natl Acad Sci USA.* 2007;**104**:6013–18.

27. Savonenko AV, Markowska AL. The cognitive effects of ovariectomy and estrogen replacement are modulated by aging. *Neuroscience.* 2003;**119**:821–30.

28. Daniel JM, Hulst JL, Berbling JL. Estradiol replacement enhances working memory in middle-aged rats when initiated immediately after ovariectomy but not after a long-term period of ovarian hormone deprivation. *Endocrinology.* 2006;**147**: 607–14.

29. Stampfer MJ. Cardiovascular disease and Alzheimer's disease: common links. *J Intern Med.* 2006;**260**:211–23.

30. Schneider JA, Arvanitakis Z, Bang W, Bennett DA. Mixed brain pathologies account for most dementia cases in community-dwelling older persons. *Neurology.* 2007;**69**:2197–204.

31. Herrington DM, Espeland MA, Crouse JR, 3rd, *et al.* Estrogen replacement and brachial artery flow-mediated vasodilation in older women. *Arterioscler Thromb Vasc Biol.* 2001;**21**:1955–61.

32. Hodis HN, Mack WJ, Lobo RA, *et al.* Estrogen in the prevention of atherosclerosis. A randomized, double-blind, placebo-controlled trial. *Ann Intern Med.* 2001;**135**:939–53.

33. Hodis HN, Mack WJ, Azen SP, *et al.* Hormone therapy and the progression of coronary-artery atherosclerosis in postmenopausal women. *N Engl J Med.* 2003;**349**: 535–45.

34. Clarkson TB. Estrogen effects on arteries vary with stage of reproductive life and extent of subclinical atherosclerosis progression. *Menopause.* 2007;**14**: 373–84.

35. Umetani M, Domoto H, Gormley AK, *et al.* 27-Hydroxycholesterol is an endogenous SERM that inhibits the cardiovascular effects of estrogen. *Nat Med.* 2007;**13**:1185–92.

36. Rossouw JE, Prentice RL, Manson JE, *et al.* Postmenopausal hormone therapy and risk of cardiovascular disease by age and years since menopause. *JAMA.* 2007;**297**:1465–77.

37. Sherwin BB, Tulandi T. "Add-back" estrogen reverses cognitive deficits induced by a gonadotropin-releasing hormone agonist in women with leiomyomata uteri. *J Clin Endocrinol Metab.* 1996;**81**:2545–9.

38. Resnick SM, Maki PM, Golski S, Kraut MA, Zonderman AB. Effects of estrogen replacement therapy on PET cerebral blood flow and neuropsychological performance. *Horm Behav.* 1998;**34**:171–82.

39. Hogervorst E, Williams J, Budge M, Riedel W, Jolles J. The nature of the effect of female gonadal hormone replacement therapy on cognitive function in post-menopausal women: a meta-analysis. *Neuroscience.* 2000;**101**:485–512.

40. LeBlanc ES, Janowsky J, Chan BKS, Nelson HD. Hormone replacement therapy and cognition: systematic review and meta-analysis. *JAMA.* 2001;**285**:1489–99.

41. Brett KM, Chong Y. *Hormone Replacement Therapy: Knowledge and Use in the United States.* Hyattsville, MD: National Center for Health Statistics, 2001.

42. Henderson VW, Paganini-Hill A, Miller BL, *et al.* Estrogen for Alzheimer's disease in women: randomized, double-blind, placebo-controlled trial. *Neurology.* 2000;**54**:295–301.

43. Mulnard RA, Cotman CW, Kawas C, *et al.* Estrogen replacement therapy for treatment of mild to moderate Alzheimer disease: a randomized controlled trial. *JAMA.* 2000;**283**:1007–15.

44. Asthana S, Baker LD, Craft S, *et al.* High-dose estradiol improves cognition for women with AD: results of a randomized study. *Neurology.* 2001;**57**:605–12.

45. Shumaker SA, Legault C, Kuller L, *et al.* Conjugated equine estrogens and incidence of probable dementia and mild cognitive impairment in postmenopausal women: the Women's Health Initiative Memory Study. *JAMA.* 2004;**291**:2947–58.

46. Rapp SR, Espeland MA, Shumaker SA, *et al.* The effect of estrogen with progestin treatment on global cognitive function in postmenopausal women: results from the Women's Health Initiative Memory Study. *JAMA.* 2003;**289**:2663–72.

47. Espeland MA, Rapp SR, Shumaker SA, *et al.* Conjugated equine estrogens and global cognitive function in postmenopausal women: the Women's Health Initiative Memory Study. *JAMA.* 2004;**291**: 2959–68.

48. Henderson VW, Espeland MA, Hogan PE, *et al.* Prior use of hormone therapy and incident Alzheimer's disease in the Women's Health Initiative Memory Study. *Neurology.* 2007;**68**(suppl. 1): A205.

49. Henderson VW. Hormone therapy and Alzheimer's disease: benefit or harm? *Expert Opin Pharmacother.* 2004;**5**:389–406.

50. Henderson VW. Estrogen-containing hormone therapy and Alzheimer's disease risk: understanding discrepant inferences from observational and experimental research. *Neuroscience*. 2006;**138**:1031–9.

51. Matthews KA, Kuller LH, Wing RR, Meilahn EN, Plantinga P. Prior to use of estrogen replacement therapy, are users healthier than nonusers? *Am J Epidemiol*. 1996;**143**:971–8.

52. Henderson VW, Benke KS, Green RC, Cupples LA, Farrer LA. Postmenopausal hormone therapy and Alzheimer's disease risk: interaction with age. *J Neurol Neurosurg Psychiatry*. 2005;**76**:103–5.

53. Brenner DE, Kukull WA, Stergachis A, *et al*. Postmenopausal estrogen replacement therapy and the risk of Alzheimer's disease: a population-based case-control study. *Am J Epidemiol*. 1994;**140**:262–7.

54. Seshadri S, Zomberg GL, Derby LE, *et al*. Postmenopausal estrogen replacement therapy and the risk of Alzheimer's disease. *Arch Neurol*. 2001;**58**:435–40.

55. Kang JH, Weuve J, Grodstein F. Postmenopausal hormone therapy and risk of cognitive decline in community-dwelling aging women. *Neurology*. 2004;**63**:101–7.

56. Carlson MC, Zandi PP, Plassman BL, *et al*. Hormone replacement therapy and reduced cognitive decline in older women: the Cache County study. *Neurology*. 2001;**57**:2210–16.

57. Henderson VW, Sherwin BB. Surgical versus natural menopause: cognitive issues. *Menopause*. 2007;**14**:572–9.

58. Resnick SM, Maki PM, Rapp SR, *et al*. Effects of combination estrogen plus progestin hormone treatment on cognition and affect. *J Clin Endocrinol Metab*. 2006;**91**:1802–10.

59. Grady D, Yaffe K, Kristof M, *et al*. Effect of postmenopausal hormone therapy on cognitive function: the Heart and Estrogen/Progestin Replacement Study. *Am J Med*. 2002;**113**:543–8.

60. Viscoli CM, Brass LM, Kernan WN, *et al*. Estrogen therapy and risk of cognitive decline: results from the Women's Estrogen for Stroke Trial (WEST). *Am J Obstet Gynecol*. 2005;**192**:387–93.

61. Almeida OP, Lautenschlager NT, Vasikaran S, *et al*. 20-week randomized controlled trial of estradiol replacement therapy for women aged 70 years and older: effect on mood, cognition and quality of life. *Neurobiol Aging*. 2006;**27**:141–9.

62. Yaffe K, Vittinghoff E, Ensrud KE, *et al*. Effects of ultra-low-dose transdermal estradiol on cognition and health-related quality of life. *Arch Neurol*. 2006;**63**:945–50.

63. Xu J, Bartoces M, Neale AV, *et al*. Natural history of menopause symptoms in primary care patients: a MetroNet study. *J Am Board Fam Pract*. 2005;**18**:374–82.

64. Henderson VW, Dudley EC, Guthrie JR, Burger HG, Dennerstein L. Estrogen exposures and memory at midlife: a population-based study of women. *Neurology*. 2003;**60**:1369–71.

65. Herlitz A, Thilers P, Habib R. Endogenous estrogen is not associated with cognitive performance before, during, or after menopause. *Menopause*. 2007;**14**:425–31.

66. Luetters C, Huang MH, Seeman T, *et al*. Menopause transition stage and endogenous estradiol and follicle-stimulating hormone levels are not related to cognitive performance: cross-sectional results from the study of women's health across the nation (SWAN). *J Women's Health*. 2007;**16**:331–44.

67. Fuh J-L, Wang S-J, Lee S-J, Lu S-R, Juang K-D. A longitudinal study of cognition change during early menopausal transition in a rural community. *Maturitas*. 2006;**53**:447–53.

68. Kok HS, Kuh D, Cooper R, *et al*. Cognitive function across the life course and the menopausal transition in a British birth cohort. *Menopause*. 2006;**13**:19–27.

69. Maki PM, Gast MJ, Vieweg A, Burriss SW, Yaffe K. Hormone therapy in menopausal women with cognitive complaints: a randomized, double-blind trial. *Neurology*. 2007;**69**:1322–30.

70. Woods NF, Mitchell ES, Adams C. Memory functioning among midlife women: observations from the Seattle Midlife Women's Health Study. *Menopause*. 2000;**7**:257–65.

71. Shaywitz SE, Naftolin F, Zelterman D, *et al*. Better oral reading and short-term memory in midlife, postmenopausal women taking estrogen. *Menopause*. 2003;**10**:420–6.

72. Phillips SM, Sherwin BB. Effects of estrogen on memory function in surgically menopausal women. *Psychoneuroendocrinology*. 1992;**17**:485–95.

73. Rocca WA, Bower JH, Ahlskog JE, *et al*. Increased risk of cognitive impairment or dementia in women who underwent oophorectomy before menopause. *Neurology*. 2007;**69**:1074–83.

74. MacLennan AH, Henderson VW, Paine BJ, *et al*. Hormone therapy, timing of initiation, and cognition in women aged older than 60 years: the REMEMBER pilot study. *Menopause*. 2006;**13**:28–36.

75. Bagger YZ, Tankó LB, Alexandersen P, Qin G, Christiansen C. Early postmenopausal hormone replacement therapy may prevent cognitive impairment later in life. *Menopause.* 2005;**12**: 12–17.

76. Toran-Allerand CD. Estrogen as treatment for Alzheimer disease [letter]. *JAMA.* 2000;**284**: 307–8.

77. Karim R, Hodis HN, Stanczyk FZ, Lobo RA, Mack WJ. Relationship between serum levels of sex hormones and progression of subclinical atherosclerosis in postmenopausal women. *J Clin Endocrinol Metab.* 2008;**93**:131–8.

78. Kritz-Silverstein D, Barrett-Connor E. Hysterectomy, oophorectomy, and cognitive function in older women. *J Am Geriatr Soc.* 2002;**50**:55–61.

Chapter 5

Animal studies that support estrogen effects on cognitive performance and the cholinergic basis of the critical period hypothesis

Robert B. Gibbs

Editors' introduction

Gibbs reviews the basic science, animal and neuro-chemical data, regarding estrogens and cognitive function. Importantly, estrogenic regulation of cognitive function is selective and does not affect all types of cognitive function but instead selectively affects specific types of behaviors. He goes on to review the impact of combination hormone therapy (HT) on cognitive performance and basic science investigations of the critical period of hormone intervention hypothesis. These findings indicate that estradiol enhancement of cognitive performance is lost over time following ovariectomy, which is consistent with Gibbs's cholinergic hypothesis and the critical window of therapeutic opportunity hypothesis (see Chapter 4). Results derived largely from rodent studies suggest that estradiol regulation of basal forebrain cholinergic neurons plays an important role in the regulation of select types of cognitive function, and may provide a mechanistic foundation for the critical period hypothesis. Gibbs proposes that identifying the specific neural circuits that account for the task-selective effects of estradiol, as well as the mechanisms by which these effects are mediated by basal forebrain cholinergic neurons, will aid in the proper use and timing of HT in postmenopausal women to sustain cognitive performance and prevent age-related cognitive decline and dementia.

Introduction

For many peri- and postmenopausal women, concerns about the risks and benefits of HT have become a major health issue. Recent scientific debate has done little to resolve the dilemma. On the one hand, animal studies clearly indicate that HT consisting of estradiol, or estradiol + progesterone, has many beneficial effects on the brain, such as protecting neurons from cardiac arrest and stroke [1], improving cognitive performance [2], and preventing or slowing age-related cognitive decline [3]. Human studies likewise have reported beneficial effects of HT on cognitive performance, particularly in younger postmenopausal women and in the area of verbal memory [4, 5]. Over a dozen retrospective and observational studies also have reported substantial reductions (up to 83%) in the risk of developing Alzheimer's-related dementia among women who received postmenopausal HT compared with those who did not [6]. In contrast, prospective, randomized trials have shown fewer benefits. The Women's Health Initiative Memory Study (WHIMS) in particular showed an increased (~two-fold) risk of dementia among women receiving combined HT (conjugated equine estrogens + medroxy-progesterone acetate) [7], and a trend towards increased risk of dementia among women receiving conjugated equine estrogens alone [8], particularly among women with lower cognitive scores at the onset of treatment (see Chapter 1). Could it be that randomization uncovered a true detrimental effect of HT that was not detected in the observational studies? Is it possible that both the WHIMS and the observational studies are correct?

One possible explanation for the disparity in findings relates to the timing of HT relative to age and the onset of menopause. We and others have hypothesized that HT must be initiated during or soon after

---

the onset of menopause in order to have beneficial effects on the brain, and to prevent age-related cognitive decline and dementia [9, 10]. In contrast, HT administered late in life may have no effect, or even adverse effects, due to physiological changes in estrogen response caused by aging and long-term hormone deprivation [11]. This "window of opportunity" for estrogen response forms the basis of the critical period hypothesis. This chapter discusses animal studies and potential mechanisms that support the critical period hypothesis, focusing primarily on the role of basal forebrain cholinergic neurons in mediating the effects of estradiol on cognitive performance.

Estradiol and cognitive performance

Numerous animal studies have demonstrated that ovariectomy impairs performance, and that estradiol treatment enhances performance, on a variety of cognitive tasks [2, 12]. It is important to note, however, that estradiol does not enhance performance on all tasks, and that the effects of estradiol are task specific. For example, our own studies have shown that estradiol significantly enhances acquisition of a delayed matching-to-position (DMP) T-maze task [9] (Fig. 5.1A). This is a spatial learning task in which rats typically use extramaze cues to identify correct vs. incorrect arm choices, and are rewarded for returning to the maze arm visited on the immediately preceding trial (i.e., a win–stay paradigm). Our studies show that animals receiving estradiol learn the task faster than ovariectomized controls, and that this reflects an increase in the rate of learning rather than a nonspecific increase in performance. We have also demonstrated robust effects of ovariectomy and estradiol treatment on a 12-arm radial maze task [13]. Like the DMP task, this is a spatial learning task but allows for a more rigorous analysis of working vs. reference memory. On this task, ovariectomy significantly impairs acquisition, particularly on the working memory component of the task, and performance is restored by estradiol treatment (Fig. 5.1B) [13]. Other studies have reported similar results using T-maze alternation and radial arm maze tasks [2, 12, 14], water maze tasks [15, 16], and place learning tasks [17, 18], all of which can be categorized as spatial learning tasks. Effects on non-spatial tasks such as visual object recognition [17, 19], and contextual and cued fear conditioning [20] also have been reported. In addition to effects on mnemonic functions,

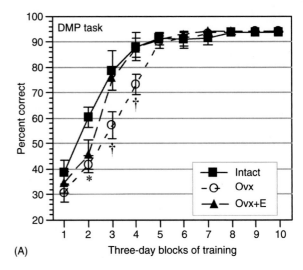

(A)

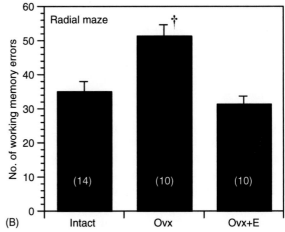

(B)

Fig. 5.1 Graphs showing that ovariectomy impairs and estradiol treatment restores acquisition of a delayed matching-to-position T-maze task (A), and a 12-arm radial maze task (B). Panel A depicts mean percent correct ± s.e.m. across ten three-day blocks of training. Panel B depicts mean total errors ± s.e.m across 42 days of training. Numbers in parentheses indicate group sizes. *Ovx differs significantly from gonadally intact rats. †Ovx differs significantly from both gonadally intact rats and from ovariectomized rats treated with estradiol. Significance defined as p < 0.05.

estradiol can also affect strategy selection, and can bias animals to use strategies based on hippocampal vs. striatal systems [21].

In contrast, ovariectomy and estradiol treatment appear to have no effect on acquisition of a configural association operant conditioning task [9]. This non-spatial task requires rats to discriminate between positive reinforcement associated with a light or tone stimulus, and the lack of reinforcement associated with simultaneous presentation of the two stimuli.

Estradiol also appears to have little effect on the reference memory component of an 8-arm or 12-arm radial maze task [22, 23], and has been shown to impair performance on a Morris water maze task [24]. This means that estradiol is not simply acting as a non-specific performance enhancer, but enhances performance within specific cognitive domains.

Task-selective effects of estradiol on cognitive performance have also been observed in monkeys. For example, in Rhesus monkeys, estradiol has been shown to modulate visuospatial attention [25]. In aged ovariectomized monkeys estradiol has been shown to enhance performance on a delayed recognition span task, a task of spatial working memory, but not on a delayed response task or a modified version of a Wisconsin Card Sorting Task, both of which are associated with prefrontal cortical function [26, 27]. The implication of these results is that estradiol affects specific neural circuits that underlie performance in a task-selective way.

Hormone treatment and age-related cognitive impairment

Studies also show that estradiol, or the combination of estradiol + progesterone, can prevent or reduce age-related cognitive decline [9]. For example, Markham *et al.* [28] showed that in rats ovariectomized at 14 months of age, long-term treatment with estradiol or with estradiol + progesterone prevented overnight forgetting on a spatial version of the Morris water maze task. Using monkeys, Rapp *et al.* [29] showed that estradiol treatment initiated following ovariectomy in middle age prevented a marked age-related impairment on a delayed response task. This suggests that under certain conditions estradiol or a combination of estradiol + progesterone may have a prophylactic effect that helps to protect the brain and prevent age-related cognitive decline. What then accounts for the negative results obtained from the WHIMS and for the mixed results obtained from other prospective clinical trials?

The critical period hypothesis

Some studies suggest that the timing of HT relative to age and the loss of ovarian function may be critical, and that a window of opportunity may exist for eliciting positive effects of HT on cognitive performance. These findings form the basis of the critical period hypothesis. Evidence in support of the critical

period hypothesis is derived from both animal and human literature. As one example, we conducted a study in which rats were ovariectomized at midlife (13 months). One group received continuous low-level estradiol treatment beginning immediately or three months following ovariectomy. Other groups received weekly administration of estradiol and progesterone (cyclically) beginning 3 months or 10 months following ovariectomy. All rats were then tested at very old age (23–25 months) using the DMP task [30]. Rats that received hormone treatment either immediately or within 3 months following ovariectomy (either estradiol alone or estradiol + progesterone) learned the task significantly faster than non-treated controls and made fewer errors (Fig. 5.2). In fact, these rats performed as well as much younger ovariectomized controls, suggesting a complete prevention of age-related cognitive impairment. In contrast, treatment initiated 10 months following ovariectomy was not as effective. This was among the first data showing that the ability of HT to enhance cognitive performance diminishes with time following ovariectomy.

Similarly, Markowska and Savonenko [31] showed that estradiol treatment initiated in middle-aged and aged rats within 6 months following ovariectomy significantly enhanced performance on a delayed alternation task, whereas treatment initiated 9 months after ovariectomy did not. Daniel *et al.* [32] likewise showed

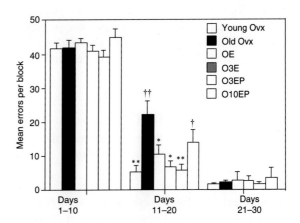

Fig. 5.2 Data showing that hormone treatments initiated in middle-aged rats either immediately (OE) or within 3 months (O3E, O3EP) following ovariectomy prevented an impairment in acquisition of the delayed matching-to-position T-maze task when the rats were old (>23 months). In contrast, treatment initiated 10 months following ovariectomy (O10EP) was less effective. See text for details. *p < 0.05; **p < 0.01 relative to aged Ovx controls. †p < 0.05; ††p < 0.01 relative to young Ovx controls. Adapted from [30].

that treating 17-month-old rats with estradiol immediately following ovariectomy enhanced performance on an eight-arm radial maze task, whereas treating rats of the same age, but 5 months following ovariectomy, was less effective. Talboom *et al.* [33] also recently showed that the effects of ovariectomy and estradiol treatment on a reference memory version of a Morris water maze task decline with age. More recently, we evaluated the effects of estradiol on DMP acquisition by middle-aged (13–15 months old) and aged (24–26 months old) rats that were ovariectomized at 3 months of age. Our data show that estradiol enhanced DMP acquisition in the middle-aged rats, but not in the aged rats. As in Talboom's study, this indicates that the ability of estradiol to enhance performance is lost with time following ovariectomy. Whether this is due primarily to age or to the prolonged loss of ovarian function is not known, but may very well be a combination of the two. Several human studies also support the idea that beneficial effects of HT on age-related cognitive decline are greatest when therapy is initiated close to menopause [34–37]. These and related studies are discussed in Chapter 6. We hypothesize that the underlying cause of this window of opportunity is related to a change in the functionality of cholinergic projection neurons located in the basal forebrain. Notably, in our rat study, the effects of estradiol on DMP acquisition were restored in aged rats by treating with donepezil, a cholinesterase inhibitor used in treating Alzheimer's-related dementia (see below). This is consistent with our cholinergic hypothesis, and raises the possibility that the 'window of opportunity' for eliciting beneficial effects of estradiol and cognitive can be restored.

The role of basal forebrain cholinergic projections

Cholinergic neurons in the medial septum, the vertical limb of the diagonal band of Broca, and the nucleus basalis magnocellularis, are the primary source of cholinergic inputs to the hippocampus and cerebral cortex [38, 39]. These neurons are well documented to play an important role in learning, memory, and attentional processes [40, 41], and there is strong evidence that impairments in basal forebrain cholinergic function contribute to age-related cognitive decline and to the behavioral and psychological symptoms of dementia [42, 43]. Many examples of decreased basal forebrain cholinergic function with age and Alzheimer's disease (AD) have been described

[44, 45]. Examples include decreases in the number and size of cholinergic neurons in the medial septum, diagonal band, and nucleus basalis magnocellularis, decreases in high affinity choline uptake in the hippocampus and frontal cortex, as well as decreases in acetylcholine synthesis, acetylcholine release, and cholinergic synaptic transmission. Moore *et al.* [46] reported a 50% reduction in potassium- and calcium-evoked acetylcholine release in the frontal cortex of 22-month-old rats relative to 4-month-old controls. Quirion *et al.* [47] likewise reported significantly less acetylcholine release in the hippocampus of aged–impaired rats (i.e., impaired on a Morris water maze task) relative to aged–unimpaired rats. Cholinergic antagonists, such as the muscarinic receptor antagonist scopolamine, produce cognitive deficits in both humans and animals similar in several respects to deficits observed with aging [48]. Conversely, cholinergic agonists such as cholinesterase inhibitors (e.g., donepezil, rivastigmine, and galantamine) and direct receptor agonists (e.g., nicotine and bethanicol), as well as agents that can indirectly enhance cholinergic function such as nerve growth factor or growth factor-producing transplants, can reduce cognitive deficits associated with aging and AD, as well as deficits caused by select cholinergic lesions [49, 50]. These studies support the idea that a decrease in the function of basal forebrain cholinergic neurons with age contributes to age-related decreases in cognitive performance.

Estradiol enhances basal forebrain cholinergic function

Many studies show that estradiol can enhance basal forebrain cholinergic function in young rats. This is demonstrated by:

- increased levels of choline acetyltransferase (ChAT), mRNA, and protein (discussed in [9, 45]); increases in high affinity choline uptake in the hippocampus and frontal cortex [51, 52]; increased acetylcholine release in the hippocampus in association with place learning [53] or in response to elevated potassium [54]; and
- increased density of cholinergic fibers in specific regions of the prefrontal cortex [55, 56].

One of the more robust effects is the enhancement of potassium-stimulated acetylcholine release. Our studies show that treating rats with physiological levels of estradiol results in a two-fold increase in potassium-stimulated acetylcholine release in the hippocampus, that the effect persists with long-term treatment, and that it is reversed when treatment is discontinued [54]. Note that estradiol affected stimulated acetylcholine release, but not basal acetylcholine release, suggesting that estradiol enhances acetylcholine release during periods of demand without affecting basal cholinergic tone. Studies show that treating rats with estradiol reduces cognitive impairments produced by the muscarinic receptor antagonist scopolamine [15, 57, 58], demonstrating the ability of estradiol to reduce or prevent cognitive impairment caused by a cholinergic deficit. Dumas *et al.* [59] reported similar results in humans, in which estradiol treatment reduced cognitive impairments produced by scopolamine and mecamilamine (a nicotinic receptor antagonist) in postmenopausal women. Further study confirmed that estradiol treatment reduced the effects of anticholinergic drugs on a test of episodic memory, but only in younger postmenopausal women (age 50–62) [60]; estradiol treatment impaired performance in older postmenopausal women (age 70–81). These data show not only that estradiol interacts with basal forebrain cholinergic function to affect cognitive performance, but that the ability of estradiol to protect against the effects of the anticholinergic drugs changes with time following menopause. This is further evidence that HT must be initiated soon following menopause in order to have a beneficial effect.

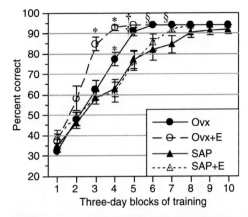

Fig. 5.3 Learning curves showing medial septal cholinergic lesions (SAP) abolish the ability of estradiol to enhance acquisition of the delayed matching-to-position T-maze task. *Differs significantly from all other groups. †Differs significantly from both the SAP and SAP+E groups. §Ovx and Ovx+E each differs significantly from the SAP group. Significance defined as $p < 0.05$. Adapted from [61].

Basal forebrain cholinergic neurons are necessary for estrogen-mediated effects on DMP acquisition

As further evidence that basal forebrain cholinergic neurons are important for mediating estradiol effects on cognitive performance, we tested whether these neurons are necessary for estradiol to enhance acquisition of the DMP task. Select cholinergic lesions were produced by discrete intraparenchymal injections of an immunotoxin (192IgG-saporin) directly into the medial septum. Destruction of the cholinergic neurons impaired DMP acquisition [61]. The lesions also completely prevented the ability of estradiol to enhance acquisition of the DMP task (Fig. 5.3). This demonstrates that cholinergic neurons in the medial septum are necessary for HT-mediated enhancement of DMP acquisition. Using a pharmacological approach,

Daniel *et al.* [62] likewise showed that intrahippocampal injections of an M2 muscarinic receptor antagonist prevented estrogen-mediated enhancement of performance on a working memory version of a water maze task. By contrast, injecting the antagonist into a cortical control site did not prevent estrogen-mediated enhancement of performance. These data demonstrate that functional cholinergic projections from the rostral basal forebrain to the hippocampus are required for estrogen to improve performance on certain tasks.

The cholinergic basis of the critical period hypothesis

Given that basal forebrain cholinergic projections are necessary, we reasoned that a gradual loss of cholinergic function post menopause might account for the presence of a critical period for eliciting positive effects of HT on cognitive performance. Notably, our studies do suggest that in rats, long-term loss of ovarian function does, in fact, have a severe negative impact on basal forebrain cholinergic neurons beyond the effects of normal aging. For example, the levels of choline acetyltransferase and trkA mRNA within cholinergic neurons of the medial septum and nucleus basalis magnocellularis of middle-aged rats killed 6 months following ovariectomy (at 19 months of age) were significantly reduced relative to age-matched gonadally intact controls [63]. TrkA is a receptor for nerve growth factor, which provides trophic support for the cholinergic neurons. In contrast, no significant decreases were observed at 3 months following ovariectomy. In addition, levels of trkA mRNA were decreased by 50%–60%, and levels of ChAT mRNA were decreased by 29%–49%, in the medial septum and nucleus basalis magnocellularis of rats killed 16–17 months following ovariectomy (at 29–30 months of age), relative to much younger ovariectomized controls [64]. This suggests that long-term loss of ovarian function has a negative impact on basal forebrain cholinergic neurons that develops gradually over time. This may account for the window of opportunity during which estrogen-containing HT remains capable of enhancing cognitive performance. Put simply, the hypothesis states that the critical period for eliciting positive effects of estradiol on cognitive performance post menopause is defined by the functionality of basal forebrain cholinergic projections. We refer to this as the *cholinergic basis of the critical period hypothesis*.

Testing the cholinergic basis of the critical period hypothesis

If our hypothesis is correct, then one would predict that enhancing cholinergic function pharmacologically may re-open the window of opportunity and restore the ability of estradiol to enhance cognitive performance in aged rats, even after prolonged loss of ovarian function. We are testing this by ovariectomizing rats at 3 months of age, and then 21 months later testing the ability to restore estradiol effects on DMP acquisition by administering daily injections of donepezil, a cholinesterase inhibitor commonly used in the treatment of AD. Preliminary results confirm that aged ovariectomized rats take much longer to reach criterion and improve more slowly than young rats, and that estradiol treatment alone produces no improvement. Donepezil alone also produced no improvement; however, rats that received both daily donepezil injections and sustained estradiol treatment took fewer days to reach criterion (Fig. 5.4) and performed consistently better than all other groups. This is exactly as predicted by the cholinergic hypothesis, and supports the idea that the loss of estradiol effect in aged ovariectomized rats is due to a reduction in basal forebrain cholinergic function. In addition, these data suggest that the ability of estradiol to enhance performance on this task can be restored in aged ovariectomized rats via the use of a cholinesterase inhibitor

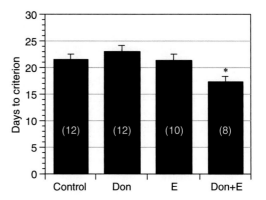

Fig. 5.4 Data showing that treating aged (>24 month old) rats that were ovariectomized at 3 months of age with donepezil restored the ability of estradiol to enhance performance on the delayed matching-to-position T-maze task. In contrast, treating the aged rats with either donepezil or with estradiol alone had no beneficial effect. Numbers in parentheses indicate group sizes. *p < 0.05 relative to controls.

commonly used in the treatment of AD. A similar effect in humans would mean that treatment with a cholinesterase inhibitor could potentially reinstate the ability of specific hormone therapies to enhance cognitive performance in postmenopausal women, even among women who have not used estrogen therapy for many years since the onset of menopause.

Other potential mechanisms

Thus far, the discussion has focused on the hypothesis that basal forebrain cholinergic neurons mediate effects of estradiol on cognitive performance and provide a mechanistic underpinning for the critical period hypothesis. Estradiol has many other effects in the brain that likely affect cognitive performance. These have been extensively reviewed [65], and are mentioned here only briefly.

Hippocampus and prefrontal cortex

Many of the effects of estrogens on cognitive performance are thought to be related to effects on hippocampal connectivity and function. For example, Fernandez *et al.* [19] recently reported that estradiol enhances object recognition in mice via a mechanism involving membrane-associated estrogen receptors and activation of the mitogen-activated protein kinases (MAPK) signaling pathway in hippocampal neurons. Estradiol has many well documented effects on hippocampal structure and function. Some of these effects include increasing the number of dendritic spines and new contacts on the apical dendrites of CA1 pyramidal cells, increasing N-methyl-D-aspartate receptor expression and responses in CA1 neurons, increasing long-term potentiation and decreasing long-term depression at CA1 synapses, increasing presynaptic proteins synaptophysin and syntaxin and postsynaptic proteins spinophilin and PSD-95 in the CA1 region, and activating microtubule associated kinases and cAMP response element binding (CREB) (reviewed in [65, 66]). Evidence suggests that some of these effects are produced via modulation of GABA-mediated inhibitory input, resulting in the disinhibition of CA1 pyramidal cells [67]. Notably, this effect is reduced by cholinergic denervation [68]. With respect to dendritic spines, both 17-alpha and 17-beta-estradiol, as well as testosterone and to a small extent dihydrotestosterone, are effective at increasing spine density on CA1 dendrites in female rats [69]. Recently, McLaughlin *et al.* [70] showed that the effects of estradiol on spine density in CA1 were reduced ten weeks following ovariectomy. In addition, studies show that the effects on spine density and N-methyl-D-aspartate (NMDA) receptor expression in the rat appear to rely on cholinergic inputs [71, 72], suggesting that effects on cholinergic function may underlie some of the effects of estrogens on hippocampal function.

Studies show that ovariectomy and estradiol treatment also affect dendritic spine density within specific regions of the prefrontal cortex. Elegant work by Luine and co-workers has shown that estradiol enhances [17] and ovariectomy impairs [73] object recognition and object placement memory in rats. The effects of ovariectomy were associated with decreased spine density within layers II/III of prefrontal cortex. Aging also is associated with impaired recognition memory, with a corresponding decrease in spine density in prefrontal cortex [74]. Whether or not these effects are associated with effects on cholinergic inputs currently is not known. Nor is it known whether the effects in the prefrontal cortex change with age and long-term ovariectomy. The recent studies by Dumas *et al.* [60] suggest that changes in the interaction between estradiol and cholinergic afferents to the prefrontal cortex are likely involved in mediating age-related changes in the effects of estradiol on cognitive performance. In the hippocampus of rats, effects on spine density on CA1 dendrites change with age such that estradiol fails to increase spine density but instead increases the quantity of NMDA receptor content per spine. Interestingly, in aged monkeys the ability of estradiol to increase spine density on CA1 dendrites is retained [65].

Neuroprotection

Estradiol also has neuroprotective effects in the brain that may affect risk for age-related cognitive impairment. Work by Wise and others has shown substantial estrogen-mediated neuroprotection of brain structures using models of stroke and cardiac arrest [1]. Estradiol also decreases beta-amyloid production in the brain, and can protect neurons from A-beta-mediated toxicity and oxidative damage [75] (also see Chapters 6 and 17). If true in humans, then early postmenopausal use of estrogen therapy may help to protect the brain not only from acute insult, but also from accumulated injury associated with prolonged cellular stress and amyloid-beta production. Some evidence, however, suggests that these neuroprotective effects may apply only to "healthy cells," and not to cells that are already damaged or in severe cellular stress. This hypothesis, called the "healthy cell bias" of estrogen action, states that estrogen has positive effects on healthy brain structures, but that once the structures are already damaged, estrogen's effects are detrimental. This is discussed further in Chapter 6. One possibility is that prolonged hypoestrogenicity biases the brain towards an "unhealthy" state. In this case, estrogen use initiated many years post menopause might have a negative effect rather than a positive effect on brain function. This fits precisely the prediction of the critical period hypothesis, and could explain why HT in the WHIMS trial had negative as opposed to positive effects on risk for dementia.

Summary

Animal studies provide compelling evidence that HT containing estrogens can significantly enhance performance on specific types of cognitive tasks. The evidence also suggests that the effects of HT change in response to both long-term loss of ovarian hormones and age, such that initiation around the time of menopause is beneficial, whereas administration many years following menopause may be ineffective or even detrimental. Data largely from rodent studies suggest that effects of estradiol on basal forebrain cholinergic neurons play an important role, and may provide a solid mechanistic underpinning to the critical period hypothesis. Cellular mechanisms affecting synaptic plasticity and neuroprotection must also play a role. The fact that, in one preliminary study, treatment with a cholinesterase inhibitor reinstated estrogen effects on DMP acquisition in aged ovari-ectomized rats raises hope that the critical period for eliciting positive effects of estradiol on cognitive per-formance can be restored, even in women that have not used HT for many years post menopause. Identi-fying the specific neural circuits that account for the task-selective effects of estradiol, as well as the mech-anisms by which these effects are mediated by basal forebrain cholinergic neurons, will greatly increase our understanding of how the proper use and timing of HT in postmenopausal women can protect cogni-tive performance and prevent age-related cognitive decline and dementia.

References

1. Suzuki S, Brown CM, Wise PM. Mechanisms of neuroprotection by estrogen. *Endocrine.* 2006;**29**(2): 209–15.

2. Daniel JM. Effects of oestrogen on cognition: what have we learned from basic research? *J Neuroendocrinol.* 2006;**18**(10):787–95.

3. Gibbs R. Preclinical data relating to estrogen's effects on cognitive performance. In Rasgon NL, ed. *The Effects of Estrogen on Brain Function.* Baltimore, MD: Johns Hopkins Press, 2006, pp. 9–45.

4. Genazzani AR, Pluchino N, Luisi S, *et al.* Estrogen, cognition and female ageing. *Hum Reprod Update.* 2007;**13**(2):175–87.

5. Sherwin BB. Estrogen and cognitive aging in women. *Neuroscience.* 2006;**138**(3):1021–6.

6. Henderson VW. Estrogen-containing hormone therapy and Alzheimer's disease risk: understanding discrepant inferences from observational and experimental research. *Neuroscience.* 2006;**138**(3): 1031–9.

7. Shumaker SA, Legault C, Rapp SR, *et al.* Estrogen plus progestin and the incidence of dementia and mild cognitive impairment in postmenopausal women: the Women's Health Initiative Memory Study: a randomized controlled trial. *JAMA.* 2003;**289**(20):2651–62.

8. Shumaker SA, Legault C, Kuller L, *et al.* Conjugated equine estrogens and incidence of probable dementia and mild cognitive impairment in postmenopausal women: the Women's Health Initiative Memory Study. *JAMA.* 2004;**291**(24):2947–58.

9. Gibbs RB, Gabor R. Estrogen and cognition: applying preclinical findings to clinical perspectives. *J Neurosci Res.* 2003;**74**:637–43.

10. Maki PM. Hormone therapy and cognitive function: is there a critical period for benefit? *Neuroscience.* 2006;**138**(3):1027–30.

11. Sherwin BB, Henry JF. Brain aging modulates the neuroprotective effects of estrogen on selective aspects of cognition in women: a critical review. *Front Neuroendocrinol.* 2008;**29**(1):88–113.

12. Dohanich GP. Gonadal steroids, learning and memory. In Pfaff DW, Arnold AP, Etgen AM, *et al.*, eds. *Hormones, Brain and Behavior.* San Diego, CA: Academic Press, 2002, pp. 265–327.

13. Gibbs RB, Johnson DA. Sex specific effects of gonadectomy and hormone treatment on acquisition of a 12-arm radial maze task by Sprague-Dawley rats. *Endocrinology.* 2008;**149**(6):3176–83.

14. Bimonte HA, Denenberg VH. Estradiol facilitates performance as working memory load increases. *Psychoneuroendocrinology.* 1999;**24**(2):161–73.

15. Packard MG. Posttraining estrogen and memory modulation. *Horm Behav.* 1998;**34**(2):126–39.

16. Bimonte HA, Hyde LA, Hoplight BJ, *et al.* In two species, females exhibit superior working memory and inferior reference memory on the water radial-arm maze. *Physiol Behav.* 2000;**70**(3/4):311–17.

17. Luine VN, Jacome LF, Maclusky NJ. Rapid enhancement of visual and place memory by estrogens in rats. *Endocrinology.* 2003;**144**(7):2836–44.

18. Li C, Brake WG, Romeo RD, *et al.* Estrogen alters hippocampal dendritic spine shape and enhances synaptic protein immunoreactivity and spatial memory in female mice. *Proc Natl Acad Sci USA.* 2004;**101**(7):2185–90.

19. Fernandez SM, Lewis MC, Pechenino AS, *et al.* Estradiol-induced enhancement of object memory consolidation involves hippocampal extracellular signal-regulated kinase activation and membrane-bound estrogen receptors. *J Neurosci.* 2008;**28**(35):8660–7.

20. Jasnow AM, Schulkin J, Pfaff DW. Estrogen facilitates fear conditioning and increases corticotropin-releasing hormone mRNA expression in the central amygdala in female mice. *Horm Behav.* 2006;**49**(2):197–205.

21. Korol DL. Role of estrogen in balancing contributions from multiple memory systems. *Neurobiol Learn Mem.* 2004;**82**(3):309–23.

22. Fader AJ, Johnson PEM, Dohanich GP. Estrogen improves working but not reference memory and prevents amnestic effects of scopolamine on a radial-arm maze. *Pharmacol Biochem Behav.* 1999;**62**(4):711–17.

23. Gibbs RB, Johnson DA. Sex-specific effects of gonadectomy and hormone treatment on acquisition

of a 12-arm radial maze task by Sprague-Dawley rats. *Endocrinology.* 2008;**149**(6):3176–83.

24. Chesler EJ, Juraska JM. Acute administration of estrogen and progesterone impairs the acquisition of the spatial Morris water maze in ovariectomized rats. *Horm Behav.* 2000;**38**(4):234–42.

25. Voytko ML. Estrogen and the cholinergic system modulate visuospatial attention in monkeys (*Macaca fascicularis*). *Behav Neurosci.* 2002;**116**(2):187–97.

26. Lacreuse A, Wilson ME, Herndon JG. Estradiol, but not raloxifene, improves aspects of spatial working memory in aged ovariectomized rhesus monkeys. *Neurobiol Aging.* 2002;**23**(4):589–600.

27. Lacreuse A, Chhabra RK, Hall MJ, *et al.* Executive function is less sensitive to estradiol than spatial memory: performance on an analog of the card sorting test in ovariectomized aged rhesus monkeys. *Behav Processes.* 2004;**67**(2):313–19.

28. Markham JA, Pych JC, Juraska JM. Ovarian hormone replacement to aged ovariectomized female rats benefits acquisition of the Morris water maze. *Horm Behav.* 2002;**42**(3):284–93.

29. Rapp PR, Morrison JH, Roberts JA. Cyclic estrogen replacement improves cognitive function in aged ovariectomized rhesus monkeys. *J Neurosci.* 2003;**23**(13):5708–14.

30. Gibbs RB. Long-term treatment with estrogen and progesterone enhances acquisition of a spatial memory task by ovariectomized aged rats. *Neurobiol Aging.* 2000;**21**:107–16.

31. Markowska AL, Savonenko AV. Effectiveness of estrogen replacement in restoration of cognitive function after long-term estrogen withdrawal in aging rats. *J Neurosci.* 2002;**22**(24):10985–95.

32. Daniel JM, Hulst JL, Berbling JL. Estradiol replacement enhances working memory in middle-aged rats when initiated immediately after ovariectomy but not after a long-term period of ovarian hormone deprivation. *Endocrinology.* 2006; **147**(1):607–14.

33. Talboom JS, Williams BJ, Baxley ER, *et al.* Higher levels of estradiol replacement correlate with better spatial memory in surgically menopausal young and middle-aged rats. *Neurobiol Learn Mem.* 2008; **90**(1):155–63.

34. Sherwin BB. The critical period hypothesis: can it explain discrepancies in the oestrogen-cognition literature? *J Neuroendocrinol.* 2007;**19**(2):77–81.

35. Zandi PP, Carlson MC, Plassman BL, *et al.* Hormone replacement therapy and incidence of Alzheimer disease in older women: the Cache County study. *JAMA.* 2002;**288**(17):2123–9.

36. Bagger YZ, Tanko LB, Alexandersen P, *et al.* Early postmenopausal hormone therapy may prevent cognitive impairment later in life. *Menopause.* 2005; **12**(1):12–17.

37. Henderson VW, Benke KS, Green RC, *et al.* Postmenopausal hormone therapy and Alzheimer's disease risk: interaction with age. *J Neurol Neurosurg Psychiatry.* 2005;**76**(1):103–5.

38. Mesulam MM. The systems-level organization of cholinergic innervation in the human cerebral cortex and its alterations in Alzheimer's disease. *Prog Brain Res.* 1996;**109**:285–97.

39. Woolf NJ. Cholinergic systems in mammalian brain and spinal cord. *Prog Neurobiol.* 1991;**37**:475–524.

40. Baxter MG, Chiba AA. Cognitive functions of the basal forebrain. *Curr Opin Neurobiol.* 1999;**9**(2): 178–83.

41. Everitt BJ, Robbins TW. Central cholinergic systems and cognition. *Annu Rev Psychol.* 1997;**48**:649–84.

42. Linstow EV, Platt B. Biochemical dysfunction and memory loss: the case of Alzheimer's dementia. *Cell Mol Life Sci.* 1999;**55**:601–16.

43. Lanari A, Amenta F, Silvestrelli G, *et al.* Neurotransmitter deficits in behavioural and psychological symptoms of Alzheimer's disease. *Mech Ageing Dev.* 2006;**127**(2):158–65.

44. Schliebs R, Arendt T. The significance of the cholinergic system in the brain during aging and in Alzheimer's disease. *J Neural Transm.* 2006;**113**(11): 1625–44.

45. Gibbs RB. Effects of estrogen on basal forebrain cholinergic neurons and cognition: implications for brain aging and dementia in women. In Morrison M, ed. *Hormones, Aging, and Mental Disorders.* Cambridge: Cambridge University Press, 2000, pp. 183–222.

46. Moore H, Stuckman S, Sarter M, *et al.* Potassium, but not atropine-stimulated cortical acetylcholine efflux, is reduced in aged rats. *Neurobiol Aging.* 1996;**17**(4): 565–71.

47. Quirion R, Wilson A, Rowe W, *et al.* Facilitation of acetylcholine release and cognitive performance by an M(2)-muscarinic receptor antagonist in aged memory-impaired. *J Neurosci.* 1995;**15**(2): 1455–62.

48. Bartus RT, Dean RL, Pontecorvo MJ, *et al.* The cholinergic hypothesis: a historical overview, current perspective, and future directions. *Ann N Y Acad Sci.* 1985;**444**:332–58.

49. Lleo A, Greenberg SM, Growdon JH. Current pharmacotherapy for Alzheimer's disease. *Annu Rev Med.* 2006;**57**:513–33.

50. Winkler J, Thal LJ, Gage FH, *et al.* Cholinergic strategies for Alzheimer's disease. *J Mol Med.* 1998;**76**(8):555–67.

51. Gibbs RB. Effects of gonadal hormone replacement on measures of basal forebrain cholinergic function. *Neuroscience.* 2000;**101**(4):931–8.

52. O'Malley CA, Hautamaki RD, Kelley M, *et al.* Effects of ovariectomy and estradiol benzoate on high affinity choline uptake, ACh synthesis, and release from rat cerebral cortical synaptosomes. *Brain Research.* 1987;**403**:389–92.

53. Marriott LK, Korol DL. Short-term estrogen treatment in ovariectomized rats augments hippocampal acetylcholine release during place learning. *Neurobiol Learn Mem.* 2003;**80**(3):315–22.

54. Gabor R, Nagle R, Johnson DA, *et al.* Estrogen enhances potassium-stimulated acetylcholine release in the rat hippocampus. *Brain Research.* 2003;**962**:244–7.

55. Kritzer MF, Kohama SG. Ovarian hormones differentially influence immunoreactivity for dopamine beta-hydroxylase, choline acetyltransferase, and serotonin in the dorsolateral prefrontal cortex of adult rhesus monkeys. *J Comp Neurol.* 1999;**409**(3):438–51.

56. Tinkler GP, Tobin JR, Voytko ML. Effects of two years of estrogen loss or replacement on nucleus basalis cholinergic neurons and cholinergic fibers to the dorsolateral prefrontal and inferior parietal cortex of monkeys. *J Comp Neurol.* 2004;**469**(4):507–21.

57. Fader AJ, Hendricson AW, Dohanich GP. Estrogen improves performance of reinforced T-maze alternation and prevents the amnestic effects of scopolamine administered systemically or intrahippocampally. *Neurobiol Learn Mem.* 1998;**69**(3):225–40.

58. Gibbs RB, Burke AM, Johnson DA. Estrogen replacement attenuates effects of scopolamine and lorazepam on memory acquisition and retention. *Horm Behav.* 1998;**34**:112–25.

59. Dumas J, Hancur-Bucci C, Naylor M, *et al.* Estrogen treatment effects on anticholinergic-induced cognitive dysfunction in normal postmenopausal women. *Neuropsychopharmacology.* 2006;**31**(9):2065–78.

60. Dumas J, Hancur-Bucci C, Naylor M, *et al.* Estradiol interacts with the cholinergic system to affect verbal memory in postmenopausal women: evidence for the critical period hypothesis. *Horm Behav.* 2008;**53**(1):159–69.

61. Gibbs RB. Estradiol enhances DMP acquisition via a mechanism not mediated by turning strategy but which requires intact basal forebrain cholinergic projections. *Horm Behav.* 2007;**52**(3):352–9.

62. Daniel JM, Hulst JL, Lee CD. Role of hippocampal M2 muscarinic receptors in the estrogen-induced enhancement of working memory. *Neuroscience.* 2005;**132**(1):57–64.

63. Gibbs RB. Impairment of basal forebrain cholinergic neurons associated with aging and long-term loss of ovarian function. *Exp Neurol.* 1998;**151**:289–302.

64. Gibbs RB. Effects of aging, ovariectomy, and long-term hormone replacement on cholinergic neurons in the medial septum and nucleus basalis magnocellularis. *J Neuroendocrinol.* 2003;**15**:477–85.

65. Spencer JL, Waters EM, Romeo RD, *et al.* Uncovering the mechanisms of estrogen effects on hippocampal function. *Front Neuroendocrinol.* 2007;**29**(2):219–37.

66. Woolley CS. Acute effects of estrogen on neuronal physiology. *Annu Rev Pharmacol Toxicol.* 2007;**47**:657–80.

67. Rudick CN, Woolley CS. Estrogen regulates functional inhibition of hippocampal CA1 pyramidal cells in the adult female rat. *J Neurosci.* 2001;**21**(17):6532–43.

68. Rudick CN, Gibbs RB, Woolley CS. A role for the basal forebrain cholinergic system in estrogen-induced disinhibition of hippocampal pyramidal cells. *J Neurosci.* 2003;**23**(11):4479–90.

69. Parducz A, Hajszan T, Maclusky NJ, *et al.* Synaptic remodeling induced by gonadal hormones: neuronal plasticity as a mediator of neuroendocrine and behavioral responses to steroids. *Neuroscience.* 2006;**138**(3):977–85.

70. McLaughlin KJ, Bimonte-Nelson H, Neisewander JL, *et al.* Assessment of estradiol influence on spatial tasks and hippocampal CA1 spines: evidence that the duration of hormone deprivation after ovariectomy compromises 17beta-estradiol effectiveness in altering CA1 spines. *Horm Behav.* 2008;**54**(3):386–95.

71. Lam TT, Leranth C. Role of the medial septum diagonal band of Broca cholinergic neurons in oestrogen-induced spine synapse formation on hippocampal CA1 pyramidal cells of female rats. *Eur J Neurosci.* 2003;**17**(10):1997–2005.

72. Daniel JM, Dohanich GP. Acetylcholine mediates the estrogen-induced increase in NMDA receptor binding in CA1 of the hippocampus and the associated improvement in working memory. *J Neurosci.* 2001;**21**(17):6949–56.

73. Wallace M, Luine V, Arellanos A, *et al.* Ovariectomized rats show decreased recognition memory and spine density in the hippocampus and prefrontal cortex. *Brain Res.* 2006;**1126**(1):176–82.

74. Wallace M, Frankfurt M, Arellanos A, *et al.* Impaired recognition memory and decreased prefrontal cortex spine density in aged female rats. *Ann N Y Acad Sci.* 2007;**1097**:54–7.

75. LeBlanc A. Estrogen and Alzheimer's disease. *Curr Opin Investig Drugs.* 2002;**3**(5):768–73.

The healthy cell bias of estrogen action through regulating glucose metabolism and mitochondrial function: implications for prevention of Alzheimer's disease

Roberta Diaz Brinton

Editors' introduction

Brinton provides a comprehensive review of the effects of estradiol on glycolytic enzymes and glucose metabolism in the brain and in neurons. Her analysis reveals a large body of corroborating evidence converging on the conclusion that estradiol promotes enhanced utilization of glucose in the brain, thereby helping neurons to meet the energy demands of neuronal activation. Seeing as how dysfunction of glucose metabolism and neuronal biogenetics are antecedents to Alzheimer's disease (AD), it is reasonable to speculate how the effects of estrogens on glucose metabolism might help stave off the disease. Her studies show, however, that as neurons become compromised such as in the context of aging and/or disease, the effects of estrogens can become deleterious and ultimately lead to the activation of apoptotic pathways and neuronal death. Hence the hypothesis that as neurons age and become increasingly stressed or compromised, the net effect of estrogens on oxidative metabolism and neuronal survival shifts from positive to negative. This healthy cell bias may explain some of the recent negative clinical results, and in particular how estrogenic therapy administered around the time of the perimenopause can be beneficial whereas the same therapy administered late in life and in the context of a developing pathology could be detrimental and result in significant cognitive decline.

Introduction

The *healthy cell bias of estrogen action* hypothesis provides a lens through which to assess the disparities in outcomes across the basic to clinical domains of scientific inquiry and on which to predict future

applications of estrogens and hormone therapeutic interventions to sustain neurological health and to *prevent* age-associated neurodegenerative diseases such as AD. The data indicate that as the continuum of neurological health progresses from healthy to unhealthy so too do the benefits of estrogens or hormone therapy (HT). If neurons are healthy at the time of estrogen exposure, their response to estrogen is beneficial for both neuronal survival and neurological function. In contrast, if neurological health is compromised, estrogen exposure over time exacerbates neurological demise. Overall, estrogen promotes the energetic capacity of brain mitochondria by maximizing aerobic glycolysis (oxidative phosphorylation coupled to pyruvate metabolism). The enhanced aerobic glycolysis in the aging brain would be predicted *to prevent conversion* of the brain to using alternative sources of fuel such as the ketone body pathway characteristic of Alzheimer's. Throughout this chapter estrogen/estrogens is used to refer to a class of hormones whereas specific estrogenic molecules are referred to by name.

Evidence for the healthy cell bias of estrogen action

Decades of basic science investigation of estrogen action in the brain and subsequent observational and clinical trials indicated the benefit of estrogenic therapies [1–4]. Embedded among these reports were suggestions that the beneficial effects of estrogen were conditional [5–11]. Results of the widely publicized Women's Health Initiative Memory Study (WHIMS) clinical trial drew substantial attention to just how

Hormones, Cognition and Dementia: State of the Art and Emergent Therapeutic Strategies, ed. Eef Hogervorst, Victor W. Henderson, Robert B. Gibbs, and Roberta Diaz Brinton. Published by Cambridge University Press.
© Cambridge University Press 2009.

conditional estrogen and HT can be [12, 13]. Analysis of the model systems used across the basic to clinical research continuum separate them into two broad classes, those that use prevention interventions in healthy organisms and those that use hormone interventions in organisms with compromised neurological function [1]. Basic science analyses that led to elucidation of the neurotrophic and neuroprotective effects of estrogen and the underlying mechanisms of action typically used a prevention experimental paradigm [1]. The prevention paradigm relies on healthy neurons/brains/animals/humans as the starting foundation, followed by exposure to estrogens/hormones, followed by exposure to neurodegenerative insult. The prevention paradigm of basic science analyses parallels the human studies of Sherwin and colleagues who investigated the cognitive impact of estrogen therapy in women with surgical or pharmacological-induced menopause [14]. Observational, retrospective and prospective, studies are also consistent with the outcomes of basic science analyses [1]. For the most part, the epidemiological observational data indicate reduction in risk of AD in women who began estrogen or hormone therapy at the time of the menopause [1, 6, 15] but see [16]. The comparable benefit seen in most observational studies and basic science analyses suggests that for the most part, the data within the observational studies were derived from women with healthy neurological status.

In contrast, studies that fall within the second class, hormone intervention in women with compromised neurological function, i.e., a treatment paradigm, exhibit a mixed profile [1]. This was first evident in the results from the Cache County trial in which risk of AD varied with age of HT initiation and duration of use [6]. A woman's sex-specific increase in risk disappeared entirely with more than ten years of treatment with most of the HT-related reduction in incidence reflecting former use. There was no effect with current hormone replacement therapy (HRT) use unless duration of treatment exceeded ten years [6]. The efficacy of estrogenic therapy (ET), which was observed in the early AD treatment trials that lasted 1.5–2 months [17], was not sustained when ET was administered for an extended period of time [18, 19]. In a randomized double-blind clinical trial of conjugated equine estrogen (CEE) therapy in a cohort of aged women ($\geq$72 years of age) diagnosed with AD, treatment with CEE resulted in a modest benefit in the short term (2 months) and adverse progression

of disease in the long term (12 months) [18, 19]. In the WHIMS cohort of women, 65–79 years of age with no indicators of neurological disease but with variable health status, no statistically significant increase in AD risk occurred in the CEE arm of the trial [12]; however, there was no benefit of CEE therapy and there was a clear decline in cognitive performance over time [12]. In contrast, the combination of CEE+MPA for five years increased the risk of developing AD by two-fold [13] and when the results of the ET and HT data were combined there was a two-fold increase in the risk of AD [13]. Subsequent post-hoc analyses of the WHIMS data suggested that women who had reported prior hormone use had a significantly lower risk of AD and all-cause dementia during the WHIMS trials [20]. Collectively, the data suggest that as the continuum of neurological health progresses from healthy to unhealthy so too do the benefits of ET or HT [1]. If neurons are healthy at the time of estrogen exposure, their response to estrogen is beneficial for both neurological function and survival. In contrast, if neurological health is compromised, estrogen exposure over time exacerbates neurological demise.

The healthy cell bias of estrogen action hypothesis predicts that ET, if initiated at the time of perimenopause when neurological health is not yet comprised, will be of benefit in terms of reduced risk for age-associated neurodegenerative diseases such as AD and Parkinson's disease. Further, 17β-estradiol (E$_2$) promotion of glycolysis and glycolytic coupled citric acid function, mitochondrial respiration and ATP generation, and antioxidant and antiapoptotic mechanisms serves as the pivotal pathway by which estrogen sustains neurological health and defense. The reliance of this pathway on Ca^{2+} signaling and on mitochondrial Ca^{2+} buffering is an Achilles heel of estrogen action in degenerating systems in which Ca^{2+} homeostasis is dysregulated. Addition of estrogen under these conditions, while of modest benefit initially (an effect likely mediated by neurons not yet affected by the disease), adds to the Ca^{2+} homeostatic challenge with predictable exacerbation of the degenerative process [10].

Estrogenic regulation of glucose metabolism: sustaining reliance of brain on glucose as primary energy fuel

Earlier work from the Simpkins group demonstrated that E$_2$ increased expression of glucose transporter subunits and increased glucose transport in blood–brain barrier endothelium [21]. Later work by Bondy and colleagues confirmed E_2 regulation of glucose transporter proteins and that regulation of glucose transporters occurs in neurons in the non-human primate brain [22]. In the frontal cortex of ovariectomized non-human primates, E_2 treatment induced two- to four-fold increases in glucose transporter proteins Glut3 and Glut4 mRNA and protein [22]. Analysis of cellular localization indicated that E_2 induced a marked rise in neuronal Glut1 mRNA levels with no appreciable effect on vascular Glut1 gene expression. Collectively, these data indicate that E_2 regulates metabolic functions sustaining the energetic demands of neuronal activation [23–28].

If E_2 is promoting glucose transport into the brain and into neural cells, then concomitant regulation of glycolytic enzymes would be anticipated. Evidence derived from rat brain indicate that, in vivo, E_2 significantly increased glycolytic enzyme activity of hexokinase (soluble and membrane-bound), phosphofructokinase, and pyruvate kinase within four hours [29]. As described above, the neuroprotective effect of E_2 is mediated by the coordinated and near simultaneous activation of both the MAPK and Akt signaling pathways through activation of PI3K in hippocampal neurons [30]. Remarkably, the anti-apoptotic effect of Akt is dependent upon hexokinase association with the voltage-dependent anion channel (VDAC) of mitochondria [31]. Hexokinases are known to bind to VDAC to directly couple intramitochondrial ATP synthesis to glucose metabolism [32]. Moreover, of the four hexokinase isoforms, only HKI and II are known to associate with mitochondria where they associate with the mitochondrial outer membrane and bind to VDAC [31]. While it is known that E_2 activates Akt [30, 33, 34] and increases HKII activity [29], it remains to be determined whether E_2 is promoting the association of HKII and VDAC in neural cells.

Functional impact of estrogen-induced glucose transporter protein would require a concomitant change in factors regulating glucose metabolism, which in turn suggests a role for insulin or its brain homolog insulin growth factor-1 (IGF-1) and its cognate receptor, IGF-1R. Bondy and colleagues found that IGF-1R mRNA was concentrated in cortical neurons in a distribution similar to Gluts 3 and 4 [22]. In the non-human primate frontal cortex, E_2-treated animals showed a significant increase in

IGF-1 mRNA without a concomitant rise in IGF-1 receptor mRNA [22]. These investigators went on to elucidate the molecular mechanisms whereby IGF-1 regulated neuronal metabolism by demonstrating that the active, phosphorylated form of Akt/PKB was selectively co-localized with the "insulin-sensitive" glucose transporter, GLUT4, in IGF-1-expressing neurons. Akt is a major target of insulin-signaling in the regulation of glucose transport via the facilitative glucose transporter (GLUT4) and glycogen synthesis in peripheral tissues. In parallel to these studies of glucose transport and metabolism, Garcia-Segura and colleagues have for many years demonstrated the synergistic coupling between ERs and IGF-1R [35–38]. Results of their analyses provide substantial evidence for the role of IGF-1, PI3K to Akt signaling pathway, estrogen receptors, and estrogen-inducible neuroprotection [37–39]. Findings of the neuroprotective actions of the synergy between the estrogen receptors and IGF-1 signaling cascades are particularly relevant to prevention of neurodegenerative diseases. Torres-Aleman and co-workers have shown that low circulating IGF-I in the brain is associated with greater accumulation of beta amyloid ($A\beta$), whereas $A\beta$ burden can be reduced by increasing serum IGF-I [40]. The inverse relationship between serum IGF-I and brain $A\beta$ levels reflects the ability of IGF-I to induce clearance of $A\beta$ from brain, likely by enhancing transport of $A\beta$ carrier proteins such as albumin and transthyretin into the brain [40].

Regulation of brain metabolism in vivo by estrogens

If estrogens are increasing glucose uptake, metabolism, and utilization in the brain then there should be evidence of increased metabolic activity in the brain following administration of estrogens. As part of a nine-year study in the Baltimore Longitudinal Study of Aging, Resnick and colleagues conducted positron emission tomography (PET) to assess regional cerebral blood flow in a small cohort of women who used ET versus women who did not. Results of this analysis showed that ET users and non-users showed significant differences in PET-regional cerebral blood flow relative activation patterns during the memory tasks. Estrogenic therapy users showed better performance on neuropsychological tests of figural and verbal memory and on some aspects of the PET activation tests. In a follow-up longitudinal study from the same cohort of healthy menopausal women, Maki and Resnick [41] found that regional cerebral blood flow was increased in ET users relative to non-users in the hippocampus, parahippocampal gyrus, and temporal lobe, regions that form a memory circuit and that are sensitive to preclinical AD [41]. Further these investigators found that the increase in regional cerebral blood flow was associated with higher scores on a battery of cognitive tests [41]. In a two-year follow-up analysis, Rasgon and colleagues detected a significant decrease in metabolism of the posterior cingulate cortex among postmenopausal women who did not receive estrogens whereas those women who used estrogens did not exhibit significant metabolic change in the posterior cingulate [42]. These findings that use of estrogens preserves regional cerebral metabolism and protects against metabolic decline in postmenopausal women, especially in the posterior cingulate cortex, is particularly important given that metabolism in this region of the brain declines in the earliest stages of AD [42, 43].

Regulation of mitochondrial function by estrogens: bioenergetic survival for the brain

Our investigation of estrogenic regulation of mitochondrial function was stimulated by our findings that E_2 prevented dysregulation of Ca^{2+} homeostasis by increasing mitochondrial sequestration of Ca^{2+} while simultaneously sustaining mitochondrial respiration [2, 25, 44]. Further, we serendipitously observed years earlier that estrogens increased ATP generation in healthy hippocampal neurons and sustained ATP generation in hippocampal neurons following exposure to $A\beta_{1-42}$ [45]. These findings coupled with our increasing awareness that signaling pathways induced by estrogens converge upon the mitochondria [25, 27, 30, 44], led us to directly investigate mitochondria as a pivotal convergence point of estrogenic action in neurons.

As a starting point, we conducted a proteomic analysis of brain mitochondria from female rats treated with E_2. Results of our proteomic analyses indicated that of the 499 detected proteins, 66 proteins exhibited a two-fold or greater change in expression [46]. Of these, 28 proteins were increased in expression following E_2 treatment whereas 38 proteins decreased relative to control. E_2 regulated protein expression and activity of key metabolic enzymes including pyruvate dehydrogenase, aconitase, and ATP-synthase [46]. Overall, E_2 induced marked changes in proteins involved in cellular energetics, free radical maintenance, metabolism, stress response, and cell survival.

In cellular energetics, E_2 induced two-fold increases in key enzymes required for glycolysis. Illustrative of this, E_2 increased expression of multiple subunits of the pyruvate dehydrogenase (PDH) enzyme complex. Pyruvate dehydrogenase is a key regulatory enzyme complex linking glycolytic metabolism to the citric acid cycle by transforming pyruvate into acetyl-CoA. Consistent with increased glycolysis, E_2 increased activity of key cytosolic glycolytic enzymes hexokinase, phosphofructokinase, and phosphoglycerate kinase in rodent brain [29]. In brain, PDH is further responsible for directing acetyl-CoA to either the tricarboxylic acid cycle (TCA, aka citric acid cycle) or to acetylcholine synthesis [47]. The mitoproteome profile induced by E_2 is reflective of enhanced glycolytic activity coupled with increased glutamatergic turnover (increased glutamate dehydrogenase and glutamate oxaloacetate transaminase-2) [46]. Together, these findings indicate that E_2 promotes enhanced utilization of glucose, the main energy source for the brain.

E_2 further increased expression and activity of proteins required for oxidative phosphorylation electron transfer, a result that was consistent with a coordinated response that optimizes glucose metabolism in brain [46]. E_2 induced significant increases in both protein expression and activity of Complex IV subunits I-IV [46], a finding consistent with previous reports [48, 49]. The E_2-induced increase is particularly relevant given that reduction in Complex IV is an early marker of AD [50]. E_2 also increased expression of ATP-synthase F1α and β [46], which is consistent with increased proteins required for mitochondrial respiration and with our previous report of increased ATP levels in primary neuronal cultures treated with CEE or with E_2 [45]. Alzheimer's pathology is accompanied by a decrease in mitochondrial respiration, in part due to a decrease in expression and activity of cytochrome C oxidase and pyruvate dehydrogenase [51, 52].

E_2 induced enhancement of energetic efficiency was paralleled by an increase in free radical defense systems. Increased expression of peroxiredoxin-V is consistent with the well documented antioxidant effects of estrogens, including increased glutaredoxin expression and manganese superoxide dismutase (MnSOD) [25, 46]. Free radical balance is maintained by reduction of the superoxide anion to hydrogen peroxidase by superoxide dismutase. The resulting hydrogen peroxide can then be removed by various peroxidases, including peroxiredoxin-V [53]. Reduction in reactive oxygen species contributes to neuroprotection and can reduce the overall stress response. In this context we identified significant alterations in the expression of two mitochondrial heat shock proteins, Hsp70 and Hsp60, which are important in the correct import of nascent proteins to the mitochondrial matrix. Many components of the mitochondrial bioenergetic network are vulnerable to oxidative stress, which can impair mitochondrial and cellular function as well as increasing apoptotic vulnerability [50, 54]. Damaged electron transport chain complexes compromise ATP synthesis and accelerate the generation of free radicals, which could cause or exacerbate neuronal degeneration [50, 54]. Estrogen-induced increase in antioxidants, reduction in free radicals, and substantially lower oxidative damage to mitochondrial DNA has been posited by Vina and colleagues to be a major contributor to the greater longevity of females relative to males [55–57].

Remarkably, E_2 regulation of mitochondrial function in neural tissue is closely paralleled in the vasculature [49, 58]. In vascular endothelium, chronic ET increased mitochondrial capacity for oxidative phosphorylation while simultaneously decreasing production of reactive oxygen species. In contrast to the emerging data regarding ERβ regulation of neural mitochondrial function, E_2 regulation of mitochondrial function in cerebral blood vessels is mediated by ERα [59]. Estrogenic regulation of mitochondrial function in both neural and vascular tissue has functional importance for coordinated responses between neural activity and vascular integrity on the one hand and sustaining neural viability on the other.

E_2 regulation of both mitochondrial and nuclear encoded gene products requires coordinated control of mitochondrial and nuclear encoded gene transcription [46, 49]. Neuronal estrogen receptors have been detected in mitochondria [49, 60–63]. In addition to classical ERs, membrane sites of estrogenic action (mER), which activate the PI3K/PKC/Src/MEK/ERK signaling pathway, activating CREB, have been identified as required for E_2 inducible neuroprotection [30, 64–66]. The simultaneous labeling of membrane, mitochondrial, and nuclear ERs within the same neuron and/or glial cell remains a challenge. While the mechanisms whereby ERs coordinate the complex signaling pathway between the three main compartments, membrane, mitochondria, and nucleus, remain to be determined [67], it is striking that ERs are perfectly positioned to coordinate events at the membrane with events in the mitochondria and nucleus [60, 61, 63, 68, 69].

Hypometabolism precedes the cognitive decline of Alzheimer's disease

Are these findings of E_2 regulation of mitochondrial function and enhancement of aerobic glycolysis relevant to AD risk? The role of mitochondria in health and disease has long been recognized [50, 70] and the evidence for mitochondrial dysfunction as a key precipitating factor in age-associated neurodegenerative diseases such as Alzheimer's and Parkinson's continues to mount [50, 52, 70–73]. The association between mitochondrial dysfunction and neurodegenerative diseases such as Alzheimer's and Parkinson's is mounting along with evidence that hypometabolism are antecedents to the cognitive deficits of Alzheimer's [43, 74–77]. There is now evidence from multiple levels of analysis and multiple experimental paradigms that range from genomic analyses in animal models and postmortem autopsy human brain to in vitro cell model systems to brain imaging in humans, that dysfunction in glucose metabolism, bioenergetics, and mitochondrial function are consistent antecedents to the development of Alzheimer pathology [43, 52, 77–82]. The decline in brain glucose metabolism and mitochondrial function can appear decades prior to diagnosis and thus may serve as a biomarker of AD risk as well as a therapeutic target.

The decrease in glucose metabolism in incipient and full-stage AD is associated with a generalized shift towards use of an alternative fuel, away from glycolytic energy production to use of peripherally derived ketone bodies and free fatty acids [79, 80, 82–85]. This shift towards an alternative fuel underlies the strategy of supplying the ketone body precursor Ketasyn™ (AC-1202) developed by Accera Biopharmaceuticals. Ketasyn™ (AC-1202) is converted by the liver into ketone bodies, which are then transported to the brain as an alternative fuel source. A Phase II clinical trial in

Alzheimer's patients and in individuals suffering from age-associated memory impairment has been completed and both groups showed improvement in memory function using the ketone body alternative fuel source (www.accerapharma.com). Under metabolically challenging conditions (i.e., starvation, aging, and neurodegeneration) neurons can utilize acetyl-CoA generated from ketone body metabolism (ketolysis), produced by the liver or under conditions of starvation in neighboring glial cells [86]. This latter pathway is much less efficient and can inhibit residual glycolysis via the Randle cycle [87]. This is evidenced by an observed 45% reduction in cerebral glucose utilization in AD patients [88], which is paralleled by decrease in the expression of glycolytic enzymes that are coupled to a decrease in the activity of the pyruvate dehydrogenase complex [89]. Further, while there is a 100:0 ratio of glucose to other substrates utilized in young controls, there is a 2:1 ratio in incipient AD patients compared to a ratio of 29:1 in healthy elderly controls [90].

Overall, E_2 promotes the energetic capacity of brain mitochondria by maximizing aerobic glycolysis (oxidative phosphorylation coupled to pyruvate metabolism). The enhanced aerobic glycolysis in the aging brain would be predicted to prevent conversion of the brain to using alternative sources of fuel such as the ketone body pathway characteristic of AD.

Remaining challenges and future directions

Major challenges for optimal ET and HT remain. Beyond the timing issue, the real and perceived risks of HT remain and were amplified by results of both the WHI and WHIMS trials. It is clear that many, *but not all*, women could potentially benefit from ET or HT intervention. Biomarkers to identify women appropriate for, and which type of, hormone regimen remain largely undeveloped beyond the hot flash. Hormone therapy interventions that selectively target the benefits of estrogen while avoiding untoward risk factors remain an unmet need in women's health. Estrogenic alternatives that activate estrogenic mechanisms in the brain but not in the breast or uterus, such as NeuroSERMs and PhytoSERMs, are promising strategies for sustaining the benefits of estrogen in the brain to prevent age-associated neurodegenerative disease.

Investigating mechanisms of estrogen action in parallel to identifying events antecedent to the development of Alzheimer's pathology that have mechanistic plausibility provides insights into the basis for disparities between basic science discovery and clinical outcomes. More generally, results of these investigations raise questions regarding applying preventive strategies to treatment modalities in the clinical realm and the reliance of healthy model systems that are abruptly exposed to neurodegenerative insults that typically develop incrementally, slowly, and accumulate over time in the preclinical discovery realm. This is particularly true for age-associated neurodegenerative diseases in which the normal aging brain undergoes dramatic changes that are either unrelated to or are the earliest signs of neurodegenerative vulnerability [78, 79, 81, 82, 91]. Efforts to bridge these gaps in women's cognitive health are emerging and hold the promise to serve as a model for mechanistic and translational neuroscience research at the bench and the bedside [92] (www.nia.nih.gov/ResearchInformation/ExtramuralPrograms/NeuroscienceOfAging/NNA_Conferences/BenchtoBedside.htm).

Acknowledgments

The many contributions of the Brinton laboratory estrogen and mitochondria research team, especially Dr. Jon Nilsen, Dr. Ronald Irwin, Dr. Shuhua Chen, Dr. Ryan Hamilton, Dr. Liqin Zhao, and Jia Yao are gratefully acknowledged. I also thank Dr. Enrique Cadenas for his critique of this manuscript and helpful discussions. This study was supported by grants from the National Institute of Mental Health (1R01 MH67159), National Institute on Aging (P01 AG026572), and the Kenneth T. and Eileen L. Norris Foundation to RDB.

References

1. Brinton RD. Investigative models for determining hormone therapy-induced outcomes in brain: evidence in support of a healthy cell bias of estrogen action. *Ann N Y Acad Sci.* 2005; **1052**:57–74.

2. Morrison JH, Brinton RD, Schmidt PJ, Gore AC. Estrogen, menopause, and the aging brain: how basic neuroscience can inform hormone therapy in women. *J Neurosci.* 2006; **26**(41):10332–48.

3. Wise PM. Estrogen therapy: does it help or hurt the adult and aging brain? Insights derived from animal models. *Neuroscience.* 2006;**138**(3):831–5.

4. Singh M, Sumien N, Kyser C, Simpkins JW. Estrogens and progesterone as neuroprotectants: what animal models teach us. *Front Biosci.* 2008;13:1083–9.

5. Nilsen J, Brinton RD. Impact of progestins on estrogen-induced neuroprotection: synergy by progesterone and 19-norprogesterone and antagonism by medroxyprogesterone acetate. *Endocrinology.* 2002;143(1):205–12.

6. Zandi PP, Carlson MC, Plassman BL, *et al.* Hormone replacement therapy and incidence of Alzheimer disease in older women: the Cache County study. *JAMA.* 2002;288(17):2123–9.

7. Resnick SM, Henderson VW. Hormone therapy and risk of Alzheimer disease: a critical time. *JAMA.* 2002;288(17):2170–2.

8. Yaffe K. Hormone therapy and the brain: deja vu all over again? *JAMA.* 2003;289(20):2717–19.

9. Sohrabji F. Estrogen: a neuroprotective or proinflammatory hormone? Emerging evidence from reproductive aging models. *Ann N Y Acad Sci.* 2005;1052:75–90.

10. Chen S, Nilsen J, Brinton RD. Dose and temporal pattern of estrogen exposure determines neuroprotective outcome in hippocampal neurons: therapeutic implications. *Endocrinology.* 2006;147 (11):5303–13.

11. Sherwin BB, Henry JF. Brain aging modulates the neuroprotective effects of estrogen on selective aspects of cognition in women: a critical review. *Front Neuroendocrinol.* 2008;29(1):88–113.

12. Shumaker SA, Legault C, Kuller L, *et al.* Conjugated equine estrogens and incidence of probable dementia and mild cognitive impairment in postmenopausal women: the Women's Health Initiative Memory Study. *JAMA.* 2004;291(24):2947–58.

13. Shumaker SA, Legault C, Rapp SR, *et al.* Estrogen plus progestin and the incidence of dementia and mild cognitive impairment in postmenopausal women: the Women's Health Initiative Memory Study: a randomized controlled trial. *JAMA.* 2003;289 (20):2651–62.

14. Sherwin BB. Estrogen and cognitive functioning in women. *Endocr Rev.* 2003;24(2):133–51.

15. Yaffe K, Sawaya G, Lieberburg I, Grady D. Estrogen therapy in postmenopausal women: effects on cognitive function and dementia. *JAMA.* 1998;279 (9):688–95.

16. Petitti DB, Crooks VC, Chiu V, Buckwalter JG, Chui HC. Incidence of dementia in long-term hormone users. *Am J Epidemiol.* 2008;167(6):692–700.

17. Fillit H, Weinreb H, Cholst I, *et al.* Observations in a preliminary open trial of estradiol therapy for senile dementia-Alzheimer's type. *Psychoneuroendocrinology.* 1986;11(3):337–45.

18. Mulnard RA, Cotman CW, Kawas C, *et al.* Estrogen replacement therapy for treatment of mild to moderate Alzheimer disease: a randomized controlled trial. Alzheimer's Disease Cooperative Study. *JAMA.* 2000;283(8):1007–15.

19. Henderson VW, Paganini-Hill A, Miller BL, *et al.* Estrogen for Alzheimer's disease in women: randomized, double-blind, placebo-controlled trial. *Neurology.* 2000;54(2):295–301.

20. Henderson VW, Hogan PE, Rapp SR, *et al.* Prior use of hormone therapy and incident Alzheimer's disease in the Women's Health Initiative Memory Study. *Neurology.* 2007;68(suppl.1):A205.

21. Shi J, Simpkins JW. 17 beta-estradiol modulation of glucose transporter 1 expression in blood-brain barrier. *Am J Physiol.* 1997;272(6 Pt 1):E1016–22.

22. Cheng CM, Cohen M, Wang J, Bondy CA. Estrogen augments glucose transporter and IGF1 expression in primate cerebral cortex. *FASEB J.* 2001;15(6):907–15.

23. Bishop J, Simpkins JW. Estradiol enhances brain glucose uptake in ovariectomized rats. *Brain Res Bull.* 1995;36(3):315–20.

24. Nilsen J, Brinton RD. Mechanism of estrogen-mediated neuroprotection: regulation of mitochondrial calcium and Bcl-2 expression. *Proc Natl Acad Sci USA.* 2003; 100(5):2842–7.

25. Nilsen J, Brinton RD. Mitochondria as therapeutic targets of estrogen action in the central nervous system. *Curr Drug Targets CNS Neurol Disord.* 2004; 3(4):297–313.

26. Simpkins JW, Wang J, Wang X, *et al.* Mitochondria play a central role in estrogen-induced neuroprotection. *Curr Drug Targets CNS Neurol Disord.* 2005;4(1):69–83.

27. Nilsen J, Chen S, Irwin RW, Iwamoto S, Brinton RD. Estrogen protects neuronal cells from amyloid beta-induced apoptosis via regulation of mitochondrial proteins and function. *BMC Neurosci.* 2006;7:74.

28. Simpkins JW, Dykens JA. Mitochondrial mechanisms of estrogen neuroprotection. *Brain Res Rev.* 2008; 57(2):421–30.

29. Kostanyan A, Nazaryan K. Rat brain glycolysis regulation by estradiol-17 beta. *Biochim Biophys Acta.* 1992;1133(3):301–6.

30. Mannella P, Brinton RD. Estrogen receptor protein interaction with phosphatidylinositol 3-kinase leads to activation of phosphorylated Akt and extracellular signal-regulated kinase 1/2 in the same population of cortical neurons: a unified mechanism of estrogen action. *J Neurosci.* 2006;26(37):9439–47.

31. Gottlob K, Majewski N, Kennedy S, *et al.* Inhibition of early apoptotic events by Akt/PKB is dependent on the first committed step of glycolysis and mitochondrial hexokinase. *Genes Dev.* 2001;**15**(11):1406–18.

32. Miyamoto S, Murphy AN, Brown JH. Akt mediates mitochondrial protection in cardiomyocytes through phosphorylation of mitochondrial hexokinase-II. *Cell Death Differ.* 2008;**15**(3): 521–9.

33. Singh M. Ovarian hormones elicit phosphorylation of Akt and extracellular-signal regulated kinase in explants of the cerebral cortex. *Endocrine Journal-UK.* 2001;**14**(3):407–15.

34. Znamensky V, Akama KT, McEwen BS, Milner TA. Estrogen levels regulate the subcellular distribution of phosphorylated Akt in hippocampal CA1 dendrites. *J Neurosci.* 2003;**23**(6):2340–7.

35. Mendez P, Wandosell F, Garcia-Segura LM. Cross-talk between estrogen receptors and insulin-like growth factor-I receptor in the brain: cellular and molecular mechanisms. *Front Neuroendocrinol.* 2006;**27**(4):391–403.

36. Mendez P, Garcia-Segura LM. Phosphatidylinositol 3-kinase and glycogen synthase kinase 3 regulate estrogen receptor-mediated transcription in neuronal cells. *Endocrinology.* 2006;**147**(6):3027–39.

37. Cardona-Gomez GP, Mendez P, DonCarlos LL, Azcoitia I, Garcia-Segura LM. Interactions of estrogen and insulin-like growth factor-I in the brain: molecular mechanisms and functional implications. *J Steroid Biochem Mol Biol.* 2002;**83**(1/5):211–17.

38. Garcia-Segura LM, Cardona-Gomez GP, Chowen JA, Azcoitia I. Insulin-like growth factor-I receptors and estrogen receptors interact in the promotion of neuronal survival and neuroprotection. *J Neurocytol.* 2000;**29**(5/6):425–37.

39. Mendez P, Azcoitia I, Garcia-Segura LM. Estrogen receptor alpha forms estrogen-dependent multimolecular complexes with insulin-like growth factor receptor and phosphatidylinositol 3-kinase in the adult rat brain. *Brain Res Mol Brain Res.* 2003; **112**(1/2):170–6.

40. Carro E, Trejo JL, Gomez-Isla T, LeRoith D, Torres-Aleman I. Serum insulin-like growth factor I regulates brain amyloid-beta levels. *Nat Med.* 2002;**8**(12):1390–7.

41. Maki PM, Resnick SM. Longitudinal effects of estrogen replacement therapy on PET cerebral blood flow and cognition. *Neurobiol Aging.* 2000;**21**(2):373–83.

42. Rasgon NL, Silverman D, Siddarth P, *et al.* Estrogen use and brain metabolic change in postmenopausal women. *Neurobiol Aging.* 2005;**26**(2):229–35.

43. Liang WS, Reiman EM, Valla J, *et al.* Alzheimer's disease is associated with reduced expression of energy metabolism genes in posterior cingulate neurons. *Proc Natl Acad Sci USA.* 2008;**105**(11):4441–6.

44. Nilsen J, Brinton RD. Mechanism of estrogen-mediated neuroprotection: regulation of mitochondrial calcium and Bcl-2 expression. *Proc Natl Acad Sci USA.* 2003;**100**(5):2842–7.

45. Brinton RD, Chen S, Montoya M, *et al.* The Women's Health Initiative estrogen replacement therapy is neurotrophic and neuroprotective. *Neurobiol Aging.* 2000;**21**(3):475–96.

46. Nilsen J, Irwin RW, Gallaher TK, Brinton RD. Estradiol in vivo regulation of brain mitochondrial proteome. *J Neurosci.* 2007;**27**(51):14069–77.

47. Holmquist L, Stuchbury G, Berbaum K, *et al.* Lipoic acid as a novel treatment for Alzheimer's disease and related dementias. *Pharmacol Ther.* 2007;**113** (1):154–64.

48. Bettini E, Maggi A. Estrogen induction of cytochrome c oxidase subunit III in rat hippocampus. *J Neurochem.* 1992;**58**(5):1923–9.

49. Stirone C, Duckles SP, Krause DN, Procaccio V. Estrogen increases mitochondrial efficiency and reduces oxidative stress in cerebral blood vessels. *Mol Pharmacol.* 2005;**68**(4):959–65.

50. Lin M, Beal M. Mitochondrial dysfunction and oxidative stress in neurodegenerative diseases. *Nature.* 2006;**443**(7113):787–95.

51. Bubber P, Haroutunian V, Fisch G, Blass JP, Gibson GE. Mitochondrial abnormalities in Alzheimer brain: mechanistic implications. *Ann Neurol.* 2005;**57**(5): 695–703.

52. Moreira PI, Santos MS, Seica R, Oliveira CR. Brain mitochondrial dysfunction as a link between Alzheimer's disease and diabetes. *J Neurol Sci.* 2007;**257**(1–2):206–14.

53. Cadenas E. Mitochondrial free radical production and cell signaling. *Mol Aspects Med.* 2004;**25**(1/2):17–26.

54. Yao J, Petanceska SS, Montine TJ, *et al.* Aging, gender and APOE isotype modulate metabolism of Alzheimer's A-beta peptides and F-isoprostanes in the absence of detectable amyloid deposits. *J Neurochem.* 2004;**90**(4):1011–18.

55. Borras C, Gambini J, Vina J. Mitochondrial oxidant generation is involved in determining why females live longer than males. *Front Biosci.* 2007;**12**:1008–13.

56. Vina J, Borras C, Gambini J, Sastre J, Pallardo FV. Why do females live longer than males? Importance of the upregulation of longevity-associated genes by oestrogenic compounds. *FEBS Lett.* 2005;**579** (12):2541–5.

57. Vina J, Sastre J, Pallardo FV, Gambini J, Borras C. Role of mitochondrial oxidative stress to explain the

different longevity between genders: protective effect of estrogens. *Free Radic Res.* 2006;**40**(12):1359–65.

58. Duckles SP, Krause DN, Stirone C, Procaccio V. Estrogen and mitochondria: a new paradigm for vascular protection? *Mol Interv.* 2006;**6**(1):26–35.

59. Razmara A, Sunday L, Stirone C, et al. Mitochondrial effects of estrogen are mediated by ERα in brain endothelial cells. *J Pharmacol Exp Ther.* 2008;**325**(3):782–90.

60. Yang SH, Liu R, Perez EJ, et al. Mitochondrial localization of estrogen receptor beta. *Proc Natl Acad Sci USA.* 2004;**101**(12):4130–5.

61. Milner TA, Ayoola K, Drake CT, et al. Ultrastructural localization of estrogen receptor beta immunoreactivity in the rat hippocampal formation. *J Comp Neurol.* 2005;**491**(2):81–95.

62. Yager JD, Chen JQ. Mitochondrial estrogen receptors – new insights into specific functions. *Trends Endocrinol Metab.* 2007;**18**(3):89–91.

63. McEwen B, Akama K, Alves S, et al. Tracking the estrogen receptor in neurons: implications for estrogen-induced synapse formation. *Proc Natl Acad Sci USA.* 2001;**98**(13):7093–100.

64. Levin ER. Cell localization, physiology, and nongenomic actions of estrogen receptors. *J Appl Physiol.* 2001;**91**(4):1860–7.

65. Wu TW, Brinton RD. Estrogen membrane receptor imaging coupled with estradiol activation of intracellular calcium rise and ERK activation in single neurons. *Society for Neuroscience Abstracts*; 2004.

66. Zhao L, Chen S, Ming Wang J, Brinton RD. 17beta-estradiol induces Ca^{2+} influx, dendritic and nuclear Ca^{2+} rise and subsequent cyclic AMP response element-binding protein activation in hippocampal neurons: a potential initiation mechanism for estrogen neurotrophism. *Neuroscience.* 2005;**132**(2):299–311.

67. Wagner BK, Kitami T, Gilbert TJ, et al. Large-scale chemical dissection of mitochondrial function. *Nat Biotechnol.* 2008;**26**(3):343–51.

68. Milner TA, Lubbers LS, Alves SE, McEwen BS. Nuclear and extranuclear estrogen binding sites in the rat forebrain and autonomic medullary areas. *Endocrinology.* 2008;**149**(7):3306–12.

69. Milner TA, McEwen BS, Hayashi S, et al. Ultrastructural evidence that hippocampal alpha estrogen receptors are located at extranuclear sites. *J Comp Neurol.* 2001;**429**(3):355–71.

70. Wallace DC. A mitochondrial paradigm of metabolic and degenerative diseases, aging, and cancer: a dawn for evolutionary medicine. *Annu Rev Genet.* 2005;**39**:359–407.

71. Murphy AN, Fiskum G, Beal MF. Mitochondria in neurodegeneration: bioenergetic function in cell life and death. *J Cereb Blood Flow Metab.* 1999;**19**(3):231–45.

72. Mattson MP. Pathways towards and away from Alzheimer's disease. *Nature.* 2004;**430**(7000):631–9.

73. Melov S. Modeling mitochondrial function in aging neurons. *Trends Neurosci.* 2004;**27**(10):601–6.

74. Martins IJ, Hone E, Foster JK, et al. Apolipoprotein E, cholesterol metabolism, diabetes, and the convergence of risk factors for Alzheimer's disease and cardiovascular disease. *Mol Psychiatry.* 2006;**11**(8):721–36.

75. Mosconi L, Sorbi S, de Leon MJ, et al. Hypometabolism exceeds atrophy in presymptomatic early-onset familial Alzheimer's disease. *J Nucl Med.* 2006;**47**(11):1778–86.

76. Reiman EM, Chen K, Caselli RJ, et al. Cholesterol-related genetic risk scores are associated with hypometabolism in Alzheimer's-affected brain regions. *Neuroimage.* 2008;**40**(3):1214–21.

77. Mosconi L, Tsui WH, Herholz K, et al. Multicenter standardized 18F-FDG PET diagnosis of mild cognitive impairment, Alzheimer's disease, and other dementias. *J Nucl Med.* 2008;**49**(3):390–8.

78. Blalock EM, Chen KC, Sharrow K et al. Gene microarrays in hippocampal aging: statistical profiling identifies novel processes correlated with cognitive impairment. *J Neurosci.* 2003;**23**(9):3807–19.

79. Blalock EM, Geddes JW, Chen KC, et al. Incipient Alzheimer's disease: microarray correlation analyses reveal major transcriptional and tumor suppressor responses. *Proc Natl Acad Sci USA.* 2004;**101**(7):2173–8.

80. Reiman EM, Chen K, Alexander GE, et al. Functional brain abnormalities in young adults at genetic risk for late-onset Alzheimer's dementia. *Proc Natl Acad Sci USA.* 2004;**101**(1):284–9.

81. Rowe WB, Blalock EM, Chen KC, et al. Hippocampal expression analyses reveal selective association of immediate-early, neuroenergetic, and myelinogenic pathways with cognitive impairment in aged rats. *J Neurosci.* 2007;**27**(12):3098–110.

82. Miller JA, Oldham MC, Geschwind DH. A systems level analysis of transcriptional changes in Alzheimer's disease and normal aging. *J Neurosci.* 2008;**28**(6):1410–20.

83. Alexander GE, Chen K, Pietrini P, Rapoport SI, Reiman EM. Longitudinal PET evaluation of cerebral metabolic decline in dementia: a potential outcome measure in Alzheimer's disease treatment studies. *Am J Psychiatry.* 2002;**159**(5):738–45.

84. Craft S. Insulin resistance and Alzheimer's disease pathogenesis: potential mechanisms and implications for treatment. *Curr Alzheimer Res.* 2007;**4**(2):147–52.

85. Ishii K, Kitagaki H, Kono M, Mori E. Decreased medial temporal oxygen metabolism in Alzheimer's disease shown by PET. *J Nucl Med.* 1996;**37**(7):1159–65.

86. Magistretti PJ, Pellerin L. Cellular bases of brain energy metabolism and their relevance to functional brain imaging: evidence for a prominent role of astrocytes. *Cereb Cortex.* 1996;**6**(1):50–61.

87. Randle PJ. Regulatory interactions between lipids and carbohydrates: the glucose fatty acid cycle after 35 years. *Diabetes Metab Rev.* 1998;**14**(4):263–83.

88. Ishii K, Minoshima S. PET is better than perfusion SPECT for early diagnosis of Alzheimer's disease. *Eur J Nucl Med Mol Imaging.* 2005;**32**(12):1463–5.

89. Blass J, Sheu R, Gibson G. Inherent abnormalities in energy metabolism in Alzheimer disease. Interaction with cerebrovascular compromise. *Ann N Y Acad Sci.* 2000;**903**:204–21.

90. Hoyer S, Nitsch R, Oesterreich K. Predominant abnormality in cerebral glucose utilization in late-onset dementia of the Alzheimer type: a cross-sectional comparison against advanced late-onset and incipient early-onset cases. *J Neural Transm Park Dis Dement Sect.* 1991;**3**(1):1–14.

91. Toescu EC, Verkhratsky A, Landfield PW. Ca^{2+} regulation and gene expression in normal brain aging. *Trends Neurosci.* 2004;**27**(10):614–20.

92. Asthana S, Brinton RD, Henderson VW, *et al.* Frontiers Proposal. National Institute on Aging. *Bench to Bedside: Estrogen as a Case Study.* AGE. 2009; in press.

7

Alternative estrogenic treatment regimens and the Kronos Early Estrogen Prevention Study – Cognitive and Affective substudy (KEEPS-CA)

Carey E. Gleason, Whitney Wharton, Cynthia M. Carlsson, and Sanjay Asthana

Editors' introduction

Few comparisons of the efficacy of different estrogenic formulations on brain function have been carried out. While most basic science studies have evaluated effects of estradiol, many of the clinical studies that have evaluated effects of hormone therapies (HT) in healthy older women have used conjugated equine estrogens (CEE). In this chapter, Gleason, Wharton, Carlsson, and Asthana review some of the cellular mechanisms by which estrogens are thought to protect the brain from age-related cognitive decline and Alzheimer's disease (AD), and discuss the pros and cons of oral vs. transdermal therapies and of estradiol vs. CEE. Their analysis identifies numerous advantages of transdermal estradiol vs. oral estrogenic therapies, primarily related to effects on liver enzymes, venus thromboembolic events, and inflammatory cytokines. Collectively, the analysis provides compelling arguments in favor of transdermal estradiol as the therapy of choice. Nevertheless, it is clear that the benefits of estradiol vs. CEE have yet to be proven, as has the efficacy of estrogenic therapies (ET) in the prevention of AD. These issues will be addressed in the recently initiated Kronos Early Estrogen Prevention Study (KEEPS) trial and the ancillary KEEPS study of cognitive aging. Details of the trial including its design and primary goals are discussed.

Introduction

Prior to the publication of the Women's Health Initiative Memory Study (WHIMS) findings [1–4], HT was thought to significantly reduce a woman's risk for dementia. This belief was based on a large body of basic science and generally supportive epidemiological evidence indicating that HT could lower the risk of Alzheimer's dementia (AD) by more than 50% (reviewed in Hogervorst *et al.* [5] and Fillit *et al.* [6].) The surprising findings from the WHIMS indicated an increased risk of dementia and cognitive decline with prolonged administration of CEE. Consequently, findings from cohort studies conducted prior to the WHIMS were attributed to inherent flaws in epidemiological research, such as a "healthy-user" bias. Still, support for potential beneficial effects of estrogens on cognition and risk for dementia continues to mount from observational (including WHIMS data [7]) and prospective cohort studies [8–10].

Recent evidence from two observational studies [11, 12] (182 and 99 women, respectively) examining effects of long-term estradiol forms of HT offered additional support for a protective effect of menopausal HT against AD. Investigators found that ET was able to protect women with a genetic risk factor for AD (APOE ε4 positive genotype) from hippocampal atrophy as measured by volumetric magnetic resonance imaging (MRI) [11, 12], and diminished hippocampal neuronal metabolism as detected with proton magnetic resonance spectroscopy (MRS) [12]. These promising findings offer the most direct link to date between menopausal HT and protection from early AD associated brain changes. Many in the scientific community agree that while the risk of dementia associated with CEE has been clarified for women over the age of 65, numerous questions remain including the question of whether other forms of HT may be useful for primary prevention of

---

dementia [13]. Further examination of the cognitive effects of other forms of HT such as estradiol based forms, and different modes of administration (i.e., transdermal vs. oral administration) are needed to inform future research in this area.

Previously, the most widely used HT formulations were the CEEs [14]. After the WHIMS, use of other formulations of HT increased. In this chapter, we discuss alternative HT regimens, after briefly summarizing evidence supporting the potential of estradiol forms of HT to favorably alter pathological processes underlying preclinical stages of AD. Lastly, we provide details of an on-going randomized, controlled clinical trial comparing the cognitive effects of CEE and estradiol HTs in menopausal women.

Neurobiological basis for estrogenic effects on Alzheimer's disease pathobiology

While estrogens' actions in the brain are varied and widespread, we present here selected mechanisms through which the estrogens could potentially alter risk for AD.

Estrogens improve cerebral blood flow

Iadecola [15] and others [16, 17] posit that cerebrovascular dysfunction and the ensuing chronic subtle hypoperfusion, combined with pathogenic processing of amyloid precursor protein (APP) play synergistic roles in the development of AD neuropathology. Whether cerebrovascular disease or pathological APP processing occurs first is unclear; however, the evidence suggests that onset of one may incite or accelerate the other (see Iadecola [15] for review). Moreover, both processes are believed to occur before neuropathological changes and clinical symptoms [18]. This suggests that interventions such as HT, that have the potential to maintain cerebrovascular health and improve cerebral perfusion prior to onset of neuropathology, hold strong promise as preventative agents [19].

The influence of estrogens on cerebral blood flow (CBF) can be attributed to multiple and well documented actions on cerebral vasculature. These effects are mediated through nuclear estrogen receptors (ER), namely ERα and ERβ [20], and non-genomic influences on signaling pathways induced through membrane receptors [21, 22] and alterations of membrane ion channels [23]. Thus, estrogens impart both rapid [21] and long-term [24] effects upon cerebral

vascular responsivity. Specific mechanisms through which estrogens increase resting dilation of cerebral blood vessels include enhanced vascular reactivity [25], possibly through improved endothelial function [26]. Both smooth muscle and the endothelial layer of cerebral vessels express ER [25]. Cerebral vascular dilation related to improved endothelial function appears to result from influences on vasoregulators, i.e., nitric oxide (NO) and prostanoids, such as prostacyclin (PGI_2) [21, 22]. The influence of PGI_2 upon vasculature appears to occur through increased endothelial nitric oxide synthase (eNOS) activity, possibly mediated by the enzyme cyclooxygenase-1 (COX-1) [27]. While endothelium vasodilatory responses are thought to largely account for the actions of estrogens on CBF, additional mechanisms have been proposed. Of particular relevance to AD-related processes, the effect of estrogens on NO production occurs in the hippocampus [28] and forebrain areas [29]. Moreover, increased vasodilation by way of effects on prostanoids appears to optimize vasodilatory responses via interactions with other vasoreactive substances [30] and changes in smooth muscle responses [31]. In addition to vascular reactivity and endothelial function, estrogens also favorably influence several processes important to cerebrovascular health, including improved mitochondrial energy metabolism [32], protection from by-products of mitochondrial metabolism (reactive oxygen species (ROS) and peroxides) [33], and reduced thromboembolic [34] and vascular inflammatory activity [35].

Effects of estrogens on Alzheimer's disease neuropathology

There is convincing evidence that estrogens exert neuromodulatory and neuroprotective effects directly relevant to AD neuropathology (for reviews see [36–38]). These include reducing inflammatory responses [39], especially to beta amyloid (Aβ) [40], improving cerebrospinal fluid (CSF) clearance of insoluble Aβ [41] while increasing amounts of non-toxic soluble Aβ [42], increasing synaptogenesis and dendritic spine density in the hippocampal CA1 neuronal field [43] and prefrontal cortex [44], and exerting antioxidant effects [45, 46].

A more comprehensive but still partial list of the neurobiological actions of estrogens is presented in Table 7.1. In summary, estrogens, particularly estradiol, exert a number of powerful neurobiological effects through which HT could favorably alter AD-related

Table 7.1 Neurobiological actions of estrogens.

Estrogens effect long-term potentiation (LTP) in the prefrontal cortex and hippocampus

- 17β estradiol deprivation disrupts synaptic plasticity associated with LTP. Replacement attenuates disruption [47]
- 17β estradiol induces expression of protein kinases and phosphatases involved in regulation of Ca^{2+} signaling [48]
- 17β estradiol up-regulates the functioning of NMDA receptor channels to activate the signaling path during LTP [49]
- Estradiol cypionate alters morphology of dendritic spines favoring expression of spines amenable to LTP-associated change [43–44]

Estrogens augment the function of multiple neurotransmitters systems

- CEE up-regulate 5-HT and catecholamines, implicated in modulation of cognition and mood in AD [50]
- Estrogens (17β estradiol, estradiol benzoate, CEE) facilitate the actions of cholinergic system (involved in attention, learning, memory, and arousal) especially in hippocampus and frontal cortices [51–54]
- 17β estradiol enhances cholinergic activity by increasing synthesis of ChAT mRNA (enzyme involved in synthesis of acetylcholine) [54]
- Estradiol benzoate deprivation reduces ChAT and trkA mRNA, and estradiol treatment reverses reduced enzymatic activity [55]
- Estradiol benzoate favorably modifies activities of both nicotinic and muscarinic cholinergic receptors [56]
- 17β estradiol upregulates neurotransmitter systems important for mood regulation: 5-HT [52], dopaminergic [57], and catecholaminergic [58]
- Complex and differential effects on multiple neurotransmitters; may be an interaction between 17β estradiol and transmitter systems [52]

Neuroprotective actions of estrogens

- 17β estradiol prevents glutamate-induced excitotoxicity [59]
- Estradiol attenuates inflammatory response in healthy tissues [39]
- 17β estradiol has both classic genomic and more rapid cell membrane-based mechanisms [60] expressed via ERα and ERβ [61]
- 17β estradiol activation of membrane receptor, ER-X, may impart neuroprotection via activation of MAPK/ERK pathways [62]
- Estradiol protects neurons from ischemic brain injury by facilitating the anti-apoptotic actions of Bcl proteins [63]
- CEE interact with the regulation of the apolipoproteins – in particular apolipoprotein E [64]
- 17β estradiol plays an antioxidant role with a number of cellular toxins, including β-amyloid (Aβ) [45]
- Estradiol and estrone protect cultured cells against damage induced by free radicals by inhibiting lipid peroxidation [46]
- 17β estradiol modifies the deleterious action of Aβ by increasing the soluble, non-toxic form of Aβ [42] and increasing clearance of toxic forms of Aβ [41]; decreasing the inflammatory reaction to Aβ [40]
- 17β estradiol has salutary effect on neurotrophins, including NGF and BDNF [65]
- 17β estradiol enhances synaptogenesis and dendritic spine density in the prefrontal cortex [66] and hippocampal CA1 field [67]
- Estrogens (17β estradiol, ethinyl estradiol, CEE) favorably effect homocysteine [68] and lipid metabolism [69]

disease processes and offer neuroprotection to women at risk for AD, particularly in the mesial temporal lobes and the prefrontal cortices.

Estradiol forms of hormone therapy may be preferable to CEE

Hormonal milieu pre- and postmenopause

Endogenous human estrogens comprise three main hormones, namely estradiol, estrone, and estriol, and their metabolites. In menstruating women, nearly 90% of circulating estradiol is produced during the follicular phase, while a small amount is derived from aromatization of testosterone and peripheral conversion of estrone. Estriol is a weak estrogen abundant during pregnancy and largely derived from estradiol and estrone metabolism in the placenta.

In the body, both estradiol and estrone primarily circulate in biologically inactive conjugated forms as sulfates and glucuronides. The free or "biologically active" forms of estrogens constitute around 2–3%

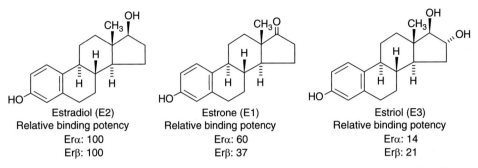

Fig. 7.1 Chemical structure and relative binding potencies for three estrogens (binding potencies from Kuiper *et al.* [71]).

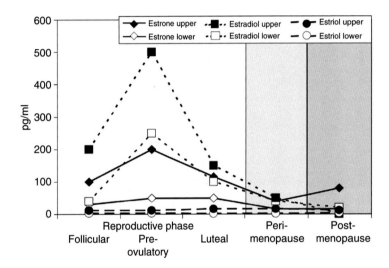

Fig. 7.2 Levels of endogenous estrogens: upper levels (solid markers) and lower levels (open markers) for three primary endogenous female hormones.

of the total body pool [70]. The chemical structure and biological potency of the three primary female hormones is depicted in Fig. 7.1.

During her reproductive life, a woman's hormonal profile follows a relatively predictable 28-day cycle. The menstrual cycle is characterized by a late follicular peak of estradiol levels; ovulatory spike of the pituitary hormones, luteinizing hormone (LH), and follicle stimulating hormone (FSH); and increasing levels of progesterone in the luteal phase. The rise in estrogens is induced by an increase in FSH at the follicular–luteal transition that is followed by a sharp decrease in FSH in the luteal phase. The drop off of FSH at the beginning of the luteal phase is associated with a sharp increase in estrogens [72].

Several authors have characterized the marked hormonal changes associated with menopause [70]. As a summary, Fig. 7.2 (adapted from Gruber *et al.* [70], Michaud *et al.* [73], Romani *et al.* [74], and Hankinson *et al.* [75]) depicts hormone levels associated with different phases of the menstrual cycle, as

well as the peri- and postmenopausal states. Estradiol is the predominant circulating hormone prior to menopause. At menopause, however, estradiol levels fall precipitously to approximately 10% of those in menstruating women, while estrone levels decline to a lesser extent [76]. Both estrone and estradiol are synthesized by peripheral conversion of adrenal androstenedione in adipose tissues and aromatization of testosterone [70], resulting in a shift in the ratio of estrone to estradiol to favor estrone in postmenopausal women. Thus, in postmenopausal women, the predominant estrogen in the body is estrone. Further, due to loss of feedback inhibition by low concentrations of estradiol and other gonadal hormones, the levels of pituitary gonadotropins increase.

Given the hormonal changes during the menstrual cycle and those occurring throughout the life-cycle, a woman's hormonal milieu is continually changing. Further, additional factors affect women's hormone profiles in a more immediate fashion. For example, estradiol is readily metabolized to estrone with some

Table 7.2 Comparison of CEE and transdermal estradiol.

	Conjugated equine estrogen	Transdermal 17β estradiol
Purity	Estrone plus at least ten other hormones; some non-human [78]	Pure 17β-estradiol
Thromboembolic events	Increased risk OR = 3.5 (1.8–6.8) [79]	Minimal or none OR = 0.9 (0.5–1.6) [79]
Hepatic 1st pass effect	Yes [80]	No [80]
Ratio of estrone to estradiol	5–7:1 [81]	1:1 [81]
Effect on binding glycoproteins (e.g., SHBG)	At least two-fold elevation [82]	No change [83]
Treatment of menopausal symptoms	Yes [84]	Yes [84]
Endothelial responsivity	No effect [85]	Beneficial [85]
β adrenoceptor reactivity	No effect [85]	Beneficial [85]
Lipid profile effects	Beneficial [86, 87]	Moderate to no effect [86, 87]
Triglycerides	No effect to harmful [87]	No effect [86, 87]
HDL	Likely beneficial [82]	No effect [86]
ER binding potency (reference is relative to 17β estradiol)	Estrone 1/3 binding potency to ERα and 2/3 to ERβ [71]	Strongest binding potency of estrogens [71]

reverse conversion, and numerous estrogenic metabolites are derived through oxidative and conjugative pathways, each exhibiting varying degrees of estrogenic properties in numerous tissues including the brain [77].

Advantages of estradiol forms over CEE

One major methodological issue related to the WHI and WHIMS is the form of HT employed in these studies. Both utilized conjugated equine estrogens (CEE), a form of HT rich in estrone and consisting of at least ten other hormones, some of which are non-human and whose neurobiology is essentially unknown [78]. At the time the WHI was initiated, CEE formulations were the most widely used forms of HT in the USA [14], and questions pertaining to cardiovascular and cognitive efficacy of CEE formulations were highly relevant. It is unclear, however, if other forms of HT have the same effects and risks as CEE therapies, especially estradiol formulations.

Among the key differences between HT preparations is the form of estrogens delivered (i.e., estrone-, estriol-, or estradiol-based HTs). There have been a number of studies comparing the route of delivery, or a combination of formulation and route of HT

administration (see below). Table 7.2 summarizes some of the findings comparing transdermal estradiol and CEE HTs. Likewise, a body of work exists from several decades ago, comparing pharmacokinetics of various forms of HT (e.g., Rauramo *et al.* [88]). However, there have been few direct comparisons of efficacy of different HT formulations, independent of route of administration (e.g., oral estradiol vs. oral estrone). Importantly, the majority of basic science evidence utilized estradiol formulations, and not CEE. For example, of the studies depicting the effect of HT on CBF presented on page 66 all used estradiol (either 17β-estradiol or estradiol benzoate), and of the findings from 59 intervention studies discussed on pages 66–7 and in Table 7.1, all but six (89.8%) used an estradiol form of HT (e.g., 17β-estradiol, estradiol benzoate, estradiol valerate, or estradiol cypionate).

In contrast to CEE, estradiol formulations are composed of 17β-estradiol and no non-human hormones. While there is bioconversion between estrone and estradiol, CEE formulations do not elevate estradiol levels to the extent seen with estradiol preparations [89]. The levels of circulating estradiol vs. estrone may be highly relevant to efficacy, as estradiol is the most potent estrogen receptor ligand, and the standard to which other ligands are compared.

For example, estrone's ER binding potency is approximately two-thirds the affinity of estradiol to the ERα, and about one-third the potency of estradiol for ERβ [71] (Fig. 7.1). Additionally, estrone and estradiol may have differential potencies for membrane mediated actions [90]. Thus, estradiol may be more efficacious than estrone formulations of HT.

If the purpose of HT is to control climacteric symptoms and prevent bone loss, the various forms of HT may be interchangeable [84]. However, if the goal of HT is to achieve a hormone state closer to that observed prior to menopause, in order to maintain neurobiological systems, administration of an estradiol HT would be preferable to CEE formulations. As noted, the predominant estrogen in premenopausal women is estradiol, the levels of which decline more than estrone levels after menopause. However, in contrast to basic science research, many clinical studies evaluating cognitive efficacy of HTs in healthy older women have utilized CEE, a preparation rich in estrone. Still, before researchers investigate the potential benefit of mimicking premenopausal hormone levels with HT, further studies are needed to ascertain whether the neurobiological systems are indeed significantly altered by the menopausal transition.

Advantages of transdermal vs. oral routes of hormone therapy administration

The route of administration is another critical factor likely to affect the results of any HT study. Oral and transdermal estrogenic preparations exhibit vastly different pharmacological profiles (reviewed by Modena et al. [91]). Oral estrogens are subject to extensive hepatic metabolism and result in estrone to estradiol ratios of approximately 5–7:1 [81]. In contrast, transdermal HT bypasses hepatic metabolism and results in a steady-state concentration of estradiol with 1:1 estrone to estradiol, closer to the ratio observed during selected phases of the menstrual cycle [81]. It is unknown whether these differences in hormone levels may result in differences in efficacy, but a recent rodent study revealed differential cognitive effects related to route of administration, such that transdermal estradiol was superior to oral preparations [92].

Transdermal HT, unlike oral preparations, does not increase binding glycoproteins, i.e., sex hormone binding globulin (SHBG) [83], resulting in higher plasma concentrations of free estradiol [93]. Additionally, oral administration of estrogens reportedly increases risk for venous thromboembolic complications by inducing pro-coagulant proteins during first-pass hepatic metabolism. For example, compared with transdermal HT, oral estrogens increase resistance to activated protein C [94], enhance fibrinolysis [95], decrease antithrombin activity by reducing tissue-type plasminogen (t-PA) concentration and plasminogen activator inhibitor (PAI-1) activity [95], and increase levels of C-reactive protein (CRP) [96]. Other advantages of transdermal estradiol over oral CEE forms of HT include greater reductions in blood pressure indices reflecting vascular sympathetic tone in healthy postmenopausal smokers, and improved beta-adrenoceptor responsivity [85]. One potential disadvantage of transdermal estradiol is relatively weaker effects on lipid profile compared to some oral forms of HT [82, 87].

Examining the effect of oral CEE vs. transdermal estradiol on hepatic and inflammatory proteins, a recent human study [80] noted that oral CEE administration resulted in hepatic portal vein levels of estrogens similar to those seen during the third trimester of pregnancy. As such, it is the mode of administration that would cause elevations in SHBG, thyroxine-binding globulin (TBG), and cortisol-binding globulin (CBG). The authors also found that oral CEE, unlike transdermal estradiol, elevated CRP, which corresponded to elevations in other inflammatory markers, interleukin 6 (IL-6) and serum amyloid A (SAA). Overall, these data confirmed findings from earlier investigations and suggested a pattern of coordinated hepatic and inflammatory responses with oral CEE not observed with transdermal estradiol. For this reason, the transdermal route has several major advantages over oral preparations and should be the preferred route of HT administration.

Micronized progesterone is preferable to medroxy-progesterone acetate

Clinical data indicate that using unopposed HT results in increased risk of endometrial cancer, but that risk returns to baseline with administration of a progestin [97]. Thus, non-hysterectomized women must receive progestin co-therapy. Of the numerous progestational agents, some synthetic progestins and their metabolites have been shown to have deleterious

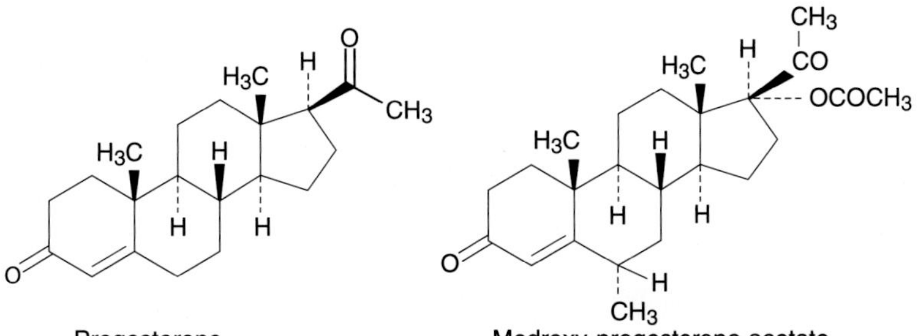

Fig. 7.3 Two common forms of progestin.

Progesterone

Medroxy-progesterone acetate

cognitive effects [98], either by exerting sedative [99] and mood effects [100], or possibly by causing faster rates of cognitive decline [101]. On the other hand, progesterone, the natural human progestin, may have important effects in the brain. Figure 7.3 details the structure of two commonly used progestinal agents. Progesterone is known to regulate synaptic density in the hippocampus, and appears to work in conjunction with estrogens across the reproductive cycle [102]. Initially, progesterone augments the effects of estradiol, but then results in a more rapid decrease in synaptic spines [103]. However, it is unknown whether synthetic forms of progestins such as medroxy-progesterone acetate (MPA) act in the same manner as the endogenous hormone. There is preliminary evidence from epidemiological studies that synthetic progestins, including MPA, can lead to decreased performance on measures of cognition [98], and a greater rate of cognitive decline [101]. Additionally, there is emerging evidence from basic science research that MPA attenuates the neuroprotective potential of estrogens and fails to protect against glutamate toxicity [104]. Greater detail on progesterone's effect on cognition in particular is provided in Chapter 11.

Prometrium® is an oral form of progesterone derived from wild yam, and is bio-identical to the progesterone produced by the human ovaries. In contrast to synthetic progestins, Prometrium® reportedly has not been shown to be associated with adverse effects related to heart disease, lipid metabolism, or thromboembolic diseases [105], and is available in a micronized formulation to increase bioavailability. While it is unknown if an exogenous progestational agent will act as the endogenous hormone, cyclic administration of a form simulating the endogenous human molecule is theoretically preferred because it more closely approximates the premenopausal hormone milieu compared to chronic dosing with MPA.

Summary of hormone therapy formulation and administration discussion

To date, no form of HT adequately simulates hormonal rhythms observed during the menstrual cycle. Unlike the cyclic hormonal changes in menstruating women, the majority of HTs are administered continuously. Additionally, plasma levels of estrone and estradiol achieved with different HTs vary dramatically with some resulting in greater elevations of estrone rather than estradiol, and with other HTs, estradiol levels far lower than those observed in menstruating women. For example, in one study higher levels of estradiol were achieved with both oral and transdermal preparations of estradiol compared to oral CEE [83]. In contrast, the greatest increases in estrone were associated with oral estradiol therapy, followed closely by CEE, and then by transdermal estradiol therapy. Figure 7.4 in part illustrates the variability in estradiol levels obtained with daily administration of either CEE or transdermal estradiol.

Kronos Early Estrogen Prevention Study – Cognitive and Affective substudy

As a follow-up to the WHI, a large, randomized controlled clinical trial, called the Kronos Early Estrogen Prevention Study (KEEPS), is evaluating the differential efficacy of CEE and transdermal estradiol on risk for heart disease in perimenopausal women following an extended therapy over four years (see Harman *et al.* [109] for a description of the study). The primary objective of KEEPS is to evaluate the differential efficacy of CEE (Premarin® 0.45 mg/day) and transdermal estradiol (Climara® 50 µg/day) versus placebo on state-of-the-art

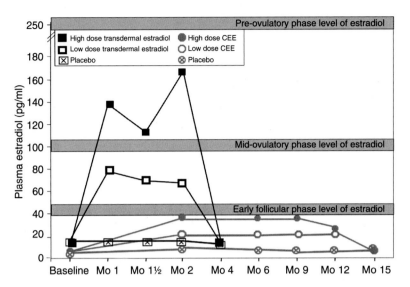

Fig. 7.4 Estradiol levels achieved with CEE and transdermal estradiol therapies. Data are adapted from three randomized, placebo-controlled clinical studies evaluating potential beneficial effects of estrogens on cognitive function of postmenopausal women with AD. In the first study [106], hysterectomized women were administered either 1.25 mg/day or 0.625 mg/day of unopposed CEE for 12 months. Findings of this study indicated that therapy with CEE was not associated with any significant improvement in cognitive function of women with AD. The second and third investigations used either 0.05 mg/day [107], or 0.1 mg/day [108] dose of transdermal estradiol for two months. Findings of both these studies indicated that short-term therapy with transdermal estradiol enhanced selective attention and verbal memory for older women with AD.

markers of progression of atherosclerosis and heart disease. Women randomized to active CEE or transdermal estradiol will receive a challenge with micronized progesterone (Prometrium® 200 mg) for the first 12 days of each month to counteract proliferative effects of estrogens on the endometrium. The secondary objectives include a systematic characterization of the effects of HT on measures of inflammation and blood hypercoagulability.

An ancillary study of KEEPS, funded by the National Institutes of Health's National Institute on Aging (NIH-NIA), called the KEEPS Cognitive and Affective substudy (KEEPS-CA) will evaluate the differential efficacy of transdermal estradiol and CEE on measures of mood and cognitive function in perimenopausal women. The collection of baseline cognitive data from over 700 women enrolled in the KEEPS-CA study was recently completed (May, 2008). The KEEPS-CA study is the first multi-site, randomized, placebo-controlled, double-blind, parallel-group design clinical study that will address major HT-related issues raised by the WHI and WHIMS. Specifically, the KEEPS-CA substudy will compare the differential efficacy of CEE and transdermal estradiol on a comprehensive battery of cognition and mood measures, sensitive to cognitive changes associated with HT in perimenopausal and recently-postmenopausal women. The hypothesis of the KEEPS-CA substudy is that, compared to CEE, treatment with transdermal estradiol will enhance cognitive function of healthy peri- and early menopausal women (i.e., decreased rate of cognitive decline or enhanced rate of cognitive

improvement compared to placebo-treated group). The battery of cognitive tests and mood inventories are administered at baseline and months 18, 36, and 48 during treatment (see Table 7.3). The evaluations at months 18 and 48 will characterize the effects of estrogenic therapy alone; thus testing will occur while subjects are not taking the progesterone challenge. The evaluation at month 36 will be timed to assess the effects of estrogens plus progesterone, and will be performed between days 6 and 12 of the progesterone challenge.

Ultimately, the KEEPS-CA substudy will build upon the knowledge gained by the WHIMS, addressing unresolved questions of pivotal clinical significance that need to be systematically evaluated in well designed human studies. The study will provide insight into: (1) whether there is cognitive benefit or harm associated with perimenopausal HT (as opposed to late postmenopausal HT investigated in the WHIMS); (2) whether there are differential cognitive effects of various estrogenic formulations (CEE vs. estradiol); (3) if there is a preferred route for administration of estrogens (oral vs. transdermal); (4) whether a cyclic micronized progestin is associated with cognitive benefit or harm; and (5) the most sensitive psychometric measures to characterize potential effects of estrogens on cognition and mood.

Given the adverse findings of the WHIMS in postmenopausal women and the fact that HT is still approved for the treatment of menopausal symptoms commonly experienced by younger perimenopausal women, it is critical that the potential cognitive effects

Table 7.3 Kronos Early Estrogen Prevention Study – Cognitive and Affective substudy (KEEPS-CA): battery of tests.

DOMAIN OR CONSTRUCT MEASURED	NEUROPSYCHOLOGICAL MEASURE	Included in WHIMS[†] or WHISCA[‡]
INTELLIGENCE: *Baseline only*	Primary Mental Abilities* – vocab [110, 111]	X
GLOBAL COGNITION:	Modified Mini-Mental State exam [112]	X
VERBAL AND VISUAL MEMORY:		
Verbal memory	California Verbal Learning Test-2* [113]	X
	NYU Paragraph Recall Test [114]	
	Prospective Memory Test [110, 111]	X
Visual memory	Benton Visual Retention Test [115]	X
LANGUAGE:		
	Controlled Oral Word Association Test FAS/Animals/Fruits/Vegetables [116]	X
ATTENTION AND EXECUTIVE FUNCTION:		
Divided attention	Trail Making Test Version A & B [116]	X
Selective attention	Stroop Test (Golden Version) [117]	X
Auditory working memory:	Letter-Number Sequencing WMS-3 [118]	X
	Digit Span WMS-3 [118]	X
Visual working memory:	Digit Symbol [119]	
COMPUTERIZED COGNITIVE TESTS:		
Visual spatial	3D Mental Rotation [120]	
Vigilance/divided attention	Visual Sensitivity Test [120]	
Selective attention	Stroop Test [120]	
MOOD:		
	Profile of Mood States [121]	
	Beck Depression Inventory [122]	
	Brief Patient Health Questionnaire [123]	
SUBJECTIVE MEMORY COMPLAINTS:	Memory Function Questionnaire [124]	

Note:
[†] Women's Health Initiative Memory Study [1–4]
[‡] Women's Health Initiative Study of Cognitive Aging [110, 125]
*Administration to match Resnick *et al.*'s WHISCA battery [110]

of HT, both beneficial and adverse, be identified in women undergoing menopausal transition. The KEEPS-CA substudy will be the first clinical study to characterize the differential effects of CEE and transdermal estradiol on cognitive function of perimenopausal women. Furthermore, as a substudy of KEEPS [109], the cognitive trial will have an unprecedented opportunity to evaluate the emerging, albeit controversial, relationship between changes in cognition induced by estrogens and markers of heart disease, atherosclerosis, lipid metabolism, and thromboembolic disease in perimenopausal women. Additionally, results of the present study will provide pivotal data and an exclusive opportunity for future studies to follow the KEEPS cohort over an extended period of 20–25 years to determine whether HT initiated during the perimenopausal period could delay or preferably prevent future development of neurodegenerative diseases such as mild cognitive impairment (MCI) and AD. Bhavnani [78] has argued that the WHI was not a true primary prevention study given the advanced age and prevalence of obesity among its participants, and the likelihood that many were beyond the opportunity to "prevent" disease. Long-term follow-up with KEEPS-CA study participants would help clarify this important question.

Summary

Until recently, there was emerging evidence that HT reduced the risk of AD by up to 50%. However, findings from the WHIMS revealed that CEE increased the risk of dementia. In order to increase the likelihood of detecting cognitive change, the WHIMS targeted older women (>65 years old), who may have been less likely to benefit from either the cognition-enhancing or neuroprotective actions of HT. To date, it is unknown if the findings of the WHIMS can be applied to a younger cohort of women. Moreover, there is a common misconception that all HTs are equally efficacious and equally harmful. In reality, the pharmacology and physiology of estrogens are complex, and it remains unknown if the findings from the WHIMS can be applied to other HT formulations and routes of administration. While there are reasons to postulate that various HTs are not bioequivalent, few studies investigating the cognitive effects of HT have incorporated factors such as formulation and route of administration of hormones into their design.

Despite the questions of generalizability of the WHIMS findings to other age groups and other HTs, postmenopausal women of all ages are discontinuing HT or opting not to initiate any form of HT due to concerns over serious adverse effects [126]. Thus, for the millions of perimenopausal women who could benefit from the relief of menopausal symptoms and who avoid all forms of HT based on a belief that they are associated with lasting deleterious effects, there is an urgent need to characterize both the beneficial and adverse effects of transdermal estradiol. The KEEPS-CA substudy will offer clarification by targeting intervention during the hypothesized "critical period" in a woman's reproductive history,

and comparing cognitive effects of two hormone formulations believed to exhibit differential efficacies.

References

1. Shumaker SA, et al. Estrogen plus progestin and the incidence of dementia and mild cognitive impairment in postmenopausal women: the Women's Health Initiative Memory Study: a randomized controlled trial. JAMA. 2003;**289**(20):2651–62.

2. Espeland MA, et al. Conjugated equine estrogens and global cognitive function in postmenopausal women: the Women's Health Initiative Memory Study. JAMA. 2004;**291**(24):2959–68.

3. Rapp SR, et al. Effect of estrogen plus progestin on global cognitive function in postmenopausal women: the Women's Health Initiative Memory Study: a randomized controlled trial. JAMA. 2003;**289**(20):2663–72.

4. Shumaker SA, et al. Conjugated equine estrogens and incidence of probable dementia and mild cognitive impairment in postmenopausal women: the Women's Health Initiative Memory Study. JAMA. 2004;**291**(24):2947–58.

5. Hogervorst E, et al. The nature of the effect of female gonadal hormone replacement therapy on cognitive function in post-menopausal women: a meta-analysis. Neuroscience. 2000;**101**(3):485–512.

6. Fillit HM. The role of hormone replacement therapy in the prevention of Alzheimer disease. Arch Intern Med. 2002;**162**(17):1934–42.

7. Henderson VW, et al. Prior use of hormone therapy and incident Alzheimer's disease in the Women's Health Initiative Memory Study. In American Academy of Neurology Annual Meeting. Boston, MA, 2007.

8. Gleason CE, et al. Hormone effects on fMRI and cognitive measures of encoding: importance of hormone preparation. Neurology. 2006;**67**(11):2039–41.

9. Yonker JE, et al. Verified hormone therapy improves episodic memory performance in healthy postmenopausal women. Neuropsychol Dev Cogn B Aging Neuropsychol Cogn. 2006;**13**(3/4):291–307.

10. Zandi PP, et al. Hormone replacement therapy and incidence of Alzheimer disease in older women: the Cache County study. JAMA. 2002;**288**(17):2123–9.

11. Hu L, et al. Evaluation of neuroprotective effects of long-term low dose hormone replacement therapy on postmenopausal women brain hippocampus using magnetic resonance scanner. Chin Med Sci J. 2006;**21**(4):214–18.

12. Yue Y, et al. Effects of long-term, low-dose sex hormone replacement therapy on hippocampus and

cognition of postmenopausal women of different apoE genotypes. *Acta Pharmacol Sin.* 2007;**28**(8):1129–35.

13. Manson JE, *et al.* Postmenopausal hormone therapy: new questions and the case for new clinical trials. *Menopause.* 2006;**13**(1):139–47.

14. Guay MP, *et al.* Changes in pattern of use, clinical characteristics and persistence rate of hormone replacement therapy among postmenopausal women after the WHI publication. *Pharmacoepidemiol Drug Saf.* 2007;**16**(1):17–27.

15. Iadecola C. Neurovascular regulation in the normal brain and in Alzheimer's disease. *Nat Rev Neurosci.* 2004;**5**(5):347–60.

16. de la Torre JC. Is Alzheimer's disease a neurodegenerative or a vascular disorder? Data, dogma, and dialectics. *Lancet Neurol.* 2004;**3**(3):184–90.

17. Nagata K, *et al.* Hemodynamic aspects of Alzheimer's disease. *Ann N Y Acad Sci.* 2002;**977**:391–402.

18. Iadecola C, *et al.* SOD1 rescues cerebral endothelial dysfunction in mice overexpressing amyloid precursor protein. *Nat Neurosci.* 1999;**2**(2):157–61.

19. Girouard H, Iadecola C. Neurovascular coupling in the normal brain and in hypertension, stroke, and Alzheimer disease. *J Appl Physiol.* 2006;**100**(1):328–35.

20. Zhao L, Brinton RD. Estrogen receptor alpha and beta differentially regulate intracellular $Ca^{(2+)}$ dynamics leading to ERK phosphorylation and estrogen neuroprotection in hippocampal neurons. *Brain Res.* 2007;**1172**:48–59.

21. Stirone C, *et al.* Estrogen receptor activation of phosphoinositide-3 kinase, akt, and nitric oxide signaling in cerebral blood vessels: rapid and long-term effects. *Mol Pharmacol.* 2005;**67**(1):105–13.

22. Chen DB, *et al.* Membrane estrogen receptor-dependent extracellular signal-regulated kinase pathway mediates acute activation of endothelial nitric oxide synthase by estrogen in uterine artery endothelial cells. *Endocrinology.* 2004;**145**(1):113–25.

23. Salom JB, *et al.* Relaxant effects of 17-beta-estradiol in cerebral arteries through $Ca^{(2+)}$ entry inhibition. *J Cereb Blood Flow Metab.* 2001;**21**(4):422–9.

24. Florian M, *et al.* Estrogen induced changes in Akt-dependent activation of endothelial nitric oxide synthase and vasodilation. *Steroids.* 2004;**69**(10):637–45.

25. Stirone C, Duckles SP, Krause DN. Multiple forms of estrogen receptor-alpha in cerebral blood vessels: regulation by estrogen. *Am J Physiol Endocrinol Metab.* 2003;**284**(1):E184–92.

26. Kublickiene K, *et al.* Small artery endothelial dysfunction in postmenopausal women: in vitro function, morphology, and modification by estrogen

and selective estrogen receptor modulators. *J Clin Endocrinol Metab.* 2005;**90**(11):6113–22.

27. Ospina JA, Duckles SP, Krause DN. 17beta-estradiol decreases vascular tone in cerebral arteries by shifting COX-dependent vasoconstriction to vasodilation. *Am J Physiol Heart Circ Physiol.* 2003;**285**(1):H241–50.

28. Grohe C, *et al.* 17 Beta-estradiol regulates nNOS and eNOS activity in the hippocampus. *Neuroreport.* 2004;**15**(1):89–93.

29. Pelligrino DA, *et al.* Cerebral vasodilating capacity during forebrain ischemia: effects of chronic estrogen depletion and repletion and the role of neuronal nitric oxide synthase. *Neuroreport.* 1998;**9**(14):3285–91.

30. Chrissobolis S, *et al.* Evidence that estrogen suppresses rho-kinase function in the cerebral circulation in vivo. *Stroke.* 2004;**35**(9):2200–5.

31. Zhang F, *et al.* 17 beta-estradiol attenuates voltage-dependent Ca^{2+} currents in A7r5 vascular smooth muscle cell line. *Am J Physiol.* 1994;**266**(4 Pt 1):C975–80.

32. Nilsen J, *et al.* Estrogen protects neuronal cells from amyloid beta-induced apoptosis via regulation of mitochondrial proteins and function. *BMC Neurosci.* 2006;**7**:74.

33. Stirone C, *et al.* Estrogen increases mitochondrial efficiency and reduces oxidative stress in cerebral blood vessels. *Mol Pharmacol.* 2005;**68**(4):959–65.

34. Ono H, *et al.* Cerebral thrombosis and microcirculation of the rat during the oestrous cycle and after ovariectomy. *Clin Exp Pharmacol Physiol.* 2002;**29**(1–2):73–8.

35. Sunday L, *et al.* Age alters cerebrovascular inflammation and effects of estrogen. *Am J Physiol Heart Circ Physiol.* 2007;**292**(5):H2333–40.

36. Sano M. Noncholinergic treatment options for Alzheimer's disease. *J Clin Psychiatry.* 2003;**64** (Suppl 9):23–8.

37. Brinton RD. Impact of estrogen therapy on Alzheimer's disease: a fork in the road? *CNS Drugs.* 2004;**18**(7):405–22.

38. McEwen B. Estrogen actions throughout the brain. *Recent Prog Horm Res.* 2002;**57**:357–84.

39. McAsey ME, *et al.* Time course of response to estradiol replacement in ovariectomized mice: brain apolipoprotein E and synaptophysin transiently increase and glial fibrillary acidic protein is suppressed. *Exp Neurol.* 2006;**197**(1):197–205.

40. Thomas T, *et al.* Estrogen and raloxifene activities on amyloid-beta-induced inflammatory reaction. *Microvasc Res.* 2001;**61**(1):28–39.

41. Li R, *et al.* Estrogen enhances uptake of amyloid beta-protein by microglia derived from the human cortex. *J Neurochem.* 2000;**75**(4):1447–54.

42. Greenfield JP, *et al.* Estrogen lowers Alzheimer beta-amyloid generation by stimulating trans-Golgi network vesicle biogenesis. *J Biol Chem.* 2002;**277**(14):12128–36.

43. Hao J, *et al.* Estrogen increases the number of spinophilin-immunoreactive spines in the hippocampus of young and aged female rhesus monkeys. *J Comp Neurol.* 2003;**465**(4):540–50.

44. Tang Y, *et al.* Estrogen replacement increases spinophilin-immunoreactive spine number in the prefrontal cortex of female rhesus monkeys. *Cereb Cortex.* 2004;**14**(2):215–23.

45. Prokai L, *et al.* Quinol-based cyclic antioxidant mechanism in estrogen neuroprotection. *Proc Natl Acad Sci USA.* 2003;**100**(20):11741–6.

46. Thibodeau PA, *et al.* In vitro pro- and antioxidant properties of estrogens. *J Steroid Biochem Mol Biol.* 2002;**81**(3):227–36.

47. Day M, Good M. Ovariectomy-induced disruption of long-term synaptic depression in the hippocampal CA1 region in vivo is attenuated with chronic estrogen replacement. *Neurobiol Learn Mem.* 2005;**83**(1):13–21.

48. Kim JS, *et al.* Enhancement of rat hippocampal long-term potentiation by 17 beta-estradiol involves mitogen-activated protein kinase-dependent and -independent components. *Neurosci Lett.* 2002;**332**(1):65–9.

49. El-Bakri NK, *et al.* Effects of estrogen and progesterone treatment on rat hippocampal NMDA receptors: relationship to Morris water maze performance. *J Cell Mol Med.* 2004;**8**(4):537–44.

50. Blum I, *et al.* The effect of estrogen replacement therapy on plasma serotonin and catecholamines of postmenopausal women. *Isr J Med Sci.* 1996;**32**(12):1158–62.

51. Tinkler GP, Voytko ML. Estrogen modulates cognitive and cholinergic processes in surgically menopausal monkeys. *Prog Neuropsychopharmacol Biol Psychiatry.* 2005;**29**(3):423–31.

52. Matsuda Y, Hirano H, Watanabe Y. Effects of estrogen on acetylcholine release in frontal cortex of female rats: involvement of serotonergic neuronal systems. *Brain Res.* 2002;**937**(1/2):58–65.

53. Daniel JM, Dohanich GP. Acetylcholine mediates the estrogen-induced increase in NMDA receptor binding in CA1 of the hippocampus and the associated improvement in working memory. *J Neurosci.* 2001;**21**(17):6949–56.

54. Gibbs RB. Basal forebrain cholinergic neurons are necessary for estrogen to enhance acquisition of a delayed matching-to-position T-maze task. *Horm Behav.* 2002;**42**(3):245–57.

55. Luine V, *et al.* Immunochemical demonstration of increased choline acetyltransferase concentration in rat preoptic area after estradiol administration. *Brain Research.* 1980;**191**:273–7.

56. Daniel JM, Hulst JL, Lee CD. Role of hippocampal M2 muscarinic receptors in the estrogen-induced enhancement of working memory. *Neuroscience.* 2005;**132**(1):57–64.

57. Sawada H, Shimohama S. Neuroprotective effects of estradiol in mesencephalic dopaminergic neurons. *Neurosci Biobehav Rev.* 2000;**24**(1):143–7.

58. Kim YJ, *et al.* Nongenomic inhibition of catecholamine secretion by 17beta-estradiol in PC12 cells. *J Neurochem.* 2000;**74**(6):2490–6.

59. Nilsen J, Brinton RD. Mechanism of estrogen-mediated neuroprotection: regulation of mitochondrial calcium and Bcl-2 expression. *Proc Natl Acad Sci USA.* 2003;**100**(5):2842–7.

60. Guerra B, *et al.* Plasma membrane oestrogen receptor mediates neuroprotection against beta-amyloid toxicity through activation of Raf-1/MEK/ERK cascade in septal-derived cholinergic SN56 cells. *J Neurochem.* 2004;**91**(1):99–109.

61. Zhao L, Wu TW, Brinton RD. Estrogen receptor subtypes alpha and beta contribute to neuroprotection and increased Bcl-2 expression in primary hippocampal neurons. *Brain Res.* 2004;**1010**(1/2):22–34.

62. Toran-Allerand CD. Estrogen and the brain: beyond ER-alpha and ER-beta. *Exp Gerontol.* 2004;**39**(11–12):1579–86.

63. Dubal DB, *et al.* Estradiol modulates bcl-2 in cerebral ischemia: a potential role for estrogen receptors. *J Neurosci.* 1999;**19**(15):6385–93.

64. Rozovsky I, *et al.* Equine estrogens induce apolipoprotein E and glial fibrillary acidic protein in mixed glial cultures. *Neurosci Lett.* 2002;**323**(3):191–4.

65. Jezierski MK, Sohrabji F. Estrogen enhances retrograde transport of brain-derived neurotrophic factor in the rodent forebrain. *Endocrinology.* 2003;**144**(11):5022–9.

66. Sakamoto H, *et al.* Dendritic growth and spine formation in response to estrogen in the developing Purkinje cell. *Endocrinology.* 2003;**144**(10):4466–77.

67. Rune GM, *et al.* Estrogen up-regulates estrogen receptor alpha and synaptophysin in slice cultures of rat hippocampus. *Neuroscience.* 2002;**113**(1):167–75.

68. Giltay EJ, *et al.* Oral and transdermal estrogens both lower plasma total homocysteine in male-to-female transsexuals. *Atherosclerosis.* 2003;**168**(1):139–46.

69. Cetinkaya MB, *et al.* Tibolone versus four estrogen replacement therapy protocols and plasma lipid levels in postmenopausal women. *Int J Gynaecol Obstet.* 2002;**79**(1):17–23.

70. Gruber C, *et al.* Production and actions of estrogens. *N Engl J Med.* 2002;**346**:340–52.

71. Kuiper GGJM, *et al.* Comparison of the ligand binding specificity and transcription tissue distribution of estrogen receptors alpha and beta. *Endocrinology.* 1997;**138**(3):863–70.

72. Miro F, *et al.* Relationship between follicle-stimulating hormone levels at the beginning of the human menstrual cycle, length of the follicular phase and excreted estrogens: the FREEDOM study. *J Clin Endocrinol Metab.* 2004;**89**(7):3270–5.

73. Michaud DS, *et al.* Reproducibility of plasma and urinary sex hormone levels in premenopausal women over a one-year period. *Cancer Epidemiol Biomarkers Prev.* 1999;**8**(12):1059–64.

74. Romani W, *et al.* The correlations between estradiol, estrone, estriol, progesterone, and sex hormone-binding globulin and anterior cruciate ligament stiffness in healthy, active females. *J Womens Health (Larchmt).* 2003;**12**(3):287–98.

75. Hankinson SE, *et al.* Plasma sex steroid hormone levels and risk of breast cancer in postmenopausal women. *J Natl Cancer Inst.* 1998;**90**(17):1292–9.

76. Rannevik G, *et al.* A longitudinal study of the perimenopausal transition: altered profiles of steroid and pituitary hormones, SHBG and bone mineral density. *Maturitas.* 1995;**21**(2):103–13.

77. Jellinck PH, Lee SJ, McEwen BS. Metabolism of dehydroepiandrosterone by rat hippocampal cells in culture: possible role of aromatization and 7-hydroxylation in neuroprotection. *J Steroid Biochem Mol Biol.* 2001;**78**(4):313–7.

78. Bhavnani BR. Estrogens and menopause: pharmacology of conjugated equine estrogens and their potential role in the prevention of neurodegenerative diseases such as Alzheimer's. *J Steroid Biochem Mol Biol.* 2003;**85**(2–5):473–82.

79. Scarabin P, *et al.* Differential association of oral and transdermal oestrogen replacement therapy with venous thromboembolism risk. *Lancet.* 2003; **362**:428–32.

80. Shifren JL, *et al.* A comparison of the short-term effects of oral conjugated equine estrogens versus transdermal estradiol on C-reactive protein, other serum markers of inflammation and other hepatic proteins in naturally menopausal women. *J Clin Endocrinol Metab.* 2008;**93**(5): 1702–10.

81. Coelingh Bennink HJ. Are all estrogens the same? *Maturitas.* 2004;**47**(4):269–75.

82. Koh KK, *et al.* Vascular effects of estrogen and cholesterol-lowering therapies in hypercholesterolemic postmenopausal women. *Circulation.* 1999;**99**(3): 354–60.

83. Nachtigall LE, *et al.* Serum estradiol-binding profiles in postmenopausal women undergoing three common estrogen replacement therapies: associations with sex hormone-binding globulin, estradiol, and estrone levels. *Menopause.* 2000; **7**(4):243–50.

84. Schindler AE. Climacteric symptoms and hormones. *Gynecol Endocrinol.* 2006;**22**(3):151–4.

85. Girdler SS, *et al.* Transdermal versus oral estrogen therapy in postmenopausal smokers: hemodynamic and endothelial effects. *Obstet Gynecol.* 2004; **103**(1):169–80.

86. Vigna GB, *et al.* Simvastatin, transdermal patch, and oral estrogen-progestogen preparation in early-postmenopausal hypercholesterolemic women: a randomized, placebo-controlled clinical trial. *Metabolism.* 2002;**51**(11):1463–70.

87. de Kraker AT, *et al.* The effects of 17 beta-oestradiol plus dydrogesterone compared with conjugated equine oestrogens plus medroxyprogesterone acetate on lipids, apolipoproteins and lipoprotein (a). *Maturitas.* 2004;**49**(3):253–63.

88. Rauramo L, Punnonen R, Gronroos M. Serum concentrations of oestrone, oestradiol and oestriol during various oestrogen treatments. *Maturitas.* 1981;**3**(2):183–6.

89. Gleason CE, *et al.* Clinical pharmacology and differential cognitive efficacy of estrogen preparations. *Ann N Y Acad Sci.* 2005;**1052**:93–115.

90. Deecher DC, *et al.* Characterization of a membrane-associated estrogen receptor in a rat hypothalamic cell line (D12). *Endocrine.* 2003;**22**(3):211–23.

91. Modena MG, *et al.* New evidence regarding hormone replacement therapies is urgently required transdermal postmenopausal hormone therapy differs from oral hormone therapy in risks and benefits. *Maturitas.* 2005;**52**(1):1–10.

92. Garza-Meilandt A, Cantu RE, Claiborne BJ. Estradiol's effects on learning and neuronal morphology vary with route of administration. *Behav Neurosci.* 2006; **120**(4):905–16.

93. Akwa Y, *et al.* Neurosteroid metabolism. 7 Alpha-hydroxylation of dehydroepiandrosterone and pregnenolone by rat brain microsomes. *Biochem J.* 1992;**288**(Pt 3):959–64.

94. Skouby SO, *et al.* A comparative study of the effect of continuous combined conjugated equine estrogen plus medroxyprogesterone acetate and tibolone on blood coagulability. *Hum Reprod.* 2007;**22**(4):1186–91.

95. Scarabin PY, *et al.* Effects of oral and transdermal estrogen/progesterone regimens on blood coagulation and fibrinolysis in postmenopausal women. A randomized controlled trial. *Arterioscler Thromb Vasc Biol.* 1997;**17**(11):3071–8.

96. Decensi A, *et al.* Effect of transdermal estradiol and oral conjugated estrogen on C-reactive protein in retinoid-placebo trial in healthy women. *Circulation.* 2002;**106**(10):1224–8.

97. Lethaby A, *et al.* Hormone replacement therapy in postmenopausal women: endometrial hyperplasia and irregular bleeding. *Cochrane Database Syst Rev.* 2004; (**3**):CD000402.

98. Paganini-Hill A, Dworsky R, Krauss RM. Hormone replacement therapy, hormone levels, and lipoprotein cholesterol concentrations in elderly women. *Am J Obstet Gynecol.* 1996;**174**(3):897–902.

99. Soderpalm AH, *et al.* Administration of progesterone produces mild sedative-like effects in men and women. *Psychoneuroendocrinology.* 2004;**29**(3):339–54.

100. Freeman EW, *et al.* A placebo-controlled study of effects of oral progesterone on performance and mood. *Br J Clin Pharmacol.* 1992;**33**(3):293–8.

101. Rice MM, *et al.* Postmenopausal estrogen and estrogen-progestin use and 2-year rate of cognitive change in a cohort of older Japanese American women: the Kame Project. *Arch Intern Med.* 2000;**160**(11):1641–9.

102. McEwen B, Woolley C. Estradiol and progesterone regulate neuronal structure and synaptic connectivity in adult as well as developing brain. *Exp Gerontol.* 1994;**29**:431–6.

103. Woolley CS. Estrogen-mediated structural and functional synaptic plasticity in the female rat hippocampus. *Horm Behav.* 1998;**34**(2):140–8.

104. Nilsen J, Brinton RD. Impact of progestins on estrogen-induced neuroprotection: synergy by progesterone and 19-norprogesterone and antagonism by medroxyprogesterone acetate. *Endocrinology.* 2002;**143**(1):205–12.

105. de Lignieres B. Oral micronized progesterone. *Clin Ther.* 1999;**21**(1):41–60; discussion 1–2.

106. Thal LJ, *et al.* Estrogen levels do not correlate with improvement in cognition. *Arch Neurol.* 2003; **60**(2):209–12.

107. Asthana S, *et al.* Cognitive and neuroendocrine response to transdermal estrogen in postmenopausal women with Alzheimer's disease: results of a placebo-controlled, double-blind, pilot study. *Psychoneuroendocrinology.* 1999;**24**(6):657–77.

108. Asthana S, *et al.* High-dose estradiol improves cognition for women with AD: results of a randomized study. *Neurology.* 2001;**57**(4):605–12.

109. Harman SM, *et al.* KEEPS: the Kronos Early Estrogen Prevention Study. *Climacteric.* 2005;**8**(1):3–12.

110. Resnick SM, *et al.* The Women's Health Initiative Study of Cognitive Aging (WHISCA): a randomized clinical trial of the effects of hormone therapy on age-associated cognitive decline. *Clin Trials.* 2004; **1**(5):440–50.

111. Wilson JR, *et al.* Cognitive abilities: use of family data as a control to assess sex and age differences in two ethnic groups. *Int J Aging Hum Dev.* 1975; **6**(3):261–76.

112. Bravo G, Hebert R. Age- and education-specific reference values for the Mini-Mental and modified Mini-Mental State Examinations derived from a non-demented elderly population. *Int J Geriatr Psychiatry.* 1997;**12**(10):1008–18.

113. Delis DC, *et al. California Verbal Learning Test-II*, 2nd edn. San Antonio, TX: The Psychological Corporation, 2000.

114. Kluger A, *et al.* Neuropsychological prediction of decline to dementia in nondemented elderly. *J Geriatr Psychiatry Neurol.* 1999;**12**(4):168–79.

115. Benton A, *et al. Contributions to Neuropsychological Assessment.* New York: Oxford University Press, 1983.

116. Spreen O, Strauss E. *A Compendium of Neuropsychological Tests*, 2nd edn. New York: Oxford University Press, 1998.

117. Golden C. *The Stroop Color and Word Test: A Manual for Clinical and Experimental Uses.* Chicago: Stoetling, 1978.

118. Wechsler D. *Wechsler Memory Scales.* 3rd edn. San Antonio, TX: The Psychological Corporation, 1997.

119. Wechsler D. *WAIS-R Wechsler Adult Intelligence Scale-III*, 3rd ed. New York, NY: Psychological Corporation, 1991. 4 puzzles (object assembly), 9 plastic cubes (block design), 2 spiral booklets, 1 object assembly layout shield, 1 digit symbol scoring stencil, 1 supplementary sheet, 1 word list, 25 record forms, 1 manual.

120. Hogervorst E, Bandelow S. *Hogervorst–Bandelow Cognitive Test Battery (HBC Test).* Unpublished manual, 2003.

121. McNair DM, Lorr M, Droppleman LF. *POMS Manual.* San Diego, CA: EdITS, 1981.

122. Beck AT, *et al.* An inventory for measuring depression. *Arch Gen Psychiatry.* 1961;**4**:561–71.

123. Spitzer RL, *et al.* Validity and utility of the PRIME-MD patient health questionnaire in assessment of 3000 obstetric-gynecologic patients: the PRIME-MD Patient Health Questionnaire Obstetrics-Gynecology Study. *Am J Obstet Gynecol.* 2000;**183**(3):759–69.

124. Gilewski MJ, Zelinski EM, Schaie KW. The Memory Functioning Questionnaire for assessment of memory complaints in adulthood and old age. *Psychol Aging.* 1990;**5**(4):482–90.

125. Resnick SM, *et al.* Effects of combination estrogen plus progestin hormone treatment on cognition and affect. *J Clin Endocrinol Metab.* 2006;**91**(5): 1802–10.

126. Hickey M, Davis SR, Sturdee DW. Treatment of menopausal symptoms: what shall we do now? *Lancet.* 2005;**366**(9483):409–21.

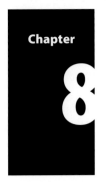

The use of transdermal 17β-estradiol in the treatment of Alzheimer's disease

Whitney Wharton, Sanjay Asthana, and Carey E. Gleason

Editors' introduction

Wharton, Asthana, and Gleason review trials that have evaluated the efficacy of estrogenic therapies in the treatment and prevention of Alzheimer's disease (AD). They point out that of three large clinical trials that used conjugated equine estrogen (CEE) therapies, all reported no cognitive benefits in women with AD. This is in contrast to several small observational and uncontrolled studies that reported positive effects of estrogens on measures of mood, memory, and dementia, as well as two more recent observational trials in which long-term treatment with estradiol appeared to protect 'at-risk' women from AD-related pathologies (hippocampal atrophy and neuronal metabolism). In addition, two recent controlled trials evaluated the effects of transdermal estradiol on cognitive function in women with AD. These trials demonstrated rapid improvement in verbal memory, which correlated positively with plasma estradiol levels, in addition to positive effects on attention, visual memory, and semantic memory. The authors' analysis highlights the need for more research on the pharmacology of estrogenic effects on cognitive function, and in particular on the benefits of transdermal estradiol vs. oral CEE-based therapies in women with AD.

Transdermal estradiol in the treatment of dementia

This chapter discusses the potential salutary effects of estrogenic therapy (ET) in postmenopausal women diagnosed with probable AD. We open with a brief discussion of normative AD participant characteristics, followed by the neurophysiology of levels of estrogens in AD patients. Additionally, estrogenic

formulations will be explored, as we highlight the fact that most basic science and animal research utilizes estradiol formulations in AD studies. Animal models and basic research studies of AD suggest a probable cognitive and neuroprotective effect of estradiol formulations of hormone therapy (HT). Later in the chapter, we focus on clinical trials that have used estradiol formulations of HT, and offer a rationale regarding why this formulation may be particularly beneficial to women diagnosed with probable AD. Although some clinical studies support this theory, three large clinical trials did not report cognitive benefits. Notably, all three of these trials used CEE formulations of HT. Additionally, clinical trials utilizing transdermal estradiol formulations in women with AD have only been conducted in studies examining short-term administration. A review of relevant literature, as well as possible explanations for conflicting findings, will be discussed. We close with potential mediating factors that may influence HT and AD research, followed by recommendations for future directions in clinical research investigating the relationship between transdermal estradiol therapies in the treatment of AD.

Introduction

Findings from the seminal Women's Health Initiative [1] (WHI) and its two ancillary studies, the WHI Memory Study [2] (WHIMS) and the WHI Study of Cognitive Aging [3] (WHISCA) have characterized the cognitive efficacy and adverse effect profile of CEE plus medroxy-progesterone acetate (MPA) in older postmenopausal women. Most relevant to the current chapter, the WHIMS found an increased risk for dementia in postmenopausal women aged 65 and older, treated with CEE and MPA. These results initiated much discussion regarding the possible limitations of HT research and sparked a misguided general distrust of all HT regimens, prompting many HT users to cease treatment. Subsequently, far fewer women considered HT to be a viable physiological and cognitive resource, including older women already diagnosed with probable AD. Unfortunately, the results of prior and recent research indicating the beneficial effects of some HTs have been overshadowed in the wake of these findings. Many studies, both preceding and since the WHI and the WHIMS, have indicated multiple physiological and cognitive salutary effects of estrogens. Moreover, findings from a number of clinical investigations suggest that estrogens can enhance cognitive functioning in women diagnosed with AD, although HT is not currently prescribed for such purposes.

At present, drugs designed to treat AD are mainly cholinesterase inhibitors, which work by preventing synaptic breakdown of acetylcholine in the brain. However, cholinesterase inhibitors alleviate only some AD symptoms and a positive treatment response is seen in a considerably small subset of the affected population. An ideal pharmacological treatment for AD should be directed towards multiple pathophysiological mechanisms, have the potential to favorably alter disease neurobiology, be associated with minimum toxicity, and result in clinically significant improvements in AD symptoms. While the current direction of HT research focuses on AD prevention as opposed to treatment, HT is still considered a potentially viable treatment option for women afflicted with AD.

Postmenopausal women diagnosed with AD are likely to be much older than the average woman treated with HT. As the WHIMS indicated, CEE is not a feasible treatment for older participants, so alternative HT options are currently being explored. Recent evidence from basic science, observational, and clinical studies suggests that other forms of HT, such as transdermal estradiol, can favorably alter the neurobiology of AD, perhaps preventing AD related changes in hippocampal volume and metabolism [4]. In this portion of the chapter, we will discuss studies that have employed transdermal estradiol as an alternative to estrone (the main estrogen found in CEE) in HT treatment for postmenopausal women, focusing on women who are diagnosed with probable AD. While many methodologies and results may be generally applicable to the larger HT population, some of the studies discussed also enrolled women with AD. It is important to note that an AD cohort may respond differently to HT than a non-AD population and may differ from the overall population in ways that would set them apart. Such differences may include age, apolipoprotein (APOE) status, supplementary medications, medication compliance, and affective symptoms or illness. The appropriateness of an AD diagnosis is an additional potentially confounding variable that must be taken into account when conducting research in the AD population.

Estrogens and Alzheimer's disease

There is compelling scientific evidence indicating the neuromodulatory and neuroprotective effect of estrogens, which is directly relevant to AD neuropathology. Estrogens exert biological actions through estrogen receptors (ERs) distributed selectively throughout the brain, including the hippocampus and hypothalamus [5, 6]. Of note, the hippocampus is a brain region selectively affected by AD pathology in addition to mediating various cognitive functions, including memory. As discussed elsewhere in this book (Chapters 17, 18, and 26), beta amyloid (Aβ) deposition is a primary feature of AD. Reduction of Aβ is a principal mechanism by which many basic scientists gauge the beneficial effects of HT, and estradiol in particular. Many studies suggest that the estrogenic component of HT is responsible for reduction of Aβ. Specifically, estrogens have been shown to reduce inflammatory responses to Aβ and improve cerebrospinal fluid (CSF) clearance of insoluble Aβ, while increasing amounts of non-toxic soluble Aβ [7]. Other mechanisms by which estrogens may produce neuromodulatory effects include exerting antioxidant effects and increasing synaptogenesis and dendritic spine density in the hippocampal CA1 neuronal field, an area known to be affected by AD. Importantly, basic science studies have primarily used estradiol as opposed to estrone.

Estradiol vs. estrone

One of the major methodological issues related to the WHI and WHIMS was the form of HT employed. Conjugated equine estrogens is the most widely used estrogenic formulation for hormone therapy in the USA. As discussed in Chapter 7, CEE is a form of HT rich in estrone sulfate and consists of at least ten other hormones, some of which are non-human and whose neurobiology is essentially unknown [4]. Estradiol is an alternative to CEE that is quickly gaining the support of scientists and clinicians. Estradiol is composed of 17β-estradiol, the most potent and natural human estrogen. In addition, the ER binding potency of estrone is approximately two-thirds the affinity of estradiol to the ERα, and about one-third the potency of estradiol for ERβ [8]. Additionally, estrone and estradiol may have differential potencies for membrane mediated actions [9]. Thus, estradiol may be more effective than estrone formulations of HT, especially in older populations.

Route of administration

Although route of HT administration is extensively covered by Dr. Carey E. Gleason elsewhere in the text, a brief review is warranted here, given its direct applicability to the clinical studies that will be addressed shortly. The CEE used in the WHI and WHIMS was an oral HT formulation. Oral estrogens are subject to extensive hepatic metabolism and result in an estrone to estradiol ratio of approximately 5:1 to 7:1 [4]. Additionally, oral administration of estrogens increases the risk of venous thromboembolic complications by inducing pro-coagulant proteins during first-pass hepatic metabolism. Some researchers have proposed that opposed CEE-induced cerebrovascular changes might underlie increased risk for dementia described by the WHIMS data [10]. In contrast to oral formulations, transdermal administration of estrogens bypasses hepatic metabolism and results in a steady-state concentration of estradiol with an estrone:estradiol ratio of 1:1, approximating that seen prior to menopause. Another advantage of transdermal estradiol is that, unlike oral preparations, it does not increase binding glycoproteins, such as sex hormone binding globulin (SHBG), which results in higher plasma concentrations of free estradiol. Thus, research findings to date suggest that not only is HT formulation influential, but the route of administration is equally critical.

Cognition and estradiol

In addition to epidemiological research, support for the neuromodulatory and neuroprotective effects of estrogen can be found within the cognitive neuropsychology research literature. More specifically, transdermal estradiol formulations appear to provide a more promising outcome with regards to potential cognitive benefits, particularly in older AD populations. For instance, bioavailable estradiol has been found to be more predictive of positive cognitive changes over time than estrone [11]. Estradiol has been linked to improved performance on tasks of attention, visuospatial ability, learning and memory, and particularly verbal ability. Interestingly, most studies utilizing estrone formulations did not find the beneficial cognitive effects seen in most of the estradiol studies. Notably, this pattern emerges in studies examining cohorts of women with and without dementia. Meta-analyses have shown that postmenopausal women with AD have lower levels of total estradiol than controls [11]. Interestingly, one study found that total estrone levels were higher in postmenopausal women with AD than age-matched, non-demented controls [12]. Although many studies have not found a direct relationship between estrone and AD, the result is important because CEE consists mainly of estrone. This result raises the possibility that CEE formulations of HT could further exacerbate an AD-associated cognitive decline rather than provide the neuroprotective effects seen with estradiol formulations [11]. In a recent, comprehensive review paper, Gleason compared the effects of various estrogenic formulations on cognition in postmenopausal women. She concluded that studies utilizing estradiol therapies were more likely to demonstrate enhanced cognitive effects, whereas investigations employing CEE tend to be contradictory [4]. In sum, a review of the scientific literature indicates that estrogens have cognitively beneficial properties both in non-demented and in AD participants. Moreover, the cognitive benefits associated with estrogens seem to be more regularly linked to estradiol formulations than CEE, which is composed of estrone.

Estradiol in animal models of Alzheimer's disease

Estrogens have been implicated in neuroprotection and treatment in animal models of AD. Like epidemiological studies, in vitro and in vivo animal studies supporting favorable neuroprotective effects of estrogens have generally been conducted using estradiol formulations, as opposed to estrone. Mouse models have shown that estradiol enhances neuroplasticity, induces anti-inflammatory and cytoprotective effects, reduces Aβ plaques from its precursor protein, and modulates glucose metabolism. In one well designed mouse model of AD, investigators found that mice deficient in estrogens exhibited greatly increased Aβ deposition and production [13]. In the same study, Yue measured estradiol levels in the brain tissue of women with and without AD. Results showed that AD patients had significantly reduced estradiol levels in the frontal cortex, a region characteristically affected in AD [13]. This finding, along with the results of similar animal, observational, and clinical AD studies, provides evidence that estradiol is a potentially viable treatment option for postmenopausal women with AD.

Observational and uncontrolled studies of estradiol in women with Alzheimer's disease

To date, observational and uncontrolled studies supporting a cognition-enhancing role of estrogens for women with AD have been corroborated by findings from basic research indicating a biological basis for multiple salutary effects of estrogens on the brain [14, 15]. In one uncontrolled study, treatment with unopposed, low-dose, micronized estradiol resulted in a significant improvement in orientation, attention, mood, and social interaction, as evidenced by improved scores on the Mini-Mental State Examination (MMSE), Randt Memory Test, and Hamilton Depression Scale for three of seven women with AD [16]. There are a small number of studies that have directly examined the therapeutic potential of different estrogenic formulations in postmenopausal women with AD, many of which have reported a beneficial effect, as well [17, 18, 19, 20, 21]. Recent evidence from two large observational studies (182 and 99 women, respectively) examining the effect of long-term estradiol forms of HT in Chinese women offers some of the strongest support for estradiol's salutary cognitive effects on AD [22, 23]. Investigators found a neuroprotective effect of estradiol in a sample of women 'at risk' for developing AD based on the APOE ε4 genotype. Results indicated that estradiol therapy protected the 'at risk' women from AD-associated changes, including hippocampal atrophy as measured by volumetric magnetic resonance imaging (MRI), and diminished hippocampal neuronal metabolism as detected with proton magnetic resonance spectroscopy (MRS). Importantly, the neuroprotective effect was limited to neurophysiology, as no difference in

cognitive performance was detected between HT users and non-users. Of note, while participants in this sample were considered 'at risk,' they were not exhibiting AD symptoms and had not been diagnosed, so deficits in cognition would not be expected. This study not only lends further support to the growing body of research showing a beneficial effect of estradiol in AD, but it also brings another important factor in AD research to the forefront, namely AD onset and progression.

While the aforementioned studies were aimed toward AD prevention as opposed to treatment, the possibility of a direct link between estradiol and an increased risk for developing AD cannot be overlooked. However, and perhaps equally as important, the abovementioned studies [22, 23] highlight a key aspect of AD research, which is the investigation of healthy vs. patient populations. The studies emphasize that the neural features of AD, such as neurofibrillary tangles and Aβ plaques, are most likely present long before the behavioral and cognitive symptoms emerge. As such, it is important that the scope of AD treatment not only be directed toward those individuals with longstanding symptomology, but also toward participants at high risk of developing AD based on APOE status and positive familial history of the disease. More specifically, researchers utilizing an 'at risk' sample might opt to focus on neurophysiological characteristics associated with AD, as opposed to cognitive symptoms, as the latter will not be affected until much later. On the other hand, investigators examining the effects of estrogens in women already diagnosed with AD might want to measure the beneficial effects of estrogens in terms of cognition, such as memory and attention, as these aspects may be more clinically relevant to a diagnosed population. Essentially, estrogens have the potential to treat a wide array of individuals, ranging from those considered 'at risk' based on a single dimension (e.g., APOE status), to those already diagnosed with probable AD for a number of years. Additionally, for patients already diagnosed with AD, clinically relevant aspects of the disease, such as HT used in conjunction with AD medications, should be explored.

Clinical estradiol research in women with Alzheimer's disease

Very few controlled clinical trials have examined the therapeutic potential of estrogens in women with AD.

83

Of these, three clinical studies have supported a cognitive benefit in women with AD [24, 25, 26]. An early, double-blind, placebo-controlled study of 14 women with AD (aged 83.7 ± 4.5 years; mean ± SD) suggested that CEE improved performance on the MMSE and the Hasegawa Dementia Scale (HDS-R). The seven women receiving 1.25 mg CEE showed significant memory score improvements in the MMSE after three weeks, while the placebo group did not display any significant change in the MMSE or HDS-R score.

In our own laboratory, we conducted a placebo-controlled, double-blind, parallel-group clinical study to evaluate the cognitive and neuroendocrine response to estradiol administration for postmenopausal women with AD [24]. Specifically, the experiment examined the effect of a transdermal 17β-estradiol patch delivering 0.05 mg per day for eight weeks. The six women who received transdermal estradiol exhibited improved performance on attention and verbal memory tasks. Women treated with transdermal estradiol made significantly more self-corrections and demonstrated overall faster task completion on the Stroop task than did controls. Cognitive improvement was directly correlated with plasma concentrations of estradiol, and observed at a dose of estradiol most commonly used in clinical practice. We observed a rapid improvement in verbal memory, suggesting that female dominant tasks may be decidedly sensitive to estradiol in this population. Importantly, verbal memory improved after only one week of estradiol treatment and scores were positively correlated to plasma estradiol levels. Conversely, language did not appear to benefit from estradiol administration, which supports the idea that the beneficial effects may be restricted to certain cognitive domains [24]. In a follow-up study, our laboratory aimed to characterize the cognitive effect of treatment with a high dose (0.10 mg per day) of 17β-estradiol to determine whether a clinically efficacious higher dose would further enhance cognition for postmenopausal women with AD. Significant effects of transdermal estradiol were observed on attention tasks (Stroop Color Word Interference Test), verbal memory (Buschke Selective Reminding Test), visual memory (Figure Copy/Memory), and semantic memory (Boston Naming Test) [25]. These results, together with those from our previously published study and other preliminary clinical trials, provide converging evidence in support of a beneficial effect of estrogens on cognition in postmenopausal women with AD. Our findings were replicated in a meta-analysis [27] and are consistent with those reported in several uncontrolled estradiol studies.

While some larger clinical trials have not supported a therapeutic role of estrogens for women with AD [28–30], the majority of these studies employed CEEs instead of estradiol. For instance, Henderson conducted a double-blind, randomized placebo-controlled study examining the effect of unopposed CEE for 16 weeks [31]. Interestingly, the same author previously reported that HT was linked to improved cognition in AD participants. The later study was intended to provide information regarding the degree to which short-term CEE administration enhances performance on cognitive tasks and global and daily function scores in participants with probable AD. However, contrary to his earlier findings, results of the well designed study showed no significant differences or statistical trends between treatment groups on any of the outcome measures, including tests of attention, verbal memory, and visuospatial ability [29]. Similarly, no significant treatment effects were observed in another comprehensive, one-year investigation examining the effects of unopposed CEE on cognition in hysterectomized women [30]. Like the WHI and WHIMS, participants were older (mean age was 75 years) than most women beginning an HT regimen and as we learned through the WHI and WHIMS, CEE does not seem to be a viable treatment option in an older cohort. Lastly, comprehensive meta-analyses conducted by Hogervorst et al. revealed that HT did produce an initial cognitive benefit in women with AD, but that this benefit was short lived, lasting on average approximately two to three months [31]. With only a limited number of published studies, notably different in methodology, definitive conclusions regarding the therapeutic potential of estrogens in AD would be premature at present.

Potential mediating variables in estrogen/ Alzheimer's disease research

Several potentially confounding variables that may clarify conflicting findings illustrated above remain unexplored. In particular, the differential effects of various hormone preparations and doses, as well as the effect of concomitant progestin therapy, hysterectomy status, prior history of HT exposure, the multiple stages of AD pathology, and APOE status should be examined. Additionally, no data exist on women with other types of dementia (e.g., vascular dementia), or age of dementia onset (e.g., early AD). Additionally, age in general is another variable that could potentially confound the effects of an investigation enrolling AD patients. As noted earlier, AD patients are generally much older than the age of menopause. It has been suggested that beginning an HT regimen many years after menopause eliminates the possible protective effects of HT. This issue is discussed at length elsewhere in this book. Moreover, although there is notable evidence for the favorable effect of some estrogenic formulations on cognition in older AD participants, the well designed and important trials examining the neurocognitive effects of CEEs cannot be ignored. But, again, we stress that these findings should *not* be generalized to all estrogens, an unfortunate consequence of which would be the failure to examine a viable treatment option for a devastating disease [4]. Furthermore, it is possible that the cognition-enhancing efficacy of estrogens may only be observed in patients with mild to moderate dementia or mild cognitive impairment, rather than those with advanced AD.

Future research investigating the potential salutary effect of estrogens in women with, and at all stages of, AD is essential. The prevalence of AD will continue to grow with the increase in the average lifespan in industrialized countries. Sixty-eight percent of individuals diagnosed with AD are women. The same 68% of women comprises roughly 5–10% of our population, and this statistic increases dramatically with age [32, 33]. This reality reinforces the immediate need for basic, translational, observational, and clinical research to develop safe and efficacious HT regimens. Based on the aforementioned results, it is likely that transdermal estradiol formulations of HT may be useful in terms of AD prevention or delaying disease progression, as well as for combating the cognitive symptoms of AD patients. While there is support for transdermal estradiol in older postmenopausal women with AD, it is unclear what proportion of women would likely benefit, and for how long the therapy should be administered. In addition, HT initiated during the menopausal transition (the 'critical period' hypothesis) has been associated with beneficial effects on AD biomarkers. Thus, it may be crucial to initiate HT several years before the onset of AD's cognitive symptoms in order to evaluate the full neuroprotective potential of estrogens. It is likely that a large-scale, longitudinal, cyclical, HT study with transdermal estradiol would offer much needed information to the field of AD and HT research. The KEEPS (Kronos Early Estrogen Prevention Study) and the KEEPS Cognitive and Affective Study (KEEPS-CA) are currently underway and are positioned to address such issues. The KEEPS and KEEPS-CA are discussed at length in Chapter 7.

References

1. Rossouw JE, Anderson GL, Prentice RL, *et al.* Risks and benefits of estrogen plus progestin in healthy postmenopausal women: principal results from the Women's Health Initiative randomized controlled trial. *JAMA.* 2002;**288**:321–33.

2. Shumaker SA, Legault C, Kuller L, *et al.* Conjugated equine estrogens and incidence of probable dementia and mild cognitive impairment in postmenopausal women: the Women's Health Initiative Memory Study. *JAMA.* 2004;**291**:2947–58.

3. Resnick SM, Maki PM, Rapp SR, *et al.* Effects of combination estrogen plus progestin hormone treatment on cognition and affect. *J Clin Endocrinol Metab.* 2006;**91**:1802–10.

4. Gleason CE, Carlsson CM, Johnson S, Atwood C, Asthana S. Clinical pharmacology and differential cognitive efficacy of estrogen preparations. *Ann N Y Acad Sci.* 2005;**1052**:93–115.

5. Shughrue PJ, Merchenthaler I. Estrogen is more than just a 'sex hormone': novel sites for estrogen action in the hippocampus and cerebral cortex. *Front Neuroendocrinol.* 2000;**21**:95–101.

6. Shughrue PJ, Merchenthaler I. Distribution of estrogen receptor beta immunoreactivity in the rat central nervous system. *J Comp Neuro.* 2001;**436**:64–81.

7. Bhavnani BR. Estrogens and menopause: pharmacology of conjugated equine estrogens and their potential role in the prevention of neurodegenerative diseases such as Alzheimer's. *J Steroid Biochem Mol Biol.* 2003;**85**:473–82.

8. Kuiper GGJM, Carlsson BO, Grandien K, *et al.* Comparison of the ligand binding specificity and transcription tissue distribution of estrogen receptors alpha and beta. *Endocrinology.* 1997;**138**:863–70.

9. Deecher DC, Swiggard P, Frail DE, *et al.* Characterization of a membrane associated estrogen receptor in a rat hypothalamic cell line (D12). *Endocrine.* 2003;**22**:211–23.

10. Yaffe K. Hormone therapy and the brain: deja vu all over again. *JAMA.* 2003;**289**:2717–19.

11. Hogervorst E, Williams J, Budge M, *et al.* The nature of the effect of female gonadal hormone replacement therapy on cognitive function in post-menopausal women: a meta-analysis. *Neuroscience.* 2000;**101** (3):485–512.

12. Cunningham C, Synncot M, Rowan M, *et al.* Oestrogen levels in demented and nondemented postmenopausal women. UK Dementia Research Group, Annual Meeting, University of Leicester, Gilbert Murray Hall, Leicester, 1994, pp. 5–6.

13. Yue X, Lu M, Lancaster T, *et al.* Brain estrogen deficiency accelerates A-beta plaque formation in an Alzheimer's disease animal model. *Proc Natl Acad Sci.* 2005;**102**:19198–203.

14. McEwen B, Alves S, Bulloch K, *et al.* Ovarian steroids and the brain: implications for cognition and aging. *Neurology.* 1997;**48**(7):S8–S15.

15. Yaffe K, Sawaya G, Lieberburg I, *et al.* Estrogen therapy in postmenopausal women: effects on cognitive function and dementia. *J Am Med Assoc.* 1998;**279**:688–95.

16. Fillit H, Weiner H, Cholst I, *et al.* Observations in a preliminary open trial of estradiol therapy for senile dementia-Alzheimer's type. *Psychoneuroendocrinology.* 1986;**11**:337–45.

17. Honjo H, Ogino Y, Naitoh K, *et al.* In vivo effects by estrone sulfate on the central nervous system-senile dementia (Alzheimer's type). *J Steroid Biochem.* 1989;**34**:521–5.

18. Ohkura T, Isse K, Akazawa K, *et al.* Low-dose estrogen replacement therapy for Alzheimer disease in women. *Menopause.* 1994;**1**:125–30.

19. Ohkura T, Isse K, Akazawa K, *et al.* Evaluation of estrogen treatment in female patients with dementia of the Alzheimer type. *Endocr J.* 1994;**41**:361–71.

20. Ohkura T, Isse K, Akazawa K, *et al.* Long-term estrogen replacement therapy in female patients with dementia of the Alzheimer type: 7 case reports. *Dementia.* 1995;**6**:99–107.

21. Henderson VW, Watt L, Buckwalter JG. Cognitive skills associated with estrogen replacement in women with Alzheimer's disease. *Psychoneuroendocrinology.* 1996;**21**(4):421–30.

22. Hu L, Yue Y, Zuo PP, *et al.* Evaluation of neuroprotective effects of long-term low dose hormone replacement therapy on postmenopausal women brain hippocampus using magnetic resonance scanner. *Chin Med Sci J.* 2006;**21**:214–18.

23. Yue Y, Hu L, Tian QJ, *et al.* Effects of long-term, low-dose sex hormone replacement therapy on hippocampus and cognition of postmenopausal women of different apoE genotypes. *Acta Pharmacologica Sinica.* 2007;**28**:1129–35.

24. Asthana S, Baker LD, Craft S, *et al.* Cognitive and neuroendocrine response to transdermal estrogen in postmenopausal women with Alzheimer's disease: results of a placebo-controlled, double-blind, pilot study. *Psychoneuroendocrinology.* 1999;**24**:657–77.

25. Asthana S, Baker LD, Craft S, *et al.* High-dose estradiol improves cognition for women with AD: results of a randomized study. *Neurology.* 2001;**57**:605–12.

26. Honjo H, Ogino Y, Tanaka K, *et al.* An effect of conjugated estrogen to cognitive impairment in women with senile dementia-Alzheimer's type: a placebo-controlled, double-blind study. *J Jap Menop Soc.* 1993;**1**:167–71.

27. Hogervorst E. The short-lived effect of hormone therapy on cognition function. In Rasgon NL, ed. *The Effects of Estrogen on Brain Function.* Baltimore, MD: John Hopkins Press, 2006, pp. 46–79.

28. Wang P, Liao S, Liu R, *et al.* Effects of estrogen on cognition, mood, and cerebral blood flow in AD. *Neurology.* 2000;**54**:2061–6.

29. Henderson VW, Paganini-Hill A, Miller BL, *et al.* Estrogen for Alzheimer's disease in women: randomized, double-blind, placebo-controlled trial. *Neurology.* 2000;**54**:295–301.

30. Mulnard RA, Cotman CW, Kawas C, *et al.* Estrogen replacement therapy for treatment of mild to moderate Alzheimer disease: a randomized controlled trial. Alzheimer's Disease Cooperative Study. *JAMA.* 2000;**283**:1007–15.

31. Hogervorst E. The short-lived effect of HRT on cognition function. In N Rasgon. Estrogen's effects on brain function. What's next? The AlzGene Database. Alzheimer Research Forum. Available at: http://www.alzgene.org. Accessed 2006.

32. Brookmeyer R, Gray S, Kawas C. Projections of Alzheimer's disease in the United States and the public health impact of delaying disease onset. *Am J Public Health.* 1998;**88**:1337–42.

33. Morrison JH, Brinton RD, Schmidt PJ, *et al.* Estrogen, menopause, and the aging brain: how basic neuroscience can inform hormone therapy in women. *Neuroscience.* 2006;**26**(41):10332–48.

Alternative modes of treatment: pulsatile estradiol treatment

Jin Li and Farook Al-Azzawi

Editors' introduction

It is increasingly clear that not all estrogenic treatment regimens are alike with respect to effects on the brain, and that alternative regimens need to be evaluated and compared. In this chapter, Li and Al-Azzawi discuss the advantages of intranasal pulsatile estradiol administration relative to oral or transdermal therapies. Pharmacokinetic analyses demonstrate the feasibility of using intranasal pulsatile estradiol treatments to produce estradiol exposures comparable to those achieved via a transdermal route. As with transdermal therapies, intranasal application avoids the negative effects on liver enzymes associated with oral treatment. Major differences in the effects of pulsatile vs. sustained estradiol administration on gene expression have been detected. In addition, there are noted potential advantages of pulsatile vs. sustained treatment such as up-regulation of estrogen receptors, initialization of estrogen receptor co-factors, repeated activation of non-genomic pathways, and lower levels of potentially active (and carcinogenic) metabolites.

Postmenopausal estrogen therapy: an overview

Estrogens are known to play an important role in diverse physiological processes of target cells through a signal transduction system based on the intracellular soluble estrogen receptor (ER) proteins [1]. It is universally acknowledged that treatment with estrogens (ET) cures symptoms of estrogen deficiency in postmenopausal women, improves mood, protects the genitourinary system, improves lipoprotein profile, and prevents bone loss. In numerous laboratory-based as well as comparative clinical studies, the

administration of estrogens in estrogen deprivation paradigms showed enhanced nitric oxide synthase activity [2], reduced vascular tone [3, 4], reduced blood pressure [5], and enhanced cardiac function with prolongation of time to develop exercise-induced ST segment depression on exercise bikes [6]. Its oral administration is associated with a first-pass effect of hepatic metabolism resulting in higher estrone (E_1) conjugates, increases sex hormone binding globulin and angiotensinogen, raises triglycerides levels, and induces hepatic synthesis of clotting factors [7]. In order to avoid these hepatic effects, the transdermal route was introduced in the form of patches and gels. These preparations mount lower serum levels of 17-β-estradiol (E_2) and E_1 with a resulting serum $E_1:E_2$ ratio of 0.8:1 as opposed to 4:1 with oral administration of E_2. The clinical corollary is that while the transdermal route is as effective in improving the clinical and biochemical picture in postmenopausal women, it has not been associated with the slight increase in the incidence of venous thrombosis noted with oral E_2. The transdermal route does not succeed all the time as an effective mode of administration of E_2 due to skin reaction to adhesives and limited capacity to absorb the hormone through the skin in some women. Other routes of administration have been sought and vaginal rings impregnated with E_2 have been used.

Pulsed estradiol therapy

The concept of pulsatile administration of E_2 to induce an intended cellular effect with minimal background serum levels has been exploited by the introduction of a nasal spray delivery system [8]. The rich blood supply of the nasal mucosa offers $160 \, mm^2$ of

Hormones, Cognition and Dementia: State of the Art and Emergent Therapeutic Strategies, ed. Eef Hogervorst, Victor W. Henderson, Robert B. Gibbs, and Roberta Diaz Brinton. Published by Cambridge University Press. © Cambridge University Press 2009.

capillary bed and ensures rapid absorption. This novel route of administration of E_2 via the nasal mucosa is made possible with the use of α-cyclodextrin, which increases the stability of E_2 in aqueous solution.

The pharmacokinetics of E_2 and E_1 were studied following intranasal administration of E_2 (100, 300, or 450 µg) once or twice 12 hours apart, and the results were compared with those for E_2 administered as a reservoir patch 50 µg twice-weekly application, or a tablet of 2 mg micronized E_2 daily. Systemic exposure to intranasally administered E_2 was dose-proportional but independent of the treatment regimen. Moreover, the dose of 300 µg gave an estimated 24 hours of systemic exposure to exogenous E_2 close to that of 50 µg twice-weekly applied reservoir patch, or the 2 mg/day tablet. The serum $E_1{:}E_2$ ratio was similar to that of the transdermal patch (0.8:1) and four-fold lower than the ratio observed with the tablet.

Following nasal application of E_2, there was an immediate rise in serum E_2 levels to around 3,500 pmol/L within 30 minutes, followed by a rapid decline to one-tenth of the peak value after two hours, reaching the pre-treatment value at 12 hours [9]. The area under the concentration versus time curve, or the area under the curve (AUC), has been calculated for the various doses of the intranasal route and compared with those determined for oral or transdermal application of the hormone. The AUC for 300 µg of intranasal E_2 is slightly lower than that for 2 mg of oral E_2, but the effectiveness of the intranasal route appears to be comparable. Interestingly, this trial showed time-independent pharmacokinetics of E_2 and E_1, indicating that E_2 and E_1 do not accumulate. Moreover, the profile of these steroids was not different when a progestogen was added. The suppressive effect of pulsed E_2 on follicle stimulating hormone (FSH) shadowed the plasma E_2 levels. However, the basal FSH level declined progressively over time, to 83% at 14 days, and 76% at 28 days after commencement of treatment. It seems that the lack of accumulation of E_2 and E_1 with the intranasal route results in a lower intra- and interindividual variation in plasma values, comparing favorably with those calculated for the oral route and transdermal patch.

The above pharmacodynamic profile is not subjected to the hepatic first-pass effect, with the important consequence of no increased synthesis of sex hormone-binding globulin, angiotensinogen, or triglycerides [8].

Clinical evaluation of transnasal estradiol

In clinical trials, E_2 delivered by nasal spray has been proven to provide the same efficacy on climacteric symptoms as classical oral and transdermal therapy, when dosages are equivalent in terms of 24-hour exposure to estrogens [10], and a pronounced effect not only on vasomotor symptoms but also a significant and clinically relevant improvement in several other quality of life dimensions [11]. In these studies, such pulsed therapy was also found to be associated with statistically significantly shorter duration of uterine bleeding, scantier amount of blood loss, and lower incidence of mastalgia compared to the oral or transdermal patches.

Estrogen receptor dynamics

The biological actions of estrogens are mediated by two genetically and functionally distinct receptors, ERα and ERβ, which share similar cellular expression profiles in target cells [12]. The estrogen receptor resides within the nucleus in an inactive form, and is bound to heat-shock proteins (HSPs). When E_2 reaches its cognate receptor within the nucleus it induces conformational changes, such that it separates from its chaperoning HSP and dimerizes, and the ligand–receptor complex seeks access to the DNA at a specific sequence, termed the estrogen response element (ERE), within target gene promoters exerting either a positive or negative effect on gene transcription. It recruits other nuclear proteins such as steroid receptor co-activator (SRC), which in turn activates the enzyme histone acetyl transferase (HAT). The activated HAT helps the DNA to unwind, to expose the ERE within its helices for binding with the ligand–receptor complex. Once binding occurs, transcription of the DNA to RNA follows.

Estrogen receptor isotypes

Estrogen receptor isotypes are ligand-activated transcriptional factors that regulate a number of cellular mechanisms, a function that depends on a number of factors. Essentially, the overall shape of ERα and ERβ is plastic and substantially influenced by the nature of the bound ligand [13]. The relevance of this observation is highlighted by the demonstration that receptor conformational changes are primary regulators of the ability of ERs to interact with transcriptional co-activators and co-repressors, the proteins responsible for manifesting the transcriptional effect of the DNA-bound receptor in the cell and tissue context [14]. It also has been determined that ER can interact with at least 50 functionally distinct co-activators and co-repressors, the relative and absolute levels of which can differ greatly between different cells [15].

Upon binding an agonist, these receptors spontaneously form ERα and ERβ homodimers, but heterodimers in cells expressing both receptor subtypes have also been identified [16]. Whereas both receptor subtypes are capable of activating transcription, ERα seems to be a more robust activator than ERβ [16]. Analysis of the ERα crystal structure of the ligand-bound ERα showed that different conformational changes occur with the receptor upon its interaction with agonist, compared with antagonist [17, 18]. Furthermore, target cells can distinguish between these neo-conformational complexes [13, 19, 20]. This is clearly observed in selective estrogen receptor modulator (SERM) interactions with ERα. For example, the antagonistic effect of tamoxifen in the breast is associated with an agonistic effect on bone turnover and lipid metabolism, and a modified agonist action on the endometrium. Although ERα and ERβ share mechanistic similarities, they play different roles in estrogenic action, a conclusion that is supported by the distinct phenotypes observed in mice in which either or both subtypes have been genetically disrupted, and the observation that ERβ-specific agonists, such as ERβ-041 [21], function as therapeutically effective treatments in animal models of inflammatory bowel disease and rheumatoid arthritis but unlike E_2 (not selective), they do not manifest agonist activity in the reproductive tract, bone, or mammary glands [22].

Ligand binding affects the stability of the ERα and accelerates its degradation, and therefore its half-life is shortened from five to eight hours to three to four hours following the binding of the ligand [23–27]. Not all liganded receptors reach the DNA, and may be retained in the nuclear matrix; indeed, some receptors remain inactive. An estradiol dose-dependent reduction in the amount of receptors occurs. In vitro, degradation of ERα and many short-lived transcriptional factors appears to be mediated by the ubiquitin-proteosome pathway [28], but the in vivo evidence is still lacking. However, in intact cells, estradiol-induced ERα degradation appears to be mediated by the 26S

proteosome pathway [29, 30]. It is plausible that such a reduction in nuclear content of estrogen receptor, and the rapid loss of the ligand, stimulates rapid regeneration of the receptor complement ready to receive the next dose.

Pulsed E_2 treatment and mammary carcinogenesis

It has been demonstrated that pulsed exposure is as efficient as continuous exposures on the expression of endogenous or transfected genes regulated by estrogens and proliferation in normal and malignant human breast cells [31]. As the pulsed estradiol administration is associated with relatively high serum levels, albeit for a short duration, it is important to compare both routes of administration with regard to the modulation of carcinogenesis. In animal models of dimethylbenzanthracine (DMBA)-induced mammary carcinogenesis, pulsed E_2 therapy administered as tail vein injections was associated with a lower incidence rate and a lower progression of tumors compared to continuous E_2 exposure. One explanation is the pharmacodynamic features of pulsed E_2 therapy where the rapid decline in serum levels of estrogens is associated with lowered levels of their metabolites. Catechol metabolites of estradiol cause oxidative damage that may contribute to carcinogenesis [32]. These findings question the widely held views of the carcinogenic feature of E_2. Indeed, the findings of the Women' Health Initiative (WHI) study have documented that conjugated equine estrogen-only therapy was not only neutral as far as breast cancer risk is concerned but actually protective [33].

Pulsed versus continuous E_2 exposure and endothelial cells

Non-genomic effects

Simoncini et al. investigated differential estrogenic signaling in human umbilical vein endothelial cells (HUVECs) following pulsed or continuous administration [34]. Their findings suggest the ER signaling to the nucleus can be recruited quickly and, once activated, transcriptional machinery can proceed independent of further ligand availability. It follows that there is no mandatory requirement for prolonged contact between hormone and cells in order to recruit the classic genomic mechanisms of gene regulation, if a sufficient exposure to E_2 is provided. Furthermore, a transient exposure to a high level of estrogens can maximize the recruitment of non-genomic pathways by ERs. Indeed, when comparing the degree of activation of the ERK1/2 and of the PI3K/Akt cascades at different time points with either transient or continuous exposure to E_2, it is clear that by concentrating the delivery of the steroid over a shorter period of time, non-genomic signaling is more strongly activated. Although the difference between pulsed and continuous treatments may not seem too marked, it must be noted that the concentrations of steroid used in inducing physiological signaling in non-malignant cells may be relevant.

Further, with pulsed administration of E_2, non-genomic signaling is repeatedly recruited during every transient exposure, thus maximizing the biological actions of these rapid mechanisms. Indeed, non-genomic signaling of steroids requires marked changes of hormone concentration to be triggered. Pulsed administration is, therefore, more effective in recruiting these pathways, as compared to administrations leading to continuous, slowly changing, levels of estrogens.

These results suggest that the kinetics of contact of the steroids with the cell receptors are important for the determination of their final biological effects, particularly for the choice between non-transcriptional or transcriptional signaling pathways.

Genomic effects [35]

The observation made in clinical trials of significantly lower frequency of mastalgia and uterine bleeding with transnasal E_2, compared with conventional oral or patch administration of estrogens [36], suggests a possible differential effect of pulsed E_2 administration on vascular biology in terms of reduced development of capillary congestion and edema in endometrial and breast tissues.

There are several published studies where microarrays have been utilized to assess the effect of estrogenic stimulation on gene expression profiles in estrogen receptor positive cells, such as the MCF-7 breast cancer cell line [37, 38]. Vascular permeability changes in response to estrogenic therapy may play a key role in the development of climacteric symptoms. Relatively few microarray studies have examined the role of estrogens in regulating gene expression in endothelial cells, and the published studies have focused on the effects of continuous treatment of E_2

after 40–60 minutes of its application [39]. The exact roles of pulsed versus continuous E_2-mediated gene regulation in the human endothelial cell model remain to be elucidated.

In pursuing this question we treated HUVECs with continuous or pulsed E_2 for five days [40]. We chose a relatively long E_2 exposure time to better replicate the clinical situation. Of the more than 22,000 genes queried on the Affymetrix 133A microarray, we identified approximately 600 genes that showed a robust pattern of regulation by either continuous or pulsed E_2, the majority of these genes (more than 60%) were up-regulated. After five days of treatment, we did not find the expression of known estrogen responsive genes to be altered as previously reported, such as ESR1 and ESR2 (ERα and ERβ, respectively), SP1 transcription factor [41], and HSP27 (heat shock protein 27) [42–44]. These genes may be modified rapidly (within a few minutes or hours) and return to pretreatment levels five days later when we collected the samples. However, the fact that the expression of more than 800 genes was identified significantly different between continuous and pulsed mode gives greater necessity for further studies. From the large set of data obtained, we focus, below, on the roles of some genes that are actively involved in tumorigenesis and cell proliferation.

In contrast to the reported proliferative effects of E_2 in normal and cancerous breast cells [31], our results showed that continuous E_2 (10^{-9} M) treatment did not induce proliferation in HUVECs, and that pulsed treatment elicited, surprisingly, an inhibitory effect on cell proliferation at the same dosage of exposure as continuous therapy. This anti-proliferative effect may explain, in part, the clinical observations. The transcriptional mechanism in endothelial cell proliferation is postulated to be multi-factorial, including insulin growth factor (IGF) receptors, tumor suppressor thrombospondin-1 (THBS1), and vascular endothelial growth factor (VEGF).

Of the signal transducer genes regulated by estrogens in our experiments, IGF1R expression of pulsed treatment is lower than continuous treatment ($p < 0.05$); while IGF2R expression of pulsed treatment is higher ($p < 0.05$). This suggests that IGF1-mediated mitogenic activity, inhibition of cell adhesion, and promotion of metastatic processes may be less activated with pulsed therapy [45, 46]. A significantly increased expression of THBS-1 and a lower VEGF expression with pulsed therapy, using real-time polymerase chain reaction (PCR), may explain inhibition of endothelial cell proliferation, which agrees with earlier reports [47, 48]. Since VEGF acts on endothelial cells by stimulating cell proliferation, migration, and tubular organization, and increases vascular permeability [49], its down-regulation may contribute to less capillary congestion and edema in endometrial and breast tissues during pulsed E_2 therapy.

Conclusion

There are three possible mechanisms to explain the effect of pulsatile E_2 treatment. First, the system, in vitro or in vivo, becomes primed to receive further signaling from the administration of estradiol, through up-regulation of ERs' production via alternative promoters. Second, initialization of receptor cofactors in target cells is achieved since the initial pulsed E_2 loads cells with non-degraded E_2. Third, it results in a low level of potentially active metabolites of E_2, which otherwise may increase hepatic globin synthesis. The principle of pulsed E_2 therapy may help unravel many aspects of the physiology of estrogens.

References

1. McDonnell DP, Norris JD. Connections and regulation of the human estrogen receptor. *Science*. 2002; **296**:1642–4.

2. Chen DB, Bird IM, Zheng J, *et al*. Membrane estrogen receptor-dependent extracellular signal-regulated kinase pathway mediates acute activation of endothelial nitric oxide synthase by estrogen in uterine artery endothelial cells. *Endocrinology*. 2004;**145**:113–25.

3. Haas E, Meyer MR, Schurr U, *et al*. Differential effects of 17beta-estradiol on function and expression of estrogen receptor alpha, estrogen receptor beta, and GPR30 in arteries and veins of patients with atherosclerosis. *Hypertension*. 2007;**49**:1358–63.

4. Girdler SS, Hinderliter AL, Wells EC, *et al*. Transdermal versus oral estrogen therapy in postmenopausal smokers: hemodynamic and endothelial effects. *Obstet Gynecol*. 2004;**103**:169–80.

5. Ashraf MS, Vongpatanasin W. Estrogen and hypertension. *Curr Hypertens Rep*. 2006;**8**:368–76.

6. Albertsson PA, Emanuelsson H, Milsom I. Beneficial effect of treatment with transdermal estradiol-17-beta on exercise-induced angina and ST segment depression in syndrome X. *Int J Cardiol*. 1996;**54**:13–20.

7. Scarabin PY, Alhenc-Gelas M, Plu-Bureau G, *et al*. Effects of oral and transdermal estrogen/progesterone regimens on blood coagulation and fibrinolysis in postmenopausal women. A randomized controlled trial. *Arterioscler Thromb Vasc Biol*. 1997;**17**:3071–8.

8. Mattsson LA, Christiansen C, Colau JC, *et al*. Clinical equivalence of intranasal and oral 17beta-estradiol for postmenopausal symptoms. *Am J Obstet Gynecol*. 2000;**182**:545–52.

9. Devissaguet JP, Brion N, Lhote O, *et al*. Pulsed estrogen therapy: pharmacokinetics of intranasal 17-beta-estradiol (S21400) in postmenopausal women and comparison with oral and transdermal formulations. *Eur J Drug Metab Pharmacokinet*. 1999;**24**:265–71.

10. Studd J, Pornel B, Marton I, *et al*. Efficacy and acceptability of intranasal 17 beta-oestradiol for menopausal symptoms: randomised dose-response study. Aerodiol Study Group. *Lancet*. 1999;**353**: 1574–8.

11. Nielsen TF, Ravn P, Pitkin J, *et al*. Pulsed estrogen therapy improves postmenopausal quality of life: a 2-year placebo-controlled study. *Maturitas*. 2006;**53**:184–90.

12. Kuiper GG, Enmark E, Pelto-Huikko M, *et al*. Cloning of a novel receptor expressed in rat prostate and ovary. *Proc Natl Acad Sci USA*. 1996;**93**:5925–30.

13. Paige LA, Christensen DJ, Gron H, *et al*. Estrogen receptor (ER) modulators each induce distinct conformational changes in ER alpha and ER beta. *Proc Natl Acad Sci USA*. 1999;**96**:3999–4004.

14. Norris JD, Paige LA, Christensen DJ, *et al*. Peptide antagonists of the human estrogen receptor. *Science*. 1999;**285**:744–6.

15. McDonnell DP. Mechanism-based discovery as an approach to identify the next generation of estrogen receptor modulators. *FASEB J*. 2006;**20**:2432–4.

16. Hall JM, McDonnell DP. The estrogen receptor beta-isoform (ERbeta) of the human estrogen receptor modulates ERalpha transcriptional activity and is a key regulator of the cellular response to estrogens and antiestrogens. *Endocrinology*. 1999;**140**:5566–78.

17. Brzozowski AM, Pike AC, Dauter Z, *et al*. Molecular basis of agonism and antagonism in the oestrogen receptor. *Nature*. 1997;**389**:753–8.

18. Shiau AK, Barstad D, Loria PM, *et al*. The structural basis of estrogen receptor/coactivator recognition and the antagonism of this interaction by tamoxifen. *Cell*. 1998;**95**:927–37.

19. McDonnell DP, Dana SL, Hoener PA, *et al*. Cellular mechanisms which distinguish between hormone- and antihormone-activated estrogen receptor. *Ann N Y Acad Sci*. 1995;**761**:121–37.

20. Wijayaratne AL, Nagel SC, Paige LA, *et al*. Comparative analyses of mechanistic differences among antiestrogens. *Endocrinology*. 1999;**140**:5828–40.

21. Harris HA, Albert LM, Leathurby Y, *et al*. Evaluation of an estrogen receptor-beta agonist in animal models of human disease. *Endocrinology*. 2003;**144**:4241–9.

22. McDonnell DP. The molecular pharmacology of estrogen receptor modulators: implications for the treatment of breast cancer. *Clin Cancer Res.* 2005;**11**:871s–7s.

23. Dauvois S, Danielian PS, White R, *et al.* Antiestrogen ICI 164,384 reduces cellular estrogen receptor content by increasing its turnover. *Proc Natl Acad Sci USA.* 1992;**89**:4037–41.

24. Eckert RL, Mullick A, Rorke EA, *et al.* Estrogen receptor synthesis and turnover in MCF-7 breast cancer cells measured by a density shift technique. *Endocrinology.* 1984;**114**:629–37.

25. Monsma FJ, Jr., Katzenellenbogen BS, Miller MA, *et al.* Characterization of the estrogen receptor and its dynamics in MCF-7 human breast cancer cells using a covalently attaching antiestrogen. *Endocrinology.* 1984;**115**:143–53.

26. Nardulli AM, Katzenellenbogen BS. Dynamics of estrogen receptor turnover in uterine cells in vitro and in uteri in vivo. *Endocrinology.* 1986;**119**:2038–46.

27. Scholl S, Lippman ME. The estrogen receptor in MCF-7 cells: evidence from dense amino acid labeling for rapid turnover and a dimeric model of activated nuclear receptor. *Endocrinology.* 1984;**115**:1295–301.

28. Ciechanover A. The ubiquitin-proteasome proteolytic pathway. *Cell.* 1994;**79**:13–21.

29. Alarid ET, Bakopoulos N, Solodin N. Proteasome-mediated proteolysis of estrogen receptor: a novel component in autologous down-regulation. *Mol Endocrinol.* 1999;**13**:1522–34.

30. El Khissiin A, Leclercq G. Implication of proteasome in estrogen receptor degradation. *FEBS Lett.* 1999;**448**:160–6.

31. Cavailles V, Gompel A, Portois MC, *et al.* Comparative activity of pulsed or continuous estradiol exposure on gene expression and proliferation of normal and tumoral human breast cells. *J Mol Endocrinol.* 2002;**28**:165–75.

32. Yager JD, Davidson NE. Estrogen carcinogenesis in breast cancer. *N Engl J Med.* 2006;**354**:270–82.

33. Stefanick ML, Anderson GL, Margolis KL, *et al.* Effects of conjugated equine estrogens on breast cancer and mammography screening in postmenopausal women with hysterectomy. *JAMA.* 2006;**295**:1647–57.

34. Simoncini T, Fornari L, Mannella P, *et al.* Differential estrogen signaling in endothelial cells upon pulsed or continuous administration. *Maturitas.* 2005; **50**:247–58.

35. Li J, Wang H, Johnson SM, *et al.* Differing transcriptional responses to pulsed or continuous estradiol exposure in human umbilical vein endothelial cells. *J Steroid Biochem Mol Biol.* 2008; **111**(1/2):41–9.

36. Lopes P, Merkus HM, Nauman J, *et al.* Randomized comparison of intranasal and transdermal estradiol. *Obstet Gynecol.* 2000;**96**:906–12.

37. Frasor J, Danes JM, Komm B, *et al.* Profiling of estrogen up- and down-regulated gene expression in human breast cancer cells: insights into gene networks and pathways underlying estrogenic control of proliferation and cell phenotype. *Endocrinology.* 2003;**144**:4562–74.

38. Inoue A, Yoshida N, Omoto Y, *et al.* Development of cDNA microarray for expression profiling of estrogen-responsive genes. *J Mol Endocrinol.* 2002; **29**:175–92.

39. Pedram A, Razandi M, Aitkenhead M, *et al.* Integration of the non-genomic and genomic actions of estrogen. Membrane-initiated signaling by steroid to transcription and cell biology. *J Biol Chem.* 2002; **277**:50768–75.

40. Li J, Wang H, Johnson SM, *et al.* Differing transcriptional responses to pulsed or continuous estradiol exposure in human umbilical vein endothelial cells. *J Steroid Biochem Mol Biol.* 2008;**111**:41–9.

41. Li C, Briggs MR, Ahlborn TE, *et al.* Requirement of Sp1 and estrogen receptor alpha interaction in 17beta-estradiol-mediated transcriptional activation of the low density lipoprotein receptor gene expression. *Endocrinology.* 2001;**142**:1546–53.

42. Zhou J, Ng S, Adesanya-Famuiya O, *et al.* Testosterone inhibits estrogen-induced mammary epithelial proliferation and suppresses estrogen receptor expression. *FASEB J.* 2000;**14**:1725–30.

43. Cappelletti V, Saturno G, Miodini P, *et al.* Selective modulation of ER-beta by estradiol and xenoestrogens in human breast cancer cell lines. *Cell Mol Life Sci.* 2003;**60**:567–76.

44. Porter W, Wang F, Duan R, *et al.* Transcriptional activation of heat shock protein 27 gene expression by 17beta-estradiol and modulation by antiestrogens and aryl hydrocarbon receptor agonists. *J Mol Endocrinol.* 2001;**26**:31–42.

45. Dunn SE, Ehrlich M, Sharp NJ, *et al.* A dominant negative mutant of the insulin-like growth factor-I receptor inhibits the adhesion, invasion, and metastasis of breast cancer. *Cancer Res.* 1998;**58**:3353–61.

46. Kahlert S, Nuedling S, van Eickels M, *et al.* Estrogen receptor alpha rapidly activates the IGF-1 receptor pathway. *J Biol Chem.* 2000;**275**:18447–53.

47. Lawler J. Thrombospondin-1 as an endogenous inhibitor of angiogenesis and tumor growth. *J Cell Mol Med.* 2002;**6**:1–12.

48. Neufeld G, Cohen T, Gengrinovitch S, *et al.* Vascular endothelial growth factor (VEGF) and its receptors. *FASEB J.* 1999;**13**:9–22.

49. Ferrara N, Davis-Smyth T. The biology of vascular endothelial growth factor. *Endocr Rev.* 1997;**18**:4–25.

Chapter 10

In search of estrogen alternatives for the brain

Liqin Zhao and Roberta Diaz Brinton

Editors' introduction

This chapter briefly reviews recent advancements in the search for a non-feminizing estrogen alternative that can mimic estrogen's positive effects on cognitive health without eliciting an undesirable impact on reproductive and cardiovascular systems. The discussion focuses on two avenues of translational development, tissue-selective and subtype-selective estrogen receptor (ER) modulators (SERMs), in particular ERβ-selective phyto-SERMs as a natural approach for potentially promoting neurological health and preventing age-associated cognitive impairment and risk of Alzheimer's disease in both genders.

Estrogen for the female brain

Postmenopausal women are prone to cognitive changes as a result of diminished serum levels of female sex hormones following menopause, which increase the risks for cognitive impairment and dementia such as Alzheimer's disease (AD). A large body of evidence suggests that estrogen therapy (ET) can potentially counteract these changes by sustaining the brain in a proactively defensive status against neurodegeneration (reviewed in Chapter 6). Until recently, this well documented concept has been complicated by the findings of the largest randomized and controlled clinical study, the Women's Health Initiative Memory Study (WHIMS), which was designed to evaluate the relationship between estrogen and cognition. It was found that ET was either to be of no benefit (estrogen-alone) or to afford a negative impact (estrogen plus progestin) on global cognition in postmenopausal women aged 65 years or older [1–4] (see also Chapters 1–5). The WHIMS results provoked in-depth debate with respect to the use of ET in women. Basic and clinical

scientists as well as the public have been asking the same question: is estrogen good or bad for the brain and what has caused the disparity in outcomes? To answer the question, scientists have been taking a careful second look at the data collected from basic science research, observational studies, and the WHIMS, and it is becoming increasingly clear that among many factors, "timing" could be a significant regulator of the health impact of ET on postmenopausal women [5–7]. Among the WHIMS study participants, women who reported using any form of ET before reaching 65 years had a 50% reduction in risk for developing AD or other types of dementia than women who did not use such a therapy by that age [5]. In contrast, women who began estrogen-alone therapy after the age of 65 years had an approximately 50% increased risk of developing dementia [5]. The risk was nearly double among women using the combined estrogen plus progestin therapy [5]. These analyses, along with many observational studies, such as the Cache County Study [8] and REMEMBER pilot study [9], support a "healthy cell bias" of estrogen action in the brain, and suggest that ET may serve as a "preventive" rather than "treatment" strategy against estrogen deficiency-related cognitive decline and neurodegenerative diseases such as AD in postmenopausal women [10, 11].

Estrogen for the male brain

In addition to the male sex hormone testosterone, 17β-estradiol may also play a role in preserving certain functions in the male brain, although it has received far less research attention than in women. This notion can be supported by three levels of research findings. First, despite possible sex differences, as in the female brain, both estrogen receptor (ER)

Hormones, Cognition and Dementia: State of the Art and Emergent Therapeutic Strategies, ed. Eef Hogervorst, Victor W. Henderson, Robert B. Gibbs, and Roberta Diaz Brinton. Published by Cambridge University Press.
© Cambridge University Press 2009.

subtypes, ERα and ERβ, are abundantly expressed throughout the male brain [12, 13]. In particular, ERs are found co-localized with testosterone receptors in the areas essential for learning and memory [14]. Second, studies in rodent models demonstrated that developmental exposure to estrogen enhanced spatial learning in male rats [15]. Estrogen treatment protected against experimentally induced brain injuries in male mice [16, 17]. Third, clinical studies suggest a positive relationship between high serum levels of estrogen and certain cognitive functions in healthy elderly men [18]. The age-related loss of testosterone is associated with an increased risk of AD and it can be modified by testosterone supplementation partially via aromatization of testosterone to estrogen [19]. In patients with prostate cancer, estrogen treatment reversed the negative impact of androgen deprivation on memory performance [20]. In comparison with a more notable benefit of testosterone on working memory, as in the female brain, estrogen appears to offer a more favorable effect on verbal memory function in the male brain [19, 20]. Another clinical observation is that a 70-year-old man has a higher level of circulating estrogen, 3.5-fold more than the level in a 70-year-old female counterpart [21]. Despite the fact that it is too premature to draw conclusions at this stage, one can conceive that an overall lesser vulnerability to AD in older men (32% of AD cases) when compared to age-matched women (68% of AD cases) may be to some extent attributed to a much higher level of estrogens in older men [22]. Taken together, these findings support a positive role of estrogens in the male brain. However, given limited data and the fact that some studies presented discrepant results [23], more research will be needed to further investigate the sex-associated effects of estrogen alone or as a result of interaction with male sex hormones on the male brain.

Tissue-selective ER modulators and cognition

Despite the fact that timely use of ET has been associated with a cognition-promoting effect in both genders, long-term administration of ET can potentially cause health risks. An increased risk of breast cancer is a major concern for women who receive ET [24]. Moreover, induction of coagulation and fibrinolysis that could lead to stroke remains another serious threat to therapy recipients [7, 25, 26]. In recent years,

substantial research has focused on the development of a safe alternative approach that is non-feminizing but can realize estrogen's health-promoting benefits and potentially be used in both women and men. To date, there are two avenues that have been vigorously pursued. One focus has been placed on the development of tissue-selective ER modulators (SERMs) [22]. These compounds are characterized by exhibiting both estrogen agonist and antagonist activity dependent upon the gene promoter and target tissue being examined. There has been success in the use of SERMs for the prevention and treatment of breast cancer and postmenopausal osteoporosis; however, their impact on cognitive activity remains to be further investigated. Some preclinical studies suggest that clinically relevant SERMs may play a protective role in the brain [27, 28], while other studies did not see such a positive association [29]. A few clinical studies have been completed and results are mixed as well. The first trial conducted by Yaffe et al., the Multiple Outcomes of Raloxifene Evaluation (MORE) study, revealed that raloxifene treatment for three years did not affect overall cognitive scores in postmenopausal women with osteoporosis [30]. Further analyses revealed a favorable effect from a high dose, but not a low dose, of raloxifene in reducing the risk of cognitive impairment in these women [31]. Two other studies found no impact from raloxifene on short-term cognitive function in postmenopausal women [32, 33]. A few more studies, including the Cognition in the Study of Tamoxifen and Raloxifene (Co-STAR) and studies on newer SERMs in older women, are reported to be ongoing or have been completed but the results have not yet been made available. In addition to the investigations in women, it is suggested that raloxifene may also have a functional impact in the male brain, as demonstrated by studies where raloxifene was found to enhance brain activation during memory performance in healthy elderly men [34, 35]. Our laboratory recently discovered that ICI 182,780, a full estrogen antagonist in reproductive tissues, and its structural analogs acted as estrogenic agonists in hippocampal neurons, offering a new avenue of research for their potential application for the brain [36, 37]. However, due to the large molecular size and unfavorable physiochemical properties that may prohibit penetration of ICI 182,780 across the blood–brain barrier [38], to make these compounds to be brain accessible will be a major challenge down the road.

ERβ as a non-feminizing target for neurotrophism and neuroprotection

In recent years, along with the basic science advancements in understanding the mechanisms of estrogen action in the brain, ER subtype-selective SERMs have emerged as another avenue of research in the search for a safe estrogen alternative strategy. It is well documented that both ERα and ERβ are abundantly expressed in both female and male brains, and their roles could be overlapping and differential. As reviewed in our recent article [39], many studies including our own demonstrate that activation of either ERα or ERβ could contribute to neuroprotective outcomes and some elements of the underlying mechanisms [40, 41]. However, ERβ appears to have a broader involvement in mediating some aspects of estrogen-induced neuroprotective activities [42]. For instance, at the subcellular level, sustaining of mitochondrial function has been suggested as a convergent mechanism conveying estrogen's proactive defensive protection against neurodegeneration [43, 44], and ERβ serves as a major player in these dynamic processes [42]. Another example relates to our recent analyses where we found that ERβ, but not ERα, mediated estrogen regulation of mechanisms required for β-amyloid degradation in hippocampal neurons (unpublished data). In addition to roles associated with neuroprotection, ERβ is indicated to be crucial to brain development, neural plasticity, and regulation of estrogen promotion of hippocampus-dependent learning and memory in both genders [45–51]. An ERβ-selective therapy could be also potentially benefit APOE4 allele carriers, a population susceptible to AD [52]. In comparison with their impact with a large degree of overlaps in the brain, ERα and ERβ play more differential roles in reproductive systems. In females, ERα serves as the primary mediator of sexual development and modulation, whereas ERβ has a much smaller impact on these processes [39]. This differential regulation presents an opportunity for an ERβ-selective therapy to minimize ERα-mediated proliferative responses known to cause elevated risks for reproductive cancers in women [39]. In males, it is suggested that ERβ, the predominant ER in the prostate gland, regulates prostate growth by down-regulating androgen receptor expression. Therefore, an ERβ-selective therapy could also be potentially beneficial as an anti-proliferative agent for preventing prostate cancer in men.

Soy foods and soy extracts are not the same

Phytoestrogens are a diverse group of plant-derived and non-steroidal structural analogs of mammalian estrogens, and can bind at weak to moderate affinities to ERs and exert estrogenic or anti-estrogenic activities (see Chapter 13). In the last decade, increasing research interests in phytoestrogens have been attributed in part to indications of health-promoting effects of soy foods that are rich in phytoestrogens in Asian populations. A number of epidemiological studies suggest that the high dietary intake of phytoestrogen-enriched soy foods (20 to 80 mg/d) in Asians [53] may contribute to the low incidence of multiple sex hormones-related disorders such as menopausal hot flashes [54] and breast cancers [55, 56] in Asian women, and prostate cancers in Asian men [57], compared to the incidence in Westerners who consume a much smaller amount of phytoestrogens (<1 mg/d) [58]. The high habitual intake of phytoestrogen-enriched soy foods has also been linked to the lower prevalence of AD in Asia compared to the Western world. A summary of 22 epidemiological studies conducted in populations across continents reveals a 2.5-fold higher prevalence rate for AD in North America and Europe than in Japan and China, although the prevalence rates for vascular dementia were similar [59]. However, these positive observational findings lack confirmation from results derived from randomized and controlled human trials, which have been found to be inconsistent and inconclusive [59]. Of a total of seven human studies on soy-derived extract supplements conducted in postmenopausal women (published in 2000–7), four studies revealed a positive impact of soy extracts on select domains of cognitive function, while the others failed to show a significant effect [59]. The discrepant outcomes could be caused in part by potentially significant differences in the constitutive composition between the natural forms of soy foods and pharmacological preparations of soy extracts, and among soy extracts obtained from various sources. At present, a great deal of soy extract products are sold over the counter and most of these are advertised as dietary supplements for use by women to lessen menopausal symptoms such as hot flashes. However, according to the Dietary Supplement Health and Education Act passed by the US Congress in 1994, these supplements are unregulated by the Food and Drug Administration (FDA), leaving the public a serious lack of information about their safety and efficacy. In addition, there is no standardization as to how these soy extract preparations are processed. Therefore, results derived from one study can refer only to the specific soy preparation tested, and cannot be extrapolated to other preparations.

Development of an ERβ-selective phytoSERM formulation

Basic science research in determining the relationship between the use of phytoestrogens and brain functions has been mostly based upon exposures to either single phytoestrogens or soy diets that resemble the natural forms of soy intake in Asians. Since phytoestrogens are weak forms of estrogen-like molecules, it is no surprise to observe a small magnitude of neuroprotection in neurons when exposed to individual naturally occurring phytoestrogens compared to neurons exposed to 17β-estradiol [60]. Our recent study demonstrates that the limited estrogenic activity from individual phytoestrogens can be modified if used in combination [61]. In this study, we comparatively analyzed a number of neural responses induced by four ERβ-selective phytoestrogens when used singly or in combination in both primary neuronal cultures and animal treatment paradigms [61]. These analyses have led to our discovery of a combined formulation composed of equivalent molars of genistein, daidzein, and equol (the so-called ERβ-selective phytoSERM formulation), which exhibited a significantly increased ERβ-binding selectivity compared to individual molecules or other combined formulations, and, at a clinically relevant dosage, exerted significant activation of estrogenic responses in both primary neurons and neural tissues, with some responses greater than those induced by other test formulations [61]. Despite potent neural activities, this formulation did not exert an impact on the uterus. In contrast, 17β-estradiol induced a two-fold increase in uterine weight [61]. In the following analyses, we compared the long-term (9 months) impact of two custom design diets, the PhytoSERM formulation-containing diet and a commercial soy extract-containing diet, on general health and cognition in both normal but ovariectomized and triple-transgenic AD female mice. Preliminary results evidently revealed that treatment with the phytoSERM formulation-containing diet significantly promoted general health and spatial working memory performance in both normal and

transgenic AD mice. In addition, the PhytoSERM diet significantly reduced mortality and delayed the onset of AD-like neuropathological changes in the AD mice (unpublished data). By comparison, treatment with the soy extract-containing diet did not exert a detectable effect or had a negative impact on the same measures (unpublished data). These preclinical analyses provide compelling evidence in support of the potential therapeutic application of this ERβ-selective phytoSERM formulation as a promising estrogen alternative approach to promote cognitive health and potentially prevent other estrogen-related disorders in humans. As important, findings from these analyses predict that an ERβ-selective phytoSERM formulation could provide significant clinical advantages over soy extracts for the following two primary reasons.

First, an ERβ-selective phytoSERM formulation with a standardized composition would address the compositional complexity and potential antagonism present in soy extracts. Soy-derived extract preparations have been the most common form used in phytoestrogen intervention studies. However, as discussed earlier, there could exist significant variations in the constitutive composition among soy extracts obtained from different sources of soy plants and manufactured sources based upon different protocols [59]. An analysis of 33 commercial soy extracts revealed that there was an abundance of peaks of unknown origin found in many of the extracts [62]. Possible antagonistic chemicals present in soy extracts could come from many sources [59]. Some newly formed substances derived from the process of extraction could pose an undesirable effect to counteract the favorable health-giving properties of others. Conceivably, the antagonistic impact of these substances could diminish the overall effect and present an undetectable or undesirable clinical outcome. These analyses underlie a critical notion that the compositional complexity of a random mixture makes its safety and efficacy unpredictable. Instead, a rationally designed formulation with a standardized composition could maximize the therapeutic potential and lead to a clinically meaningful effect.

Second, inclusion of equol in a formulation would address the inter-individual variations in daidzein metabolism, and potentially benefit both equol producers and non-producers. Soy-derived phytoestrogens commonly exist as inactive but water-soluble glucosides (genistin and daidzin), which are converted to estrogenically active aglycons (genistein and daidzein) by intestinal glucosidases prior to absorption [63]. Unlike genistein and daidzein, equol is not of plant origin, yet can be exclusively produced through the metabolism of daidzein catalyzed by intestinal microbial flora following the intake of soy products [63]. In comparison with daidzein, equol has been demonstrated as a much stronger ER binder and more potent transcriptional inducer [64]. Interestingly, wide variations in the ability to produce equol from daidzein metabolism exist between rodents and humans, and across human populations. It has been found that almost all rodents can produce equol in large quantities. However, only about 20–35% of Western adults have such equol-producing phenotype [65, 66]. Based on this fact, it can be speculated that the equol-producing phenotype could serve as a critical modulator of human response to phytoestrogen treatment, that is, an enhanced response could occur in equol-producers as compared to non-producers. To date, a number of clinical studies have confirmed this hypothesis [67–69]. It may also hold true for a strong link between the many health benefits associated with phytoestrogen intake and the high prevalence of equol-producing phenotype in Asian populations, with approximately 55–60% as equol-producers [70, 71]. Therefore, the failure to take the inter-individual variations in equol-producing phenotype into account could be another major cause of the disparity in clinical outcomes across studies. One way to minimize these variations, while attaining equol-inducible health effects in both phenotypes, is to administer equol exogenously so that it can be accessible in both equol-producers and non-producers.

Conclusion

A large body of evidence indicates that estrogens may play a protective role in both female and male brains. On the other hand, long-term use of estrogens may cause health risks, notably in the reproductive and cardiovascular systems. In the last several years, in the search for a non-feminizing estrogen alternative that can mimic estrogen's cognition-promoting effects without eliciting adverse impact, two avenues of translational research have vigorously been pursued. Characterization of the neural activities in both preclinical and clinical settings revealed that some clinically relevant tissue-selective SERMs may induce some positive result. However, it is still premature to

draw a definite conclusion. Our recent finding that ICI 182,780 acts as an estrogen agonist in primary neurons offers a new translational opportunity. Another avenue of research has been based upon recent advancements in understanding ER subtypes in mediating estrogen's effects in specific tissues. Recent studies provide compelling evidence in support of ERβ as a non-feminizing therapeutic target for promotion of neurotrophism and neuroprotection. Our preclinical studies in both normal aging and transgenic AD animal models predict that an ERβ-selective phytoSERM formulation with a standardized composition could provide significant therapeutic advantages over commercial soy-based extracts whose uses have not been regulated. Results from these studies strongly suggest the necessity for further clinical validation.

Acknowledgments

The authors gratefully acknowledge the grant support from the Alzheimer Association to LZ, and the National Institute of Mental Health Chemical Synthesis and Drug Supply Program, the Kenneth T. and Eileen L. Norris Foundation, and Bensussen Gift Fund to RDB.

References

1. Shumaker SA, Legault C, Rapp SR, et al. Estrogen plus progestin and the incidence of dementia and mild cognitive impairment in postmenopausal women: the Women's Health Initiative Memory Study: a randomized controlled trial. *JAMA*. 2003;**289**:2651–62.

2. Shumaker SA, Legault C, Kuller LH, et al. Conjugated equine estrogens and incidence of probable dementia and mild cognitive impairment in postmenopausal women: the Women's Health Initiative Memory Study. *JAMA*. 2004;**291**:2947–58.

3. Espeland MA, Rapp SR, Shumaker SA, et al. Conjugated equine estrogens and global cognitive function in postmenopausal women: the Women's Health Initiative Memory Study. *JAMA*. 2004;**291**: 2959–68.

4. Rapp SR, Espeland MA, Shumaker SA, et al. Effect of estrogen plus progestin on global cognitive function in postmenopausal women: the Women's Health Initiative Memory Study: a randomized controlled trial. *JAMA*. 2003;**289**:2663–72.

5. American Academy of Neurology. Estrogen use before 65 linked to reduced risk of Alzheimer's disease. Available at: http://www.aan.com/press/indexcfm?

fuseaction=releaseview&release=471. Accessed July 3, 2008.

6. Manson JE, Allison MA, Rossouw JE, *et al.* Estrogen therapy and coronary-artery calcification. *N Engl J Med.* 2007;**356**:2591–602.

7. Rossouw JE, Prentice RL, Manson JE, *et al.* Postmenopausal hormone therapy and risk of cardiovascular disease by age and years since menopause. *JAMA.* 2007;**297**:1465–77.

8. Zandi PP, Anthony JC, Hayden KM, *et al.* Reduced incidence of AD with NSAID but not H2 receptor antagonists: the Cache County Study. *Neurology.* 2002;**59**:880–6.

9. MacLennan AH, Henderson VW, Paine BJ, *et al.* Hormone therapy, timing of initiation, and cognition in women aged older than 60 years: the REMEMBER pilot study. *Menopause.* 2006;**13**:28–36.

10. Brinton RD. Estrogen therapy for prevention of Alzheimer's disease not for rehabilitation following onset of disease: the healthy cell bias of estrogen action. In Baudry M, Bi R, Schreiber SS, eds. *Synaptic Plasticity: Basic Mechanisms to Clinical Applications.* New York: Taylor & Francis Group, 2004, pp. 131–57.

11. Brinton RD. Investigative models for determining hormone therapy-induced outcomes in brain: evidence in support of a healthy cell bias of estrogen action. *Ann N Y Acad Sci.* 2005;**1052**:57–74.

12. Prewitt AK, Wilson ME. Changes in estrogen receptor-alpha mRNA in the mouse cortex during development. *Brain Res.* 2007;**1134**:62–9.

13. Zhang JQ, Cai WQ, Zhou de S, *et al.* Distribution and differences of estrogen receptor beta immunoreactivity in the brain of adult male and female rats. *Brain Res.* 2002;**935**:73–80.

14. Yaden BC, Krishnan GV, Bryant HU, *et al.* Discovery and characterization of selective ERbeta agonist. *The Endocrine Society 87th Annual Meeting*, San Diego. 2005, pp. 3–295.

15. Corrieri L, Della Seta D, Canoine V, *et al.* Developmental exposure to xenoestrogen enhances spatial learning in male rats. *Horm Behav.* 2007;**51**:620–5.

16. Toung TJ, Traystman RJ, Hurn PD. Estrogen-mediated neuroprotection after experimental stroke in male rats. *Stroke.* 1998;**29**:1666–70.

17. McCullough LD, Alkayed NJ, Traystman RJ, *et al.* Postischemic estrogen reduces hypoperfusion and secondary ischemia after experimental stroke. *Stroke.* 2001;**32**:796–802.

18. Hogervorst E, De Jager C, Budge M, *et al.* Serum levels of estradiol and testosterone and performance in different cognitive domains in healthy elderly men and women. *Psychoneuroendocrinology.* 2004;**29**:405–21.

19. Cherrier MM, Matsumoto AM, Amory JK, *et al.* The role of aromatization in testosterone supplementation: effects on cognition in older men. *Neurology.* 2005; **64**:290–6.

20. Beer TM, Bland LB, Bussiere JR, *et al.* Testosterone loss and estradiol administration modify memory in men. *J Urol.* 2006;**175**:130–5.

21. Sayed Y, Taxel P. The use of estrogen therapy in men. *Curr Opin Pharmacol.* 2003;**3**:650–4.

22. Zhao L, O'Neill K, Brinton RD. Selective estrogen receptor modulators (SERMs) for the brain: current status and remaining challenges for developing NeuroSERMs. *Brain Res Brain Res Rev.* 2005;**49**: 472–93.

23. Taxel P, Stevens MC, Trahiotis M, *et al.* The effect of short-term estradiol therapy on cognitive function in older men receiving hormonal suppression therapy for prostate cancer. *J Am Geriatr Soc.* 2004;**52**:269–73.

24. Ravdin PM, Cronin KA, Howlader N, *et al.* The decrease in breast-cancer incidence in 2003 in the United States. *N Engl J Med.* 2007;**356**:1670–4.

25. Wassertheil-Smoller S, Hendrix SL, Limacher M, *et al.* Effect of estrogen plus progestin on stroke in postmenopausal women: the Women's Health Initiative: a randomized trial. *JAMA.* 2003;**289**: 2673–84.

26. Hendrix SL, Wassertheil-Smoller S, Johnson KC, *et al.* Effects of conjugated equine estrogen on stroke in the Women's Health Initiative. *Circulation.* 2006; **113**:2425–34.

27. Littleton-Kearney MT, Ostrowski NL, Cox DA, *et al.* Selective estrogen receptor modulators: tissue actions and potential for CNS protection. *CNS Drug Rev.* 2002; **8**:309–30.

28. Dhandapani KM, Brann DW. Protective effects of estrogen and selective estrogen receptor modulators in the brain. *Biol Reprod.* 2002;**67**:1379–85.

29. LaFerla FM. Calcium dyshomeostasis and intracellular signalling in Alzheimer's disease. *Nat Rev Neurosci.* 2002;**3**:862–72.

30. Yaffe K, Krueger K, Sarkar S, *et al.* Cognitive function in postmenopausal women treated with raloxifene. *N Engl J Med.* 2001;**344**:1207–13.

31. Yaffe K, Krueger K, Cummings SR, *et al.* Effect of raloxifene on prevention of dementia and cognitive impairment in older women: the Multiple Outcomes of Raloxifene Evaluation (MORE) randomized trial. *Am J Psychiatry.* 2005;**162**:683–90.

32. Buckwalter JG, Geiger AM, Parsons TD, *et al.* Cognitive effects of short-term use of raloxifene: a randomized clinical trial. *Int J Neurosci.* 2007;**117**: 1579–90.

33. Haskell SG, Richardson ED. The effect of raloxifene on cognitive function in postmenopausal women: a randomized clinical trial. *Conn Med.* 2004;**68**:355–8.

34. Goekoop R, Duschek EJ, Knol DL, *et al.* Raloxifene exposure enhances brain activation during memory performance in healthy elderly males; its possible relevance to behavior. *Neuroimage.* 2005;**25**:63–75.

35. Goekoop R, Barkhof F, Duschek EJ, *et al.* Raloxifene treatment enhances brain activation during recognition of familiar items: a pharmacological fMRI study in healthy elderly males. *Neuropsychopharmacology.* 2006;**31**:1508–18.

36. Zhao L, Jin C, Mao Z, *et al.* Design, synthesis, and estrogenic activity of a novel estrogen receptor modulator – a hybrid structure of 17beta-estradiol and vitamin E in hippocampal neurons. *J Med Chem.* 2007;**50**:4471–81.

37. Zhao L, O'Neill K, Brinton RD. Estrogenic agonist activity of ICI 182,780 (Faslodex) in hippocampal neurons: implications for basic science understanding of estrogen signaling and development of estrogen modulators with a dual therapeutic profile. *J Pharmacol Exp Ther.* 2006;**319**:1124–32.

38. Howell A, Osborne CK, Morris C, *et al.* ICI 182,780 (Faslodex): development of a novel, "pure" antiestrogen. *Cancer.* 2000;**89**:817–25.

39. Zhao L, Brinton RD. Estrogen receptor beta as a therapeutic target for promotion of neurogenesis and prevention of neurodegeneration. *Drug Dev Res.* 2006;**66**:103–17.

40. Zhao L, Brinton RD. Estrogen receptor alpha and beta differentially regulate intracellular Ca$^{(2+)}$ dynamics leading to ERK phosphorylation and estrogen neuroprotection in hippocampal neurons. *Brain Res.* 2007;**1172**:48–59.

41. Zhao L, Wu T-W, Brinton RD. Estrogen receptor subtypes alpha and beta contribute to neuroprotection and increased Bcl-2 expression in primary hippocampal neurons. *Brain Res.* 2004;**1010**:22–34.

42. Simpkins JW, Yang SH, Sarkar SN, *et al.* Estrogen actions on mitochondria – physiological and pathological implications. *Mol Cell Endocrinol.* 2008;**290**(1/2):51–9.

43. Simpkins JW, Dykens JA. Mitochondrial mechanisms of estrogen neuroprotection. *Brain Res Rev.* 2008;**57**:421–30.

44. Nilsen J, Brinton RD. Mitochondria as therapeutic targets of estrogen action in the central nervous system. *Curr Drug Targets CNS Neurol Disord.* 2004;**3**:297–313.

45. Wang L, Andersson S, Warner M, *et al.* Estrogen receptor (ER) beta knockout mice reveal a role for ERbeta in migration of cortical neurons in the developing brain. *Proc Natl Acad Sci USA.* 2003; **100**:703–8.

46. Wang L, Andersson S, Warner M, *et al.* Morphological abnormalities in the brains of estrogen receptor beta knockout mice. *Proc Natl Acad Sci USA.* 2001;**98**:2792–6.

47. Rissman EF, Heck AL, Leonard JE, *et al.* Disruption of estrogen receptor beta gene impairs spatial learning in female mice. *Proc Natl Acad Sci USA.* 2002;**99**: 3996–4001.

48. Day M, Sung A, Logue S, *et al.* Beta estrogen receptor knockout (BERKO) mice present attenuated hippocampal CA1 long-term potentiation and related memory deficits in contextual fear conditioning. *Behav Brain Res.* 2005;**164**:128–31.

49. Liu F, Day M, Muniz LC, *et al.* Activation of estrogen receptor-beta regulates hippocampal synaptic plasticity and improves memory. *Nat Neurosci.* 2008;**11**:334–43.

50. Fan X, Warner M, Gustafsson JA. Estrogen receptor beta expression in the embryonic brain regulates development of calretinin-immunoreactive GABAergic interneurons. *Proc Natl Acad Sci USA.* 2006;**103**:19338–43.

51. Walf AA, Frye CA. Rapid and estrogen receptor beta mediated actions in the hippocampus mediate some functional effects of estrogen. *Steroids.* 2008; **73**:997–1007.

52. Wang JM, Irwin RW, Brinton RD. Activation of estrogen receptor alpha increases and estrogen receptor beta decreases apolipoprotein E expression in hippocampus in vitro and in vivo. *Proc Natl Acad Sci USA.* 2006;**103**:16983–8.

53. Rice MM, LaCroix AZ, Lampe JW, *et al.* Dietary soy isoflavone intake in older Japanese American women. *Public Health Nutr.* 2001;**4**:943–52.

54. Maskarinec S. The effect of phytoestrogens on hot flashes. *Nutrition Bytes.* 2003;**9**:Article 5.

55. Ziegler RG. Phytoestrogens and breast cancer. *Am J Clin Nutr.* 2004;**79**:183–4.

56. Henderson BE, Bernstein L. The international variation in breast cancer rates: an epidemiological assessment. *Breast Cancer Res Treat.* 1991;**18**(Suppl 1):S11–7.

57. Goetzl MA, Van Veldhuizen PJ, Thrasher JB. Effects of soy phytoestrogens on the prostate. *Prostate Cancer Prostatic Dis.* 2007;**10**:216–23.

58. de Kleijn MJ, van der Schouw YT, Wilson PW, *et al.* Intake of dietary phytoestrogens is low in postmenopausal women in the United States: the Framingham study. *J Nutr.* 2001;**131**:1826–32.

59. Zhao L, Brinton RD. WHI and WHIMS follow-up and human studies of soy isoflavones on cognition. *Expert Rev Neurother.* 2007;**7**:1549–64.

60. Zhao L, Chen Q, Brinton RD. Neuroprotective and neurotrophic efficacy of phytoestrogens in cultured hippocampal neurons. *Exp Biol Med.* 2002;**227**:509–19.

61. Zhao L, Mao Z, Brinton RD. A select combination of clinically relevant phytoestrogens enhances estrogen receptor beta-binding selectivity and neuroprotective activities in vitro and in vivo. *Endocrinology.* 2009;**150**:770–83.

62. Setchell KD, Brown NM, Desai P, *et al.* Bioavailability of pure isoflavones in healthy humans and analysis of commercial soy isoflavone supplements. *J Nutr.* 2001;**131**(4 Suppl):1362S–75S.

63. Setchell KD, Borriello SP, Hulme P, *et al.* Nonsteroidal estrogens of dietary origin: possible roles in hormone-dependent disease. *Am J Clin Nutr.* 1984;**40**:569–78.

64. Morito K, Hirose T, Kinjo J, *et al.* Interaction of phytoestrogens with estrogen receptors alpha and beta. *Biol Pharm Bull.* 2001;**24**:351–6.

65. Setchell KD, Brown NM, Lydeking-Olsen E. The clinical importance of the metabolite equol – a clue to the effectiveness of soy and its isoflavones. *J Nutr.* 2002;**132**:3577–84.

66. Atkinson C, Frankenfeld CL, Lampe JW. Gut bacterial metabolism of the soy isoflavone daidzein: exploring the relevance to human health. *Exp Biol Med.* 2005; **230**:155–70.

67. Frankenfeld CL, McTiernan A, Thomas WK, *et al.* Postmenopausal bone mineral density in relation to soy isoflavone-metabolizing phenotypes. *Maturitas.* 2006;**53**:315–24.

68. Niculescu MD, Pop EA, Fischer LM, *et al.* Dietary isoflavones differentially induce gene expression changes in lymphocytes from postmenopausal women who form equol as compared with those who do not. *J Nutr Biochem.* 2007;**18**:380–90.

69. Wu J, Oka J, Ezaki J, *et al.* Possible role of equol status in the effects of isoflavone on bone and fat mass in postmenopausal Japanese women: a double-blind, randomized, controlled trial. *Menopause.* 2007;**14**:866–74.

70. Akaza H, Miyanaga N, Takashima N, *et al.* Comparisons of percent equol producers between prostate cancer patients and controls: case-controlled studies of isoflavones in Japanese, Korean and American residents. *Jpn J Clin Oncol.* 2004;**34**:86–9.

71. Arai Y, Uehara M, Sato Y, *et al.* Comparison of isoflavones among dietary intake, plasma concentration and urinary excretion for accurate estimation of phytoestrogen intake. *J Epidemiol.* 2000;**10**: 127–35.

Progesterone regulation of neuroprotective estrogen actions

Christian J. Pike and Jenna C. Carroll

Editors' introduction

Estrogen-based therapies often include a progestin to antagonize tumorigenic effects of estrogens in the uterus. While much has been learned about the functional and neuroprotective effects of estrogens in the brain, far less is known about the effects of progestins, particularly specific progestins like progesterone and medroxy-progesterone acetate, used either alone or in combination with estrogenic therapies. In this chapter, Pike and Carroll review many of the effects on cell survival and function, first of estrogens, and then of progestins. While not all progestins are alike, the authors find that prolonged exposure to progestins often will decrease the protective effects of estradiol on cell survival and function. Evidence suggests that a cyclical regimen of estradiol and progesterone may be most efficacious. Ultimately, the development of neural selective estrogen receptor modulators (SERMs) with the potential to circumvent the need for, and hence the negative neural consequences of, progesterone will be an important advance to estrogen-based therapies.

Introduction

Abundant evidence implicates the sex steroid depletion associated with menopause as a risk-factor for the development of Alzheimer's disease (AD) in women, and the use of estrogen-based hormone therapy (HT) with reducing this risk [1, 2]. These observations in women are complemented by findings from experimental paradigms that demonstrate a range of neural actions of estrogens, and to a lesser extent progestins, which predict a protective role against development of AD-related neuropathology. However, the recent Women's Health Initiative (WHI) clinical trial surprisingly found neutral

or adverse rather than protective effects with respect to cognition and dementia in postmenopausal women treated with the most commonly utilized HT composed of conjugated equine estrogen (CEE) + medroxy-progesterone acetate (MPA) [3]. The WHI findings have led both clinical and basic researchers to re-examine the role of sex steroid hormones in AD. In the past few years, numerous issues have been raised that may significantly affect the efficacy of HT and may underlie the current confusion in our understanding of the relationship between sex steroid hormones and AD. In this chapter, we discuss one of these issues: the interactions between estrogens and progestins and how these interactions affect neuroprotective actions.

We will review and discuss basic research findings concerning the neural actions of estrogens and progestins, both alone and in combination, that are relevant to their proposed protective role against age-related cognitive decline and development of AD. Although beneficial actions of estrogens in the brain are well established, the direct neural effects of progestins and how they modulate estrogenic actions are not well understood. The consensus of basic research findings suggest that both estrogens and progestins have independent protective actions, but that these benefits are often negated rather than enhanced by combined treatment. Greater understanding of these hormone interactions is essential in order to optimize HT for effective use in the prevention of AD and related neurodegenerative disorders.

Beneficial effects of estrogens in the brain

The two primary classes of female sex steroid hormones, estrogens and progestins, have been well recognized not only for their classic roles in reproductive functions, but also for their actions on other hormone-responsive tissues such as bone and the cardiovascular system. The brain, with its broad distribution of estrogen receptors (ER) and progesterone receptors (PR) and diverse responses to estrogens and progestins, is increasingly appreciated as a hormone-responsive tissue. Estradiol, the primary endogenous estrogen, induces a wide range of beneficial actions in the brain that enhance neural functions and protect the brain, suggesting that estrogens may provide a possible therapeutic avenue for AD [4]. In parallel, estradiol also increases rodent behavioral performance in tasks dependent upon hippocampus and frontal cortex, such as delayed-match-to-position, T-maze, spontaneous alternation in the Y-maze, radial arm maze, and Morris water maze [5]. Estrogenic effects on cognition likely are mediated by several mechanisms, with the most significant actions involving synaptic plasticity. For example, estradiol increases the number of dendritic spines and spine synapses [6], synaptic excitability [7], enhances long-term potentiation [8], cholinergic function [9], and neurogenesis [10].

In addition to regulating cognition and neural plasticity, estrogens can also increase resilience against neurodegenerative diseases including AD. For example, estradiol can reduce astrogliosis associated with injury and brain aging [11] and inhibit the hyperphosphorylation of tau [12] that is linked to neurofibrillary tangle formation. For the purposes of this review, we will focus primarily on two important protective actions of estrogens, promotion of neuron viability and decreased accumulation of β-amyloid (Aβ), the protein widely implicated as a causal factor in AD pathogenesis.

Estrogens regulate neuron viability

Estrogens increase neuron viability in numerous cell culture and animal models of injury [4]. In primary neuronal, explant, organotypic, and neural cell line cultures, physiological concentrations of estradiol reduce injury associated with several types of toxic insults including serum deprivation, oxidative stress, glutamate, and Aβ. Similarly, estradiol provides protection against neuronal injury in vivo from a variety of challenges, including animal models of excitotoxic injury, stroke, and idiopathic Parkinson's disease. The broad range of neuroprotective actions suggests that estrogens may be important modulators of neuron viability in homeostatic conditions as well as under challenge from toxic conditions associated with age-related neurodegenerative diseases.

Several cellular and molecular mechanisms contribute to estrogenic neuroprotection. For example, in some paradigms estradiol neuroprotection appears to be mediated by non-classical steroid hormone mechanisms involving rapid induction of cell signaling pathways including protein kinase C, extracellular signal regulated kinase, and phosphoinositol-3-kinase. Through both rapid signaling pathways and classic genomic signaling, estradiol can also increase neuron viability by altering expression of proteins involved in regulation of cell death including pro- and anti-apoptotic members of the Bcl-2 family [13]. Both ER subtypes, ERα and ERβ, are implicated in mediating estrogenic neuroprotection. Further, increasing evidence suggests that these protective pathways may be activated not only by gonadally derived and exogenously applied hormone but also by de novo estrogen synthesis in the brain.

Estrogens regulate β-amyloid accumulation

In addition to widespread neuroprotective actions potentially relevant to many neurodegenerative conditions, estrogens also exert protective actions that are relatively disease specific. In the case of AD, an important protective estrogenic action is inhibition of Aβ accumulation. Alzheimer's disease pathogenesis is thought to be initiated and driven, at least in part, by elevated levels of Aβ that both aggregate into toxic soluble oligomers and deposit into extracellular plaques in hippocamal formation, frontal cortex, and other brain regions involved in learning and memory. In neuronal cell culture, estradiol reduces levels of secreted Aβ by altering the processing and/or trafficking of the amyloid precursor protein [14]. In animal models, depletion of endogenous estrogens and progestins by ovariectomy (OVX) in guinea pigs resulted in a significant increase in soluble Aβ levels in brain [15]. Estradiol treatment of OVX guinea pigs reduced Aβ levels, thus establishing a role for estrogens as endogenous regulators of Aβ accumulation. Similar results have been observed in several transgenic mouse models of AD [16, 17, 18]; however, experimental manipulation of estrogen status does not affect Aβ accumulation in all AD mouse models [19, 20, 21]. It is unclear why levels of estrogens are associated with Aβ accumulation in some models but not others. There are several factors that vary across the studies and may contribute to the inconsistent findings, including differences in animal models and strains, quantification of Aβ, and parameters of estradiol treatments (e.g., dose, timing). Perhaps most intriguing is the potential role of circulating versus brain levels of hormones. Although estrogens and progestins are produced predominantly in the ovaries, *de novo* steroidogenesis in the brain is also an important source of estrogens, progestins, and other hormones [22]. Yue and colleagues [21] reported that although OVX-induced hormone depletion did not affect Aβ levels in the APP23 mouse model, inhibiting neural production of estrogens by introducing aromatase knockout into the APP23 mice resulted in elevated Aβ levels. Thus, estrogenic regulation of Aβ may depend primarily upon brain levels of estrogens, which may depend on both ovarian and brain steroid production.

Effects of progestins in the brain

Since levels of both estrogens and progestins naturally fluctuate in women across the ovarian cycle, understanding estrogenic actions must include consideration of progestins. Further, estrogen-based HT typically includes a progestin component to antagonize tumorigenic effects of estrogens in uterus. Thus, although HT effects are typically attributed to the estrogenic component, progestins also contribute to HT responses. Unfortunately, in contrast to the well established effects of estradiol in the brain, the neural actions of progesterone are rather poorly understood. In the past few years, an increasing focus on progestin neurobiology has begun to define its effects on cognition and neural plasticity and to elucidate its neural cell signaling pathways [23]. Here, we briefly review the emerging literature linking progestins with regulation of two key parameters of AD neuropathology: neuron viability and accumulation of Aβ.

Progestins regulate neuron viability

The actions of progestins in the brain have been perhaps most studied in various in vitro and in vivo models of neuroprotection [24]. Like estradiol, progesterone has been reported to induce neuroprotection directly in some but not all cell culture models of neurodegeneration. For example, in cultured hippocampal neurons, progesterone but not MPA reduced excitotoxicity induced by glutamate exposure [25].

Also similar to estradiol, progesterone induces several neuroprotective cell signaling pathways, including activation of Akt [26] and ERK [25, 27], and up-regulation of anti-apoptotic protein Bcl-2 [25].

In animal models, progestins induce neuroprotection against several but not all challenges. Progesterone treatment has been shown to reduce neural injury and/or neuron death associated with traumatic brain injury [28, 29], spinal cord injury [30], ischemia [31, 32], and seizure models [33]. However, conflicting studies suggest an absence of progesterone neuroprotection in some related injury models, which hints that progesterone likely exerts less general and or less robust neuroprotection than does estradiol. Furthermore, similar to findings in cell culture studies, protective effects of progesterone in vivo are mimicked by only some progestins, findings that may provide mechanistic insight [34]. For example, the protective effects of progesterone, certain progesterone metabolites, and some progestins against neural injury induced by pilocarpine, kainate, and other seizure-inducing toxins likely reflects anxiolytic effects resulting from modulation of the GABA$_A$ receptor. The extent to which these pathways of progesterone neuroprotection may synergize with protective estrogen-mediated cell signaling remains to be fully elucidated.

Progestin regulation of β-amyloid accumulation

In contrast to the established Aβ-lowering effects of estradiol, the effect of progestins on Aβ accumulation is largely unknown. Because OVX-induced depletion of estrogens and progestins in wild type rodents and some mouse models of AD results in elevated Aβ levels, it is reasonable to speculate that the loss of endogenous progesterone may contribute to disruption in steady state Aβ levels. Further, estradiol treatment of OVX rodents often only partially reverses the increase in Aβ, perhaps suggesting that progesterone may be needed to complement estradiol action and fully reduce Aβ levels. However, in the only published study to directly assess the effect of progesterone on Aβ accumulation, our research group found no evidence that progesterone directly regulates Aβ levels. We observed that OVX was associated with a robust increase in Aβ accumulation in the hippocampal formation and frontal cortex in the 3xTg-AD mouse model of AD, but that continuous progesterone

103

treatment for three months in OVX female mice did not significantly affect Aβ accumulation [16]. Interestingly, in this same study we found that progesterone reduces a related form of AD neuropathology, tau hyperphosphorylation. Using the antibody AT-8 that recognizes a specific pathology-associated type of phosphorylated tau, we found that progesterone treatment in OVX 3xTg-AD mice strongly reduced tau pathology to levels even below those in gonadally intact 3xTg-AD mice [16]. Certainly, additional studies are necessary to more thoroughly investigate the potential role of progesterone in regulating Aβ and tau pathologies.

Interactive effects of estrogens and progestins in the brain

Because HT usually consists of both estrogenic and progestin components, clinical and basic science researchers have increasingly realized the importance of understanding not only the individual actions of estrogens and progestins but also their interactive effects. As outlined above, compelling experimental evidence indicates numerous protective actions of estradiol and progesterone when delivered independently. Comparatively less is known about interactions between estrogens and progestins when they are administered together, but accumulating observations indicate that progestins often antagonize rather than synergize with protective estrogenic actions. For example, clinical observations suggest that the progestin MPA may negate beneficial effects of CEE on cognitive function in elderly women [35]. As discussed below, data from cell culture and animal models create a pattern suggesting that the continuous combined treatment of estrogens and progestins, which is common to current HT regimens, often fails to maximize the neuroprotective potential of these hormones.

Interactive effects of estrogens and progestins: neuron viability

Although several basic science studies have investigated interactive effects of estradiol and progesterone on beneficial neural effects, relatively few focused specifically on neuron viability. One example is a recent study by our research group in which we compared the effects of estradiol, progesterone, and MPA, alone and in combination, on neuronal death induced by the excitotoxic agent kainate. Young adult female Sprague-Dawley rats were OVX and treated continuously with hormones for two weeks, then lesioned by systemic kainate exposure. In comparison to the OVX group, OVX animals treated with estradiol showed a significant increase in survival of hilar neurons. In contrast, neither progesterone nor MPA treatments significantly affected neuron survival. Significantly, when estradiol treatment was combined with either progesterone or MPA, significant neuroprotection was no longer observed [33]. Our research group recently replicated this finding in middle-aged, reproductively senescent rats. We observed that in middle-aged (14 months old) female rats, continuous estradiol treatment for two weeks significantly increased neuron survival relative to the matched, vehicle-treated OVX group. Consistent with our observations in young adult rats, progesterone treatment in OVX rats was not neuroprotective, and when replaced in combination with estradiol, it blocked the neuroprotective effect of estradiol [52]. Interestingly, acute co-treatment with progesterone did not reduce neuroprotection induced by acute estradiol treatment in a similar lesion model [36], suggesting that timing parameters (e.g., length of treatment and continuous versus cyclic exposure) may be key determinants of hormone interactions.

Our observations in the kainate lesion model parallel findings from other paradigms in which continuous progestin treatment often antagonizes beneficial neural actions of estrogens. For example, continuous progesterone treatment for four months in aged female rats blocked estradiol up-regulation of the neurotrophic factors brain derived neurotrophic factor, nerve growth factor, and neurotrophin 3 [37]. In a similar treatment paradigm with middle-aged rats, progesterone inhibited estradiol-mediated increases in spatial memory performance [38]. A partial list of studies that investigated interactive effects of estradiol and progesterone on beneficial neural actions in animal models is shown in Table 11.1. Taken together, these studies suggest that in several paradigms, progestins can block the protective effects of estrogens. The mechanisms underlying progestin antagonism of estrogen protection are not known. However, recent cell culture data from our laboratory demonstrate that progesterone strongly reduces neuronal expression of both ERα and ERβ, which is paralleled in

Table 11.1 Comparison of neural effects induced by estradiol versus estradiol with progesterone in animal models.

Reference	Experimental model	Hormone treatments (timing and duration)	Estradiol effect	Estradiol + progesterone effect
Woolley and McEwen, 1993 [39]	3-month-old rats	Acute; 1 day	Increase spine density	Block estradiol effect
Garcia-Segura et al., 1998 [49]	2-month-old rats	Acute; 1 day	Increase Bcl-2 expression	Block estradiol effect
Gibbs, 2000 [43]	~3-month-old rats	Continuous and cyclic; 2 weeks	Increase ChAT activity and high affinity choline uptake	Cyclic progesterone: increase estradiol effect; continuous progesterone: block estradiol effect
Bimonte-Nelson, Nelson, and Granholm, 2004 [37]	24-month-old rats	Continuous; 4 months	Increase neurotrophin expression	Block estradiol effect
Rosario, Ramsden, and Pike, 2006 [50]	3-month-old rats	Continuous; 2 weeks	Increase neuron viability	Block estradiol effect
Bimonte-Nelson et al., 2006 [38]	12-month-old rats	Estradiol: continuous, cyclic. Progesterone: continuous; 4 months	Increase spatial memory	Block estradiol effect
Harburger, Bennett, and Frick, 2007 [51]	22-month-old mice	Acute; 1 day	Increase spatial memory	Block estradiol effect
Carroll et al., 2007 [16]	6-month-old AD mice	Continuous; 3 months	Decrease β-amyloid accumulation	Block estradiol effect

a time-dependent manner by decreases in estradiol-mediated genomic action and neuroprotection [53].

Importantly, progestins can also interact with estrogens in an additive manner to increase beneficial neural signaling. One example of this is hormonal regulation of spine density in the hippocampus, which is important to synaptic connectivity and hippocampal function. In female rats, spine density fluctuates across the estrus cycle and is significantly reduced by OVX, implicating regulatory roles for estrogens and or progestins [39]. Ovariectomized rats treated with estradiol show increased spine density. Interestingly, brief treatment (2–6 hours) with progesterone augments the estradiol increase in spine density, but more prolonged progesterone treatment (18 hours) blocks the beneficial estradiol effect [39]. Perhaps not unexpectedly, other in vitro and in vivo studies evaluating interactive effects of estradiol and progesterone on spine density have reported both additive and antagonistic results [40, 41, 42].

Additional studies in animal models also support the concept that progestins can positively or negatively affect beneficial actions of estrogens depending in part on parameters of hormone treatment. An example concerns functional regulation by estrogens of cholinergic pathways including projections from basal forebrain to cortex and hippocampus, pathways that exhibit decreased function in AD. Several studies by Gibbs and colleagues have demonstrated that OVX decreases behavioral and biochemical properties of this pathway and that short-term treatment with estradiol and progesterone can improve cholinergic function [9] (discussed in Chapter 5). In one study of estradiol and progesterone interactions [43], Gibbs found that maximal hormone benefit on cholinergic function resulted from cyclic administration of estradiol and progesterone, exceeding the individual benefits of estradiol and progesterone. Of particular interest was his observation that continuous combined treatment with estradiol and progesterone typically yielded

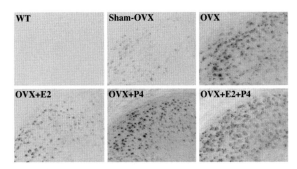

Fig. 11.1 β-amyloid (Aβ) accumulation in female 3xTg-AD mice is regulated by estradiol (E$_2$) and progesterone. Ovariectomy (OVX) induced hormone depletion increases Aβ accumulation, an effect that is reversed by continuous treatment with estradiol (OVX+E$_2$) but not progesterone (OVX+P4). The protective effect of estradiol is antagonized by continuous co-treatment with progesterone (OVX+E$_2$+P4). Images show Aβ immunoreactivity in subiculum of non-transgenic, wild-type (WT), and 3xTg-AD animals at age six months.

the lowest function. In summary, studies on the interaction between estrogens and progestins in animal models suggest that neural benefits of hormone treatment may be maximized by repeated brief cycles of estrogens and progestins and minimized by continuous combined treatment.

Interactive effects of estrogens and progestins: β-amyloid accumulation

Although relatively little information exists on the interactions between estrogens and progestins on regulation of AD-related neuropathology such as Aβ accumulation, recent findings from our research group appear consistent with the concept that continuous progestins can antagonize protective estrogenic actions. In a recently published study, we investigated the individual and combined effects of estradiol and progesterone on the development of neuropathology and behavioral deficits in the 3xTg-AD mouse model of AD [16]. Young adult (3 months of age) female 3xTg-AD mice were OVX and treated continuously for three months with hormone treatments or placebo, then were assessed for Aβ accumulation, tau hyperphosphorylation, and hippocampal-dependent behavioral impairments. We observed that OVX-induced depletion of sex steroid hormones in female 3xTg-AD mice significantly increased Aβ accumulation and worsened memory performance. Treatment of OVX 3xTg-AD mice with estradiol, but not progesterone, prevented these effects. The most

significant finding of this study was that combining progesterone with estradiol treatment blocked the Aβ-lowering effect of the estrogen (Fig. 11.1). Progesterone significantly reduced tau hyperphosphorylation to levels even lower than sham OVX animals when delivered either alone or in combination with estradiol. Thus, consistent with findings in other animal models, these data suggest that although progesterone can exert independent protective actions it can also attenuate effects of estradiol relevant to protection from development of AD.

Future directions

Findings from the WHI trial strongly challenged the notion that estrogen-based HT can effectively reduce the risk of AD and improve age-related deficits in cognition. In response to these data, both basic science and clinical researchers continue to rigorously reanalyze not only the guiding hypothesis that estrogens exert clinically significant protective neural actions in aging women, but also the underlying mechanisms of hormone action and interaction that undoubtedly impact HT efficacy. In this chapter, we have reviewed just one of these critical mechanistic issues, the interactions between estrogens and progestins in promoting neural function and protecting against age-related neurodegenerative diseases such as AD. Experimental data clearly support independent effects of both estrogens and progestins. However, a significant concern is our relative lack of knowledge about how estrogens and progestins interact and the consequences on hormone protective effects. A common but not universal observation has been that prolonged, continuous exposure to progestins can attenuate protective estrogenic actions. However, more limited but nonetheless compelling observations suggest that repeated intermittent progestin delivery not only avoids reduction of estrogenic action but also may enhance it. In order to optimize HT, we suggest two areas that future basic research should pursue that build upon the emerging concepts of estrogen–progestin interactions.

Cyclic versus continuous progestin treatment

Natural or synthetic progestins are viewed as a necessary component of HT owing to their ability to reduce the risk of endometrial cancer associated with the use of estrogens. Given the apparent necessity of progestins in HT, one area of future research must include optimization of HT administration that maximizes benefits and minimizes deleterious consequences associated with estrogen and progestin interactions. Clues provided by the research described above support a strategy of cyclic hormone delivery rather than the continuous, combined treatment that is currently common to HT. The cyclic versus continuous treatment strategy is a key design feature of two ongoing clinical studies of HT, the Kronos Early Estrogen Prevention Study (KEEPS) (discussed in Chapter 7) and the Early versus Late Intervention Trial with Estradiol (ELITE).

Although clinical investigation is certainly needed, also lacking is sufficient understanding of estrogen and progestin interactions at a basic neurobiological level to rationally design cyclic hormone regimens with desired protection against AD-relevant endpoints. Towards this end, our laboratory and others have formed a multi-group collaborative research team that is investigating timing and dosing parameters in cyclic and continuous estradiol, progesterone, and clinically relevant progestin treatment regimens in young adult and aged wild type rats and 3xTg-AD mice. Of particular interest is an ongoing study in which we are comparing the effects of continuous and cyclic progesterone paired with continuous estradiol in female 3xTg-AD mice on measures of Aβ accumulation, tau hyperphosphorylation, and behavior. Our prior data found that continuous progesterone blocked the Aβ-lowering effect of estradiol. However, we hypothesize that cyclic progesterone may further support Aβ reductions while also inhibiting tau phosphorylation. We believe that the continued evaluation of hormone treatments in animal models of AD will yield important insights into the design of future HT regimens that will safely and effectively reduce the development of AD in postmenopausal women.

Neuroactive selective estrogen receptor modulators (SERMs)

An alternative strategy to circumvent the apparent negative neural consequences of progesterone is to pursue the development of new synthetic estrogens that selectively target the brain and thus would have limited deleterious effects systemically. There are already numerous estrogenic compounds in experimental and clinical use. These compounds, collectively termed SERMs, exhibit tissue-specific agonist and antagonist effects on ER-dependent estrogenic actions. Conceptually, an ideal SERM would mimic protective neural actions of estrogens but not act on peripheral estrogen-responsive tissues such as the breast and uterus. Although a "neuroSERM" has yet to be developed [44], the SERM raloxifene, which has estrogen agonist effect in bone but not breast, may protect against the development of dementia [45]. Two interesting SERMs are propylpyrazole triol (PPT) and diarylpropionitrile (DPN), which exhibit relative selectivity for ERα and ERβ, respectively. Recent work has shown that both PPT and DPN mimic estrogenic neuroprotection in cultured neurons [46, 47]. In female 3xTg-AD mice, PPT but not DPN was comparable to estradiol in reducing the acceleration of Aβ accumulation and behavioral deficits caused by OVX [48]. These findings provide initial evidence of beneficial actions of SERMs in protecting the brain and support the continued development and investigation of neuroactive SERMs as an alternative strategy to HT in preventing and perhaps treating age-related neurodegenerative disorders.

In summary, recent controversies with the clinical use of HT have resulted in a re-evaluation of many important parameters associated with hormone action and treatment. Important issues include but are not limited to a critical window of therapeutic opportunity, formulation of HT, routes of administration, and interactive effects of estrogens and progestins. Accumulating evidence demonstrates that although estradiol and progesterone can independently induce a broad range of actions that are beneficial and protective to the brain, their combined use often results in diminished rather than enhanced actions. By focusing on endpoints such as neuron viability and Aβ accumulation that are relevant to brain aging and AD pathogenesis, it is anticipated that future research will be able to optimize combined estrogen- and progesterone-based HT and develop novel estrogenic SERM compounds that will prove effective in improving cognition and reducing neurodegenerative disease in aging women.

Acknowledgment

This work was supported by NIH grant P01 AG026572 (Roberta Diaz Brinton), Project 5 (CJP). JCC was supported by NIH grant AG032233.

References

1. Henderson VW, Paganini-Hill A, Miller BL, *et al.* Estrogen for Alzheimer's disease in women: randomized, double-blind, placebo-controlled trial. *Neurology.* 2000;**54**(2):295–301.

2. Simpkins JW, Yang SH, Wen Y, Singh M. Estrogens, progestins, menopause and neurodegeneration: basic and clinical studies. *Cell Mol Life Sci.* 2005;**62**(3):271–80.

3. Shumaker SA, Legault C, Rapp SR, *et al.* Estrogen plus progestin and the incidence of dementia and mild cognitive impairment in postmenopausal women: the Women's Health Initiative Memory Study: a randomized controlled trial. *JAMA.* 2003;**289**(20):2651–62.

4. Wise PM. Estrogens and neuroprotection. *Trends Endocrinol Metab.* 2002;**13**(6):229–30.

5. Sherwin BB, Henry JF. Brain aging modulates the neuroprotective effects of estrogen on selective aspects of cognition in women: a critical review. *Front Neuroendocrinol.* 2008;**29**(1):88–113.

6. Woolley CS, McEwen BS. Estradiol regulates hippocampal dendritic spine density via an N-methyl-D-aspartate receptor-dependent mechanism. *J Neurosci.* 1994;**14**(12):7680–7.

7. Wong M, Moss RL. Long-term and short-term electrophysiological effects of estrogen on the synaptic properties of hippocampal CA1 neurons. *J Neurosci.* 1992;**12**(8):3217–25.

8. Bi R, Broutman G, Foy MR, Thompson RF, Baudry M. The tyrosine kinase and mitogen-activated protein kinase pathways mediate multiple effects of estrogen in hippocampus. *Proc Natl Acad Sci USA.* 2000;**97**(7):3602–7.

9. Gibbs RB. Oestrogen and the cholinergic hypothesis: implications for oestrogen replacement therapy in postmenopausal women. *Novartis Found Symp.* 2000;**230**:94–107; discussion 107–11.

10. Galea LA, Spritzer MD, Barker JM, Pawluski JL. Gonadal hormone modulation of hippocampal neurogenesis in the adult. *Hippocampus.* 2006;**16**(3):225–32.

11. Struble RG, Nathan BP, Cady C, Cheng X, McAsey M. Estradiol regulation of astroglia and apolipoprotein E: an important role in neuronal regeneration. *Exp Gerontol.* 2007;**42**(1/2):54–63.

12. Goodenough S, Schleusner D, Pietrzik C, Skutella T, Behl C. Glycogen synthase kinase 3beta links neuro-protection by 17beta-estradiol to key Alzheimer processes. *Neuroscience.* 2005;**132**(3):581–9.

13. Green PS, Simpkins JW. Neuroprotective effects of estrogens: potential mechanisms of action. *Int J Dev Neurosci.* 2000;**18**(4/5):347–58.

14. Gandy S, Petanceska S. Regulation of Alzheimer beta-amyloid precursor trafficking and metabolism. *Adv Exp Med Biol.* 2001;**487**:85–100.

15. Petanceska SS, Nagy V, Frail D, Gandy S. Ovariectomy and 17beta-estradiol modulate the levels of Alzheimer's amyloid beta peptides in brain. *Exp Gerontol.* 2000;**35**(9/10):1317–25.

16. Carroll JC, Rosario ER, Chang L, *et al.* Progesterone and estrogen regulate Alzheimer-like neuropathology in female 3xTg-AD mice. *J Neurosci.* 2007;**27**(48):13357–65.

17. Levin-Allerhand JA, Lominska CE, Wang J, Smith JD. 17Alpha-estradiol and 17beta-estradiol treatments are effective in lowering cerebral amyloid-beta levels in AbetaPPSWE transgenic mice. *J Alzheimers Dis.* 2002;**4**(6):449–57.

18. Zheng H, Xu H, Uljon SN, *et al.* Modulation of A(beta) peptides by estrogen in mouse models. *J Neurochem.* 2002;**80**(1):191–6.

19. Green PS, Bales K, Paul S, Bu G. Estrogen therapy fails to alter amyloid deposition in the PDAPP model of Alzheimer's disease. *Endocrinology.* 2005;**146**(6):2774–81.

20. Heikkinen T, Kalesnykas G, Rissanen A, *et al.* Estrogen treatment improves spatial learning in APP + PS1 mice but does not affect beta amyloid accumulation and plaque formation. *Exp Neurol.* 2004;**187**(1):105–17.

21. Yue X, Lu M, Lancaster T, *et al.* Brain estrogen deficiency accelerates A-beta plaque formation in an Alzheimer's disease animal model. *Proc Natl Acad Sci USA.* 2005;**102**(52):19198–203.

22. Baulieu EE, Robel P, Schumacher M. Neurosteroids: beginning of the story. *Int Rev Neurobiol.* 2001;**46**:1–32.

23. Brinton RD, Thompson RF, Foy MR, *et al.* Progesterone receptors: form and function in brain. *Front Neuroendocrinol.* 2008;**29**(2):313–39.

24. Schumacher M, Guennoun R, Stein DG, De Nicola AF. Progesterone: therapeutic opportunities for neuroprotection and myelin repair. *Pharmacol Ther.* 2007;**116**(1):77–106.

25. Nilsen J, Brinton RD. Impact of progestins on estradiol potentiation of the glutamate calcium response. *Neuroreport.* 2002;**13**(6):825–30.

26. Singh M. Ovarian hormones elicit phosphorylation of Akt and extracellular-signal regulated kinase in explants of the cerebral cortex. *Endocrine.* 2001;**14**(3):407–15.

27. Nilsen J, Brinton RD. Divergent impact of progesterone and medroxyprogesterone acetate (Provera) on nuclear mitogen-activated protein kinase signaling. *Proc Natl Acad Sci USA.* 2003;**100**(18):10506–11.

28. Roof RL, Duvdevani R, Braswell L, Stein DG. Progesterone facilitates cognitive recovery and reduces secondary neuronal loss caused by cortical contusion injury in male rats. *Exp Neurol.* 1994;**129**(1):64–9.

29. Stein DG, Wright DW, Kellermann AL. Does progesterone have neuroprotective properties? *Ann Emerg Med.* 2008;**51**(2):164–72.

30. Labombarda F, Gonzalez SL, Deniselle MC, *et al.* Effects of injury and progesterone treatment on progesterone receptor and progesterone binding protein 25-Dx expression in the rat spinal cord. *J Neurochem.* 2003;**87**(4):902–13.

31. Gibson CL, Constantin D, Prior MJ, Bath PM, Murphy SP. Progesterone suppresses the inflammatory response and nitric oxide synthase-2 expression following cerebral ischemia. *Exp Neurol.* 2005;**193**(2):522–30.

32. Murphy SJ, Littleton-Kearney MT, Hurn PD. Progesterone administration during reperfusion, but not preischemia alone, reduces injury in ovariectomized rats. *J Cereb Blood Flow Metab.* 2002;**22**(10):1181–8.

33. Rhodes ME, Frye CA. Progestins in the hippocampus of female rats have antiseizure effects in a pentylenetetrazole seizure model. *Epilepsia.* 2004;**45**(12):1531–8.

34. Singh M. Progestins and neuroprotection: are all progestins created equal? *Minerva Endocrinol.* 2007;**32**(2):95–102.

35. Rice MM, Graves AB, McCurry SM, *et al.* Postmeno-pausal estrogen and estrogen-progestin use and 2-year rate of cognitive change in a cohort of older Japanese American women: the Kame Project. *Arch Intern Med.* 2000;**160**(11):1641–9.

36. Azcoitia I, Fernandez-Galaz C, Sierra A, Garcia-Segura LM. Gonadal hormones affect neuronal vulnerability to excitotoxin-induced degeneration. *J Neurocytol.* 1999;**28**(9):699–710.

37. Bimonte-Nelson HA, Nelson ME, Granholm AC. Progesterone counteracts estrogen-induced increases in neurotrophins in the aged female rat brain. *Neuroreport.* 2004;**15**(17):2659–63.

38. Bimonte-Nelson HA, Francis KR, Umphlet CD, Granholm AC. Progesterone reverses the spatial memory enhancements initiated by tonic and cyclic oestrogen therapy in middle-aged ovariectomized female rats. *Eur J Neurosci.* 2006;**24**(1):229–42.

39. Woolley CS, McEwen BS. Roles of estradiol and progesterone in regulation of hippocampal dendritic spine density during the estrous cycle in the rat. *J Comp Neurol.* 1993;**336**(2):293–306.

40. Murphy DD, Segal M. Progesterone prevents estradiol-induced dendritic spine formation in cultured hippocampal neurons. *Neuroendocrinology.* 2000; **72**(3):133–43.

41. Silva I, Mello LE, Freymuller E, Haidar MA, Baracat EC. Estrogen, progestogen and tamoxifen increase synaptic density of the hippocampus of ovariectomized rats. *Neurosci Lett.* 2000;**291**(3):183–6.

42. Frankfurt M, Gould E, Woolley CS, McEwen BS. Gonadal steroids modify dendritic spine density in ventromedial hypothalamic neurons: a Golgi study in the adult rat. *Neuroendocrinology.* 1990; **51**(5):530–5.

43. Gibbs RB. Effects of gonadal hormone replacement on measures of basal forebrain cholinergic function. *Neuroscience.* 2000;**101**(4):931–8.

44. Brinton RD. Requirements of a brain selective estrogen: advances and remaining challenges for developing a NeuroSERM. *J Alzheimers Dis.* 2004; **6**(6 Suppl):S27–35.

45. Yaffe K, Krueger K, Cummings SR, *et al.* Effect of raloxifene on prevention of dementia and cognitive impairment in older women: the Multiple Outcomes of Raloxifene Evaluation (MORE) randomized trial. *Am J Psychiatry.* 2005;**162**(4):683–90.

46. Zhao L, Wu TW, Brinton RD. Estrogen receptor subtypes alpha and beta contribute to neuroprotection and increased Bcl-2 expression in primary hippocampal neurons. *Brain Res.* 2004;**1010**(1/2): 22–34.

47. Cordey M, Pike CJ. Neuroprotective properties of selective estrogen receptor agonists in cultured neurons. *Brain Res.* 2005;**1045**(1/2):217–23.

48. Carroll JC, Pike CJ. Selective estrogen receptor modulators differentially regulate Alzheimer-like changes in female 3xTg-AD mice. *Endocrinology.* 2008;**149**(5):2607–11.

49. Garcia-Segura LM, Cardona-Gomez P, Naftolin F, Chowen JA. Estradiol upregulates Bcl-2 expression in adult brain neurons. *Neuroreport.* 1998;**9**(4):593–7.

50. Rosario ER, Ramsden M, Pike CJ. Progestins inhibit the neuroprotective effects of estrogen in rat hippocampus. *Brain Res.* 2006;**1099**(1):206–10.

51. Harburger LL, Bennett JC, Frick KM. Effects of estrogen and progesterone on spatial memory consolidation in aged females. *Neurobiol Aging.* 2007;**28**(4):602–10.

52. Carroll JC, Rosario ER, Pike CJ. Progesterone blocks estrogen neuroprotection from kainate in middle-aged female rats. *Neurosci Lett.* 2008;**445**(3):229–32.

53. Jayaraman A, Pike CJ. Progesterone attenuates oestrogen neuroprotection via downregulation of oestrogen receptor expression in cultured neurones. *J Neuroendocrinol.* 2009;**21**(1):77–81.

Clinical data of estrogen's effects in the central nervous system: estrogen and mood

Bevin N. Powers, Katherine E. Williams, Tonita E. Wroolie, Anna Khaylis, and Natalie L. Rasgon

Editors' introduction

In this chapter, Rasgon and colleagues first review the neurochemical basis underlying estrogen therapy use in mood disorders. They follow with an analysis of changes in estrogen and mood during different hormonal states associated with the menstrual cycle, birthing, and menopause. Results of their analysis indicate that a considerable body of basic science findings support the assertion that estrogens are prime regulators of the neurobiology of mood in women. However, there is discordance between results of animal and human studies. The source of disparity between the basic and clinical science outcomes remains undetermined but indicates the need for larger clinical trials and longitudinal studies that could identify women who are likely to respond well to estrogen monotherapy and estrogen augmentation to antidepressant treatments.

Introduction

Compared to men, women are twice as likely to suffer from uni-polar depression during the reproductive years. The relationship between estrogens and mood regulation was recognized during the end of the last century when psychological symptoms after oophorectomy were noted [1]. Although cross-sectional research has yet to clearly demonstrate an association between severity of mood symptoms and serum estrogens levels, some neurobiological studies in animals and humans suggest that estrogen status may influence mood across the female lifespan in some women. The objectives of this chapter are to (1) clarify what is currently known about the neurobiology of estrogens in relation to mood and (2) critically evaluate the existing literature regarding the use of estrogens, either alone or in combination with progesterone, for the treatment of depression in women.

Theoretical rationale for use of estrogens in mood disorders
Estrogens and serotonin

An important theoretical reason for investigation into the use of estrogens in mood disorders is the clearly documented effect of estrogens on multiple areas of serotonergic neurotransmission. Neurobiological animal studies show that estrogens increase serotonin synthesis by increasing the production of tryptophan hydroxylase (TPH), an enzyme responsible for converting tryptophan to 5-hydroxytryptophan (5-HT).

Estrogens appear to affect multiple levels of the serotonergic system [2, 3]. Both increases in serotonin transport mechanisms and binding sites [4] lead to higher overall serotonin levels in the brain [5]. Several early animal studies showed that rats treated with 17β-estradiol increased serotonin transporter (SERT) binding. For example, Rehavi *et al.* [6] found increased uptake levels of radiolabeled imipramine and serotonin in the frontal cortex and hypothalamus of ovariectomized rats treated with 17β-estradiol for 12 days. Acutely ovariectomized rats treated with estradiol benzoate were also shown to have increased SERT binding sites in the lateral septum, basolateral amygdala, ventromedial nucleus of the hypothalamus and ventral nuclei, and decreased binding sites in periaqueductal central gray matter [7]. Similarly one study found increased tritiated platelet imipramine binding sites and improved depression scores with estradiol treatment in surgically menopausal women [4].

Hormones, Cognition and Dementia: State of the Art and Emergent Therapeutic Strategies, ed. Eef Hogervorst, Victor W. Henderson, Robert B. Gibbs, and Roberta Diaz Brinton. Published by Cambridge University Press.
© Cambridge University Press 2009.

In accordance with animal models, 17β-estradiol is shown to up-regulate 5HT2A receptor binding in post-menopausal women. In one very small clincal trial by Moses-Kolko et al. [8], five euthymic postmenopausal women (not on hormone therapy for at least three months) were administered unopposed transdermal 17β-estradiol (1 mg/day) for 8–14 weeks followed by transdermal estradiol and micronized progesterone (100 mg twice a day) for an additional 2–6 weeks. These women underwent positron emission tomography (PET) imaging at baseline, after 8–14 weeks of unopposed estradiol, and again following 2–6 weeks of estradiol with progesterone. Treatment with 17β-estradiol alone led to significant increases in receptor binding potential in several regions, including the superior frontal gyrus, ventrolateral prefrontal cortex, inferior parietal lobe, and temporopolar cortex. Treatment with combined 17β-estradiol and progesterone led to widespread increases in receptor binding potential throughout the brain, including the frontal, parietal, temporal, occipital, insular parahippocampal, and posterior cingulate cortices. Compared with estradiol treatment alone, combined treatment enhanced receptor binding in medial and lateral orbitofrontal cortex, superior frontal gyrus, parahippocampal gyrus, and precuneus and superior parietal lobe [8].

Another study examined brain imaging and cognitive testing in ten postmenopausal women (at least one year after cessation of menses) with no history of psychiatric illness and free of hormone therapy for at least two months [9]. After administration of trans-dermal 17β estradiol (0.075–0.15 mg) for an average of ten weeks, comparisons of PET imaging before and after hormone therapy showed increased 5HT2A receptor binding in the right prefrontal cortex. Although 17β-estradiol treatment was associated with improved category verbal fluency and Trail Making Test A performances, no associations were seen with mood. However, this sample consisted of women who were not depressed. Studies of women with depressive symptoms would be needed to draw conclusions regarding the relationship between estradiol, 5HT receptor changes, and mood improvement.

Estrogen and norepinephrine

Research has shown that estrogens impact brain levels and metabolism of various other neurotransmitters known to have a role in regulating emotion pathways, namely norepinephrine [10]. The effect of estrogens on the noradrenergic system was investigated in earlier animal and human studies. Long-term 17β-estradiol exposure was shown to affect noradrenergic down-regulation, in a manner resembling the pattern of antidepressant drug treatment in humans [11]. Ovariectomy in rats, however, was found to influence up-regulation of adrenergic receptors in the hypothalamus, corpus callosum, and anterior pituitary [12]. Estradiol may also reduce tonic presynaptic inhibition of alpha-2 autoreceptors, facilitating norepinephrine release [13].

Estrogens and brain derived neurotrophic factor

Brain derived neurotrophic factor (BDNF) is shown to promote the growth and maintenance of serotonergic fibers [14, 15]. Because of BDNF's ability to enhance serotonin synthesis, it is thought to have antidepressant properties [16]. Amplified GABA production as a result of amplified BDNF may result in greater inhibitory input into pyramidal neurons. Conversely, decreased BDNF decreases GABA production and leads to greater excitatory cell amplitude. Length of hypoestrogenic state, and both acute and chronic estrogen administration, appear to contribute to estradiol properties that influence BDNF mRNA expressive behavior. Brain derived neurotrophic factor mRNA levels measured in normally cycling female rats were found to be significantly decreased in the medial prefrontal cortex and the hippocampal dentate gyrus (DG) granular cell layer during proestrus when estrogen levels peak. In acutely ovariectomized rats, immediate administration of estradiol led to a decrease in the hippocampal BDNF mRNA expression over time, whereas neither acute nor chronic estrogen affected BDNF expression in chronically ovariectomized rats [17]. This finding may contribute to understanding the efficacy of estrogens during the critical period in perimenopause. There appears to be a "window of opportunity" for estrogen therapy to be clinically effective during the early stages of menopause, when 17β-estradiol levels start to decline. Its clinical usefulness appears to decline in women who have been in menopause for a long period of time, similar to the effect seen in chronically ovariectomized rats.

Relationship of estrogen changes to mood disorders in women

Data from both in vitro and in vivo studies suggest that estrogens have neurobiological effects in animals and in humans. With further examination, data also suggest that a subgroup of women may be particularly vulnerable to the varying levels of estrogen on mood and have better responses to estrogen in depression treatment.

Premenstrual syndrome and premenstrual dysphoric disorder

Ever since Frank's description in 1930 of "premenstrual tension", [18] various methods of balancing hormones have been a standard approach in the treatment of premenstrual syndrome (PMS) and premenstrual dysphoric disorder (PMDD). Early treatments such as venipuncture, cathartics, and ovarian irradiation were used with the intention of ridding the body of excess estrogens. These treatments evolved into augmentation with progesterone in order to correct a hypothesized progesterone deficiency [19]. Over the past two decades, however, no diagnoses-related differences have been observed in mean serum levels of estrogens and/or progesterone across the menstrual cycle in patients with PMS when compared to normal controls [20, 21, 22].

Researchers have since re-evaluated the effects of estrogens in PMS and PMDD. Currently, severe emotional and physical symptoms experienced by women are attributed to a sensitivity to endogenous and/or exogenous estrogens [23]. For example, during the luteal phase of the menstrual cycle when plasma 17β-estradiol levels were at their highest, women reported more symptoms, such as breast swelling, breast tenderness, increased irritability, fatigue, and depression [24]. Women who were randomly assigned to Premarin® 0.625 mg also reported increased mental and physical symptoms during the luteal phase of the menstrual cycle [25].

The role of estrogen therapy in the treatment of PMS seems to be most effective when used continuously in doses high enough to suppress ovulation, rather than just during the luteal phase [26, 27]. An increase in PMS complaints may also be associated with additional cylical progesterone when it is used to prevent endometrial hyperplasia [28]. However, the most commonly used and effective treatments for PMS are selective serotonin reuptake inhibitors (SSRIs) [29]. A recently released oral contraceptive containing 30 µg of estradiol and 3 mg of drospirenone, a spironolactne derivative, was shown to be effective in treating PMS/PMDD in several placebo controlled studies [30, 31, 32].

Postpartum depression

Approximately 10% of women suffer from postpartum depression. After giving birth, women experience significant hormonal variations. Therefore, many researchers have tried to account for postpartum depression by correlating mood and hormone levels, or rate of change of hormone levels. Despite finding no differences in estrogen levels in depressed and non-depressed subjects in a recent study [33], women with a history of postpartum depression may have a particular hormonal sensitivity leaving them vulnerable to depression after giving birth. Bloch et al. [34] conducted a small study in which euthymic women were divided into two groups; one group of women with a history of postpartum depression (no other depressive episodes) and the other without this history. All the women were exposed to a gonadotropin releasing hormone (GnRH) agonist initially to induce a state of hypogonadism. Following this, a pregnant state was simulated by administering estrogen and progesterone in supraphysiological doses for eight weeks. Estradiol and progesterone were then withdrawn under double-blind conditions. Of the eight women with a previous history of postpartum depression, five reported increased symptoms of depression, compared to no women in the comparison group. Although the depressive symptoms were mild (no woman experienced an Edinburgh Depression Score greater than 10) the onset of depression symptoms was nonetheless observed in the women with a past history of postpartum depression.

Estrogen therapy in the treatment of postpartum depression

Several animal and human studies have investigated the use of estradiol for the treatment of postpartum depression. Ovariectomized female rats were injected with 17β-estradiol and progesterone daily to simulate a 23-day gestational period. One group of these female rats continued to receive 17β-estradiol injections after the simulated pregnancy, while the other group of female rats did not. The group that did not receive 17β-estradiol afterwards experienced hormonal withdrawal and exhibited depressive-like symptoms (they demonstrated less activity and resistance on a forced swimming test). Reinstatement of 17β-estradiol injections appeared to improve these depressive-like symptoms [35].

Ahokas et al. [36] evaluated the serum concentrations of 17β-estradiol in 23 women who suffered from postpartum depression. They found that the 17β-estradiol levels were lower than the threshold value for gonadal failure (less than 110 pmol/L) in 16 of the 23 women. Administration of sublingual 17β-estradiol 1–8 mg/day was dispensed for eight weeks and then doses were titrated to achieve a serum concentration of 400 pmol/L (average dose was 4.8 mg/day). At three months cyclical progesterone was added. Dramatic improvement in symptoms was reported within the first week of treatment. Twenty-one out of 23 women showed at least a 50% reduction in initial depressive symptoms and 9 out of 23 scored under 7 on the Montgomery Asberg Depression Rating Scale (MADRS). By the end of the eight-week trial, all women had a score ≤7 on the MADRS. Furthermore, the decrease in depressive symptoms coincided with a rise in serum estradiol levels.

In one double-blind, placebo-controlled study, Gregoire et al. [37] examined 61 women who met criteria for severe depression within three months postpartum. Some but not all women were taking antidepressants, but no significant antidepressant use differences were found between active group (16/34) and control group (10/27). Thirty-four women received transdermal 17β-estradiol (200 µg/day) alone for three months followed by cyclical dydrogesterone (10 mg/day) for 12 days each month for an additional three months. The remaining 27 women received placebo patches and tablets according to the same schedule. Depressive symptoms were assessed using the Edinburgh Postnatal Depression Scale (EPDS). There was a rapid improvement in depressive symptoms in the treatment group even during the first month. The placebo group improved over four months but on average, their EPDS ratings did not fall below the criteria for major depression. Although these studies demonstrate treatment effects of estrogen in postpartum depression, clearly there is a need for further investigation. Positron emission tomography imaging techniques may offer additional information regarding the association between postpartum depression and serotonin receptor function.

Estrogen in perimenopause and menopause

Perimenopause is the period of transition from regular menstrual cycles to amenorrhea [29]. During this transition, intermittent ovulation causes hormone levels to fluctuate erratically and menses to become irregular. Postmenopause usually occurs between the age of 45 and 55. The World Health Organization

and the Stages of Reproductive Aging Workshop (STRAW, [38]) define menopause transition as "the time of an increase in follicle-stimulating hormone and increased variability in cycle length, two skipped menstrual cycles with 60 or more days of amenorrhea (absence of menstruation), or both. The menopausal transition concludes with the final menstrual period (FMP) and the beginning of postmenopause." However, postmenopause is not recognized until 12 months of amenorrhea. During this process, ovarian follicles deteriorate (apoptosis) coinciding with a decrease in estrogen levels and an increase in luteinizing hormone (LH) and follicle stimulating hormone (FSH) levels [39, 29]. The mean levels of serum estradiol are approximately 5 to 35 ng/dL (50 to 350 pg/mL) in premenopausal women; however, after menopause the levels decrease to about 1.3 ng/dL (13 pg/mL). Estrone levels in postmenopause decrease to approximately 40 to 110 ng/dL to 3 ng/dL [40].

Physical and/or psychological symptoms are associated with hormonal fluctuations. The most common physical symptoms reported in menopause transition are vasomotor symptoms (hot flashes/flushes and night sweats). Hot flashes are experienced as a spontaneous sensation of warmth sometimes preceded or accompanied by palpitations, perspiration, nausea, dizziness, anxiety, headache, weakness, or a feeling of suffocation. Other commonly reported physiological symptoms include sleep disturbance, vaginal dryness and painful intercourse, urinary problems, cognitive complaints, sexual dysfunction, and uterine bleeding [41]. Psychological complaints include depression, irritability, and anxiety. Many epidemiological studies and clinic-based surveys indicate that while not all perimenopausal women experience clinically significant depression, a significant number of women do [42]. Specific risk factors influence whether or not women will develop psychiatric symptoms during menopause [39]. These risk factors include stress, poor health, a personal or family history of affective disorders or mental illness, and a history of mood changes during periods of hormonal fluctuations [29, 43].

During an exploratory study of the relationship between premenstrual symptoms and mood symptoms during perimenopause, it was found that perimenopausal mood symptoms were associated with reported premenstrual dysphoria [44]. Women with a history of premenstrual dysphoria reported more psychiatric symptoms during menopause transition, particularly depression, and, in fact, approximately one third of them met the criteria for a depressive disorder [44].

A five-year longitudinal study of 2,565 women, between the ages of 45 and 55 years, the Massachusetts Women's Health Study, found that the most predictive variable of subsequent depression was a history of depression [45]. Although these researchers did not find an overall increased risk of depression with natural menopause transition, they did find that a longer transition into menopause (at least 27 months) was associated with increased depression risk. The relationship between depression and a lengthy perimenopausal period was thought to be due to increased menopausal symptoms rather than menopause transition itself. Similarly, Rapkin et al. [29], found an increased vulnerability to mood disorders and/or anxiety with a lengthier menopause transition. However, in a four-year longitudinal study, Freeman et al. [46] found an increased risk of depression in women without a history of depression during menopause transition compared to postmenopause after controlling for other adjustment factors such as history of depression, severe PMS, age, poor sleep, employment status, and race. Depressive symptoms were shown to increase during perimenopause even in women without a prior history of depression.

Women appear to be even more vulnerable to depression during the late perimenopausal period. In a prospective evaluation of 29 asymptomatic regularly cycling premenopausal women monitored for an average of five years until at least six months of amenorrhea, Schmidt et al. [47] found a 14-fold increase in depression onset in the 24 months surrounding the last menstrual period. The premise that a shorter perimenopause phase is correlated with fewer mood symptoms is additionally supported by the finding that women with rapidly increasing FSH were less likely to report depressive symptoms [46]. Additionally, these researchers found an association between rising 17β-estradiol levels and depression, further suggesting that the fluctuation of hormone levels plays a role in dysphoric mood during menopausal transition. The correlation between mood and behavior is complex and not fully explained by simple increases or decreases in absolute hormone levels. Freeman et al.'s [46] findings, in which depressive symptoms increased during menopause transition, when hormone levels fluctuated rapidly, and

decreased in postmenopause, as hormone levels stabilized, support this concept.

Furthermore, depression or a history of depression may lessen the length of a woman's reproductive period. In the three-year longitudinal Harvard Study of Moods and Cycles, women with a history of major depression were shown to be 1.2 times more likely to experience an earlier perimenopause compared to women who did not report depression in their lifetime [48]. Moreover, women who reported more severe depression had a greater risk of transitioning into perimenopause earlier compared to non-depressed women. Additionally, women who used antidepressants and suffered from depression had three times the risk of early entry into menopause. Interestingly, women with a history of depression were shown to have higher levels of FSH and LH and lower levels of estradiol at the beginning of the study and at interim assessments. This study suggests that ovarian function declines earlier in women with a history of depression.

Estrogen monotherapy for affective disorders in peri- and postmenopausal women

Klaiber et al. [49] performed one of the initial double-blind, placebo-controlled studies examining the use of estrogen therapy in 40 peri- and postmenopausal women who reported a history of severe recurrent major depression that was historically unresponsive to all treatments, including electroconvulsive therapy (ECT). Conjugated estrogens in supraphysiological doses (5–25 mg/day, about 5 to 20 times the usual postmenopausal replacement dose) or placebo was administered for three months. The mean decrease in the Hamilton Depression Rating Scale (Ham-D) score for the estrogen group (n = 23) and placebo group (n = 17) was 9.2 and 0.1, respectively. Furthermore, the Ham-D scores decreased by 15 points in six of the 23 women in the estrogen group, while no one in the placebo group experienced a decrease of 10 or more points. There was no significance between age and menopausal status related to the amount of noted improvement. Although many of the women improved considerably with estrogen treatment, most of the women in the study remained symptomatic [49].

Following the original study by Klaiber et al. [49], numerous studies regarding the use of adjunctive estrogen or hormone therapy in postmenopausal depression have yielded contradictory results. The conflicts among studies [49, 50, 51] are likely the result of differences in study design (retrospective versus prospective), differences in hormone therapy preparations (e.g., estrogen or estrogen plus progesterone, and type of estrogen), heterogeneity of clinical populations with respect to severity of depressive illness, phase of menopause, and type of antidepressants used (e.g., tricyclics versus SSRIs). Meta-analytic studies provide some understanding of the differential findings regarding the effects of estrogens on mood among studies. One meta-analytic study evaluated 111 hormone therapy studies [52] and found no real association between hormone therapy and improvement of mood in women who experienced natural menopause. On the other hand, women who had undergone surgical menopause did have some positive effects [53]. Interestingly, observational and non-double-blind studies show increased reporting in mood improvement with HT, whereas double-blind studies have more mixed results [53]. Four of five observational or non-double-blind studies reported mood improvement with HT use [53], whereas only four of seven double-blind studies indicated mood improvement.

One meta-analysis of 26 studies suggested that HT was effective in reducing menopausal depressed mood [54]. The overall effect size for HT in this meta-analysis was 0.68, indicating that the average treatment patient had a less depressed mood than 76% of the control patients. When specific hormone treatments were analyzed separately it was shown that estrogens alone had a greater effect size than progesterone alone, or estrogens and progesterone combined. Androgen alone or in combination with estrogen resulted in an even greater decline in depressed mood. Additionally, perimenopausal women showed a greater response to treatment than postmenopausal women.

Shortly after Zweifel and O'Brien's analysis [54], two double-blind, placebo-controlled studies were published that assessed the efficacy of 17β-estradiol as a monotherapy for depression. First, Schmidt et al. [55], administered 50 μg of transdermal 17β-estradiol or placebo patches to 34 perimenopausal women with either major depressive disorder (MDD) or minor depression. Sixteen women were treated with 17β-estradiol for the first three weeks and then all of the women received 17β-estradiol from week three through six. During the initial three weeks, 80% of

those receiving estradiol had either a full or partial therapeutic response, whereas only 22% of the placebo group had any response. Nineteen of 24 women with minor depression responded, and six out of seven women with a current diagnosis of MDD responded, to treatment. The presence of hot flashes and sleep disturbance was not related to mood improvements. However, in women who experienced anhedonia and anxiety, a greater medication response was seen in the women who did not have hot flashes as compared to the depressed women with hot flashes. These findings indicate that hormone therapy may have an antidepressant effect unrelated to its effects on the physical manifestations of perimenopause; however, confirmation with larger sample populations is necessary to derive this conclusion [55].

In a second double-blind, placebo-controlled clinical trial, 17β-estradiol treatment was shown to improve depression in a population of perimenopausal women [56]. Perimenopausal women with MDD (n = 26), dysthymia (n = 11), or minor depressive disorder (n = 13) were administered either 100 mg transdermal 17β-estradiol or placebo for 12 weeks and depression was monitored with the Montgomery-Asberg Depression Rating Scale (MADRS). Remission of depression was significantly higher in the 17β-estradiol group (67%) compared to the placebo group (20%; p < 0.001) after 12 weeks. Furthermore, the antidepressant benefits held over a four-week washout period in light of an increase in somatic complaints. Improvement rates among 17β-estradiol users were similar regardless of initial diagnosis.

In contrast, a prospective study examining affective and somatic complaints in postmenopausal women attending a health clinic found that the use of estrogen therapy was associated with significantly lower somatic depressive complaints but only marginally lower affective depression scores on the Zung self-rating scale for depression [57]. Because this measure has both somatic and affective subscales, the authors controlled for each component in their analysis. They found that controlling for mood, the benefit of ET remained significant with respect to somatic symptoms, whereas controlling for somatic levels eliminated the effects of ET on affective depression levels. These findings suggest that ET use may reduce sub-syndromal depression via improvement in somatic rather than affective depressive symptoms.

In 2003, an open-label study conducted by Cohen et al. [58] utilized a similar population of women and explored the effect of transdermal 17β-estradiol (100 μg/day) on depression over a four-week period. Twenty-two perimenopausal (n = 10) and postmenopausal (n = 12) women were followed: of which 12 satisfied the criteria for MDD, seven of the women met the criteria for minor depression, and three met the criteria for dysthmic disorder. Interestingly, the perimenopausal women showed the most response to 17β-estradiol treatment. Six of the nine perimenopausal study completers achieved remission assessed by the MADRS and Beck Depression Inventory (BDI) scales, whereas depression in only two of the eleven postmenopausal study completers remitted. The results from this study suggest that mood disturbances in perimenopausal women are directly related to the reproductive cycle and may be responsive to ET [58]. Consistent with animal data previously discussed, the length of hypoestrogenic status may correlate to the responsiveness to acute estrogen treatment. In animal models, the effect of estrogens on the serotonin system seems to be strongly associated with the length of time since ovariectomy, and acute and persistent estradiol replacement.

Estrogen as an adjunctive treatment for mood disorders in peri- and postmenopausal women

Selective serotonin reuptake inhibitors have been particularly useful in symptom reduction among perimenopausal or menopausal women with mood disorders [59]. It has been suggested that estrogens augment the effects of traditional antidepressants, such as SSRIs, during the perimenopausal period [29]. Menopause is often associated with decreased levels of estrogens, and given that estrogens modulate serotonergic function in the central nervous system, these decreased levels may affect the response to serotonergic antidepressants. This was supported by a study that examined the serotonin agonist meta-chlorophenylpiperazine (m-CPP) in 18 healthy postmenopausal women not on estrogen therapy, and 15 healthy menstruating women [60]. After administration of m-CPP and prior to administration of estrogen therapy, postmenopausal women exhibited a significantly blunted prolactin peak as well as decreased cortisol peak when compared to healthy menstruating women in response to an m-CPP challenge. After one month of estrogen (estraderm 0.1 mg) treatment, cortisol and prolactin response to m-CPP levels significantly increased [60].

In addition to human and animal neurobiological studies, clinical trials also support the hypothesis that estrogens augment the treatment effects of antidepressants. For example, one study compared antidepressant response rates and tolerability in younger (<44 years; n = 91) and older women (>50 years; n = 24) who met DSM-IV criteria for MDD versus a comparison group of 86 age-matched men [61]. Compared to the older women, younger women had significantly lower Hamilton Depression Rating Scale (HDRS) scores after eight weeks of antidepressant treatment and exhibited significantly higher rates of remission. The findings in the male control group were not consistent with this pattern, highlighting the role of estrogenic function in gender specific antidepressant response.

Several studies suggest that this augmentation effect of estrogen therapy may be specific to SSRIs. In a large clinical trial of 235 men and 400 women with chronic major depression or "double depression" (major depressive episodes superimposed on dysthymic disorder), Kornstein et al. [62] found that pre- and postmenopausal women and men had differential responses to sertraline and imipramine. Premenopausal women responded significantly better to sertraline than to imipramine, whereas postmenopausal women had similar rates of response to the two medications. Furthermore, women were significantly more likely to show a favorable response to sertraline than to imipramine, whereas the opposite pattern was true for men. The findings from the study suggest that female sex hormones alter treatment response by possibly enhancing the effect of SSRIs or inhibiting response to tricyclic antidepressants (TCAs) [62].

Clinical studies also suggest that estrogens may not be as beneficial in augmenting the effects of TCAs. Two early studies examined the use of estrogens to augment TCAs and did not find any additional benefits. In one study, 11 women who had been previously unresponsive to treatment received augmentation with estrogens after two weeks of treatment with imipramine alone [51]. After four weeks, HDRS scores did not improve. Moreover, manic symptoms may be induced by the use of estrogens in addition to antidepressant therapies [51, 63, 64]. Consequently, further research is needed before the use of estrogens as an effective augmentation to TCAs among unresponsive patients can be endorsed. Future studies should examine age, estrogen status, length of time in perimenopause, and measurement of TCA levels.

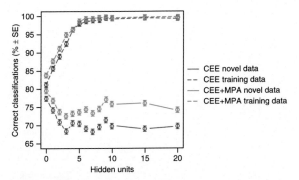

Fig. 2.1 Artificial neural network model accuracy (percent correct classifications ± SE) on training and novel data for the CEE-alone and CEE+MPA trials for 3MS examination changes of four points or more as a function of hidden unit number.

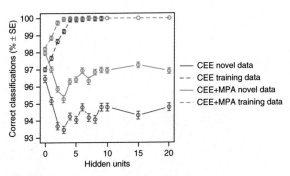

Fig. 2.3 Artificial neural network model accuracy (percent correct classifications ± SE) on training and novel data for the CEE-alone and CEE+MPA trials for the clinical diagnosis outcome as a function of hidden unit number.

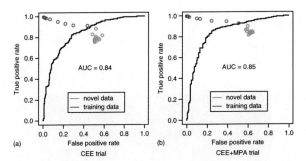

Fig. 2.2 The full logistic regression model ROC compared to ANN model performance for 3MS examination changes of four points or more.

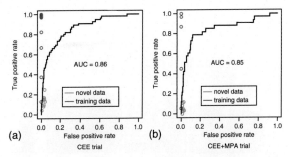

Fig. 2.4 The full logistic regression model ROC compared to ANN model performance on the clinical diagnosis outcome.

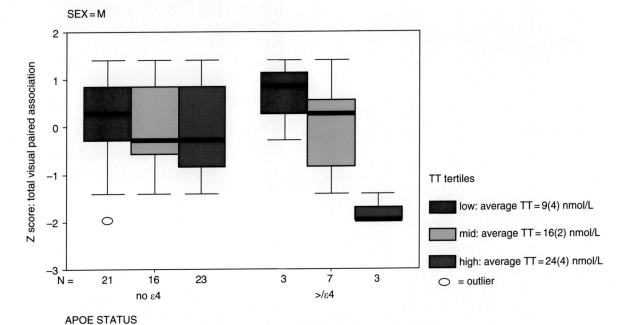

Fig. 18.4 Foresight MRC Challenge data showed that verbal memory had negative associations with higher testosterone levels in men (Hogervorst, 2002). Further analyses showed that in healthy older men (74 (6) years of age), visual memory performance showed an interaction of APOE × TT (beta = 0.96, $p < 0.05$, which was independent of age, education, SHBG, TT, TT^2, FAI, APOE, and BMI). Men who carried the ε4 allele had worse visual memory performance when they had higher total testosterone (TT) levels.

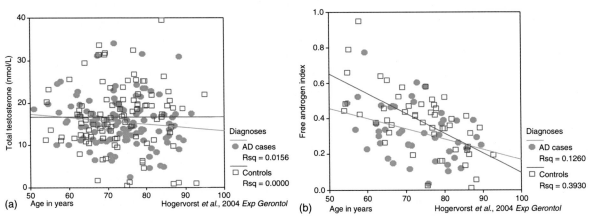

Fig. 18.2 (a) Levels of total testosterone with age of men with Alzheimer's disease and controls. (b) Levels of bio-available or free testosterone (free androgen index or FAI = TT/SHBG) with age of men with Alzheimer's disease and controls.

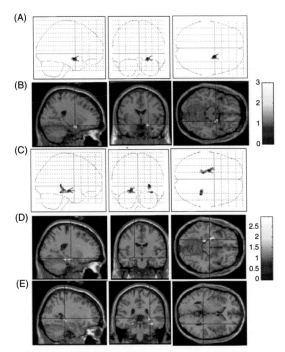

Fig. 22.3 Effects of testosterone on glucose metabolism in the hippocampus and amygdala during performance of a verbal memory task. This figure shows within-subject changes in relative brain activity with testosterone supplementation compared with placebo. Brain areas showing significant changes are labeled with the anatomical location by Brodmann area and Talairach coordinates (x, y, z). Panel A shows glass-brain sagittal, coronal, and axial projections of all medial temporal regions showing significant (p < 0.01) decreases in glucose metabolism with testosterone supplementation compared with placebo. Panel B highlights treatment-related decrease in right entorhinal cortex/amygdala (22, −2, −10). Panel C shows glass-brain projections of all medial temporal regions demonstrating trends (p < 0.05) of increased glucose metabolism with testosterone supplementation compared with placebo. Panel D highlights treatment-related increase in the left entorhinal cortex, Brodmann area 28 (−20, −14, −9) in the crosshairs. Panel E highlights treatment-related increase in the right posterior hippocampus (30, −33, 3) in crosshairs, and the coronal view also shows increase in the right parahippocampal gyrus, Brodmann area 36 (36, −36, −12). Maki, P. M. *et al. Journal of Clinical Endocrinology and Metabolism.* 2007 Nov;92(11):4107–14. © 2007, The Endocrine Society.

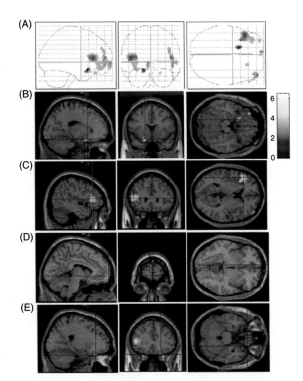

Fig. 22.4 Effects of testosterone on glucose metabolism in the prefrontal cortex during performance of a verbal memory task. This figure shows within-subject increases in relative brain activity with testosterone supplementation compared with placebo. Brain areas showing significant increases are labeled with the anatomical location by Brodmann Area and Talairach coordinates (x, y, z). Panel A shows glass-brain sagittal, coronal, and axial projections of all prefrontal areas showing significant increases in glucose metabolism with testosterone supplementation compared with placebo. Panel B highlights the left medial frontal gyrus, subgenual, Brodmann area 25 (−16, 13, −16), in the crosshairs, and the axial view also shows left superior frontal gyrus, Brodmann area 10 (−32, 60, −3). Panel C highlights the left inferior frontal cortex, Brodmann area 45 and 46 (−46, 28, 8), in the crosshairs, and the axial view also shows increase in the right middle frontal gyrus Brodmann area 46 (48, 55, 5). Panel D highlights the left superior frontal gyrus, Brodmann area 10 (−6, 66, −7). Panel E highlights the right orbitofrontal cortex, Brodmann area 47 (22, 30, −23). Maki, P. M. *et al. Journal of Clinical Endocrinology and Metabolism.* 2007 Nov;92(11): 4107–14. © 2007, The Endocrine Society.

Preliminary data suggest that ET augmentation in peri-and postmenopausal women with no or partial response to SSRIs may be more promising. In a post hoc analysis of a six-week, placebo-controlled clinical trial with fluoxetine (20 mg/day) with women over the age of 60 and a diagnosis of MDD, Schneider *et al.* [65] found that 20% of 358 patients were taking concurrent HT and that improvements in Ham-D scores were greater on average in patients who were on fluoxetine + ET versus fluoxetine + placebo (40.1% vs. 17.0%, respectively).

Conversely, in a retrospective study of women aged 45 years and older with MDD, Amsterdam *et al.* [50] found no difference in response to fluoxetine (20 mg/day) among women on HT (n = 40) compared to women not on HT (n = 132). Data from two multi-center clinical trials with sertraline were analyzed to determine the effects of combined ET and sertraline [66]. Women over the age of 60 (n = 127) were administered sertraline while simultaneously taking estrogen therapy (without progesterone), no significant differences on Ham-D or Ham-A scores were found between the women taking sertraline alone compared to the women taking both sertraline and ET. However, the women taking adjunctive ET reported significantly greater global improvement and quality of life. Furthermore, women between the ages of 60 and 64 were more likely to exhibit improvements in response to sertraline than older women.

Other studies suggest that ET may augment the antidepressant response to fluoxetine in treatment-resistant MDD [67]. During an eight-week clinical trial, six women were administered 17β-estradiol in addition to fluoxetine. This study found that one woman remitted, and five had a partial response. Furthermore, there was a mean decrease of 12.6 points in Ham-D ratings over the course of the trial. Interestingly, a drastic decrease in Ham-D scores was noted after the first week of ET treatment. This acceleration effect was replicated in another study [68]. Twenty-two postmenopausal women with MDD in a ten-week double-blind, placebo-controlled clinical trial were treated with sertraline and randomized to either transdermal estrogen or placebo patches. All women received 50 mg/day of sertraline for one week and this increased to 100 mg/day at week two. Estrogen or placebo patches were initated concurrently with the sertraline. Both groups showed significant improvements in HDRS scores by the end of the trial, although the women receiving sertraline with ET improved significantly more rapidly than the women receiving sertraline with placebo. These findings suggest that ET may play a role in accelerating the antidepressant response in postmenopausal women with MDD.

Conclusion

Multiple animal and human studies support the contribution of estrogens in the neurobiology of mood in women; however, further investigation of ET use in women during periods of hormonal changes is necessary to further understand mood instability during peri- and postmenopause. Results previously obtained from animal and human basic neurobiological and clinical studies have yielded discordant findings, and support the demand for larger clinical trials and longitudinal studies that could potentially define women who are likely to respond well to estrogen monotherapy and estrogen augmentation to antidepressant treatments. The Women's Health Initiative's (WHI) findings firmly maintain the importance of defining the risks and benefits of estrogen treatment and identifying subsets of women whose mood symptoms are distinctively dependent upon estrogen status. Studies with homogeneous populations may assist in this determination.

References

1. Stoppe G, Doren M. Critical appraisal of effects of estrogen replacement therapy on symptoms of depressed mood. *Arch Women Ment Health.* 2002;5(2):39–47.

2. Cone RI, Davis GA, Goy RW. Effects of ovarian steroids on serotonin metabolism within grossly dissected and microdissected brain regions of the ovariectomized rat. *Brain Res Bull.* 1981;7:639–44.

3. Biegnon A. Effects of steroid hormones on the serotonergic system. In Whitaker-Azmida PM, Peroutka SJ, eds. *The Neuropharmacology of Serotonin.* New York Academy of Sciences, 1990, pp. 427–31.

4. Sherwin BB, Suranyi-Cadotte BE. Up-regulatory effect of estrogen on platelet 3H-imipramine binding sites in surgically menopausal women. *Biol Psychiatry.* 1990;28(4):339–48.

5. Guicheney P, Leger D, Barrat J, *et al.* Platelet serotonin content and plasma tryptophan in peri- and postmenopausal women: variations with plasma oestrogen levels and depressive symptoms. *Eur J Clin Invest.* 1988;18(3):297–304.

6. Rehavi M, Sepcuti H, Weizman A. Upregulation of imipramine binding and serotonin uptake by estradiol in female rat brain. *Brain Res.* 1987;**410**:135–9.

7. McQueen JK, Wilson H, Fink G. Estradiol-17 beta increases serotonin transporter (SERT) mRNA levels and the density of SERT-binding sites in female rat brain. *Brain Res Mol Brain Res.* 1997;**45**(1):13–23.

8. Moses-Kolko EL, Greer PJ, Smith G, *et al.* Widespread increases of cortical serotonin type 2A receptor availability after hormone therapy in euthymic postmenopausal women. *Fertil Steril.* 2003;**80**:554–9.

9. Kuyaga A, Epperson N, Zoghbi S, *et al.* Increase in prefrontal cortex serotonin 2A receptors following estrogen treatment in postmenopausal women. *Am J Psych.* 2003;**160**:1522–4.

10. Ball P, Knuppen R, Haupt M, Breuer H. Interactions between estrogens and catechol amines. 3. Studies on the methylation of catechol estrogens, catechol amines and other catechols by the catechol-O-methyltransferases of human liver. *J Clin Endocrinol Metab.* 1972;**34**(4):736–46.

11. Biegnon A, Reches A, Synder L, *et al.* Serotonergic and noradrenergic receptor in the rat brain: modulation by chronic exposure to ovarian hormones. *Life Sci.* 1983;**32**:2015–21.

12. Petrovic SI, McDonald JK, DeCastro G, *et al.* Regulation of anterior pituitary and brain beta-adrenergic receptors by ovarian steroids. *Life Sci.* 1983;**37**:1563–70.

13. Etgen AM, Karkanias GB. Estrogen regulation of noradrenergic signaling in the hypothalamus. *Psychoneuroendocrinology.* 1994;**19**(5/7):603–10.

14. Mamounas LA, Blue ME, Siuciak JA, *et al.* Estradiol-17β increases serotonin transporter (SERT) mRNA levels and the density of SERT-biding sites in female rat brain. *Molecular Brain Res.* 1997;**45**:13–23.

15. Mamounas LA, Altar CA, Blue ME, *et al.* BDNF promotes the regenerative sprouting, but not survival, of injured serotonergic axons in the adult rat brain. *J Neurosci.* 2000;**20**(2):771–82.

16. Siuciak JA, Clark MS, Rind HB, *et al.* BDNF induction of tryptophan hydroxylase mRNA levels in the rat brain. *J Neurosci Res.* 1998;**52**(2):149–58.

17. Cavus I, Duman RS. Influence of estradiol, stress, and 5-HT2A agonist treatment on brain-derived neurotrophic factor expression in female rats. *Biol Psychiatry.* 2003;**54**(1):59–69.

18. Frank RT. Hormonal causes of premenstrual tension. *Arch Neurol Psychiatry.* 1931;**26**:1053–7.

19. Severino SK, Moline ML. *Premenstrual Syndrome. A Clinicians Guide.* New York: Guilford Press, 1989.

20. Watts JF, Butts WR, Edwards RI, *et al.* Hormonal studies in women with premenstrual tension. *Br J Obstet Gynecol.* 1985;**92**:247–55.

21. Rubinow DR, Hoban MC, Grover GN, *et al.* Changes in plasma hormones across the menstrual cycle in patients with menstrually related mood disorder and in control subjects. *Am J Obstet Gynecol.* 1988;**158**:5–11.

22. Dennerstein L, Brown JB, Gotts G, *et al.* Menstrual cycle hormonal profiles of women with and without premenstrual syndrome. *J Psychosom Obstet Gynecol.* 1993;**14**:259–68.

23. Schmidt PJ, Nieman LK, Danaceau MA, *et al.* Differential behavioral effects of gonadal steroids in women with and in those without premenstrual syndrome. *N Engl J Med.* 1998;**338**:209–16.

24. Hammarback S, Damber JF, Backstrom T. Relationship between symptom severity and hormone changes in women with premenstrual syndrome. *J Clin Endocrinol Metab.* 1989;**68**:125–30.

25. Dhar V, Murphy GE. Double blind randomized crossover trial of luteal phase estrogens (Premarin) in the premenstrual syndrome (PMS). *Psychoneuroendocrinology.* 1990;**15**:489–93.

26. Smith RN, Studd JW, Zamblera D, *et al.* A randomized comparison over 8 months of 100 micrograms and 200 micrograms twice weekly doses of transdermal oestradiol in the treatment of severe premenstrual syndrome. *Br J Obstet Gynaecol.* 1995;**102**(6):475–84.

27. Backstrom T, Hansson-Malmstrom Y, Lindhe BA, *et al.* Oral contraceptive in premenstrual syndrome: a randomized comparison of triphasic and monophasic preparations. *Contraception.* 1992;**46**(3):253–68.

28. Watson NR, Studd JW, Savvas M, *et al.* Treatment of severe premenstrual syndrome with oestradiol patches and cyclical oral norethisterone. *Lancet.* 1989;**23**:730–2.

29. Rapkin AJ, Mikacich JA, Moatakef-Imani B, *et al.* The clinical nature and formal diagnosis of premenstrual, postpartum, and perimenopausal affective disorders. *Curr Psychiatry Rep.* 2002;**4**(6):419–28.

30. Freeman EW, Kroll R, Rapkin A, *et al.* Evaluation of a unique oral contraceptive in the treatment of premenstrual dysphoric disorder. *J Womens Health Gend Based Med.* 2001;**20**:561–96.

31. Pearlstein TB, Bachmann GA, Zacur HA, Yonkers KA. Treatment of premenstrual dysphoric disorder with a new drospirenone-containing oral contraceptive formulation. *Contraception.* 2005;**72**(6):414–21.

32. Yonkers KA, Brown C, Pearlstein TB, *et al.* Efficacy of a new low-dose oral contraceptive with drospirenone in premenstrual dysphoric disorder. *Obstet Gynecol.* 2005;**106**:492–501.

33. Hendrick V, Altshuler L, Suri R. Hormonal chanages in the postpartum and implications for postpartum depression. *Psychosomatics*. 1998;**39**:93–101.

34. Bloch M, Schmidt PJ, Danaceau M, *et al.* Effects of gonadal steroids in women with a history of postpartum depression. *Am J Psych*. 2000;**157**:924–30.

35. Galea LA, Wide JK, Alasdair MB. Estradiol alleviates depressive-like symptoms in a novel animal model of post-partum depression. *Behav Brain Res*. 2001;**122**:1–9.

36. Ahokas A, Kaukoranta J, Wahlbeck K, Aito M. Estrogen deficiency in severe postpartum depression: successful treatment with sublingual physiologic 17beta-estradiol: a preliminary study. *J Clin Psychiatry*. 2001;**62**(5):332–6.

37. Gregoire AJP, Kumar R, Everitt B, *et al.* Transdermal oestrogen for treatment of severe postnatal depression. *Lancet*. 1996;**347**:930–3.

38. Soules MR, Sherman S, Parrott E *et al.* Stages of Reproductive Aging workshop (STRAW). *J Womens Health Gend Based Med*. 2001;**10**(9):843–8.

39. Steiner M, Dunn E, Born L. Hormones and mood: from menarche to menopause and beyond. *J Affect Disord*. 2003;**74**(1):67–83.

40. Judd HL. Transdermal estradiol. A potentially improved method of hormone replacement. *J Reprod Med*. 1994;**39**(5):343–52.

41. Nelson HD, Vesco KK, Haney E *et al.* Nonhormonal therapies for menopausal hot flashes systematic review and meta-analysis. *JAMA*. 2006;**295**:2057.

42. Schmidt PJ, Roca CA, Bloch M, *et al.* The perimenopause and affective disorders. *Semin Reprod Endocrinol*. 1997;**15**(1):91–100.

43. Banger M. Affective syndrome during perimenopause. *Maturitas*. 2002;**41**(Suppl 1):S13–8.

44. Novaes C, Almeida OP, de Melo NR. Mental health among perimenopausal women attending a menopause clinic: possible association with premenstrual syndrome? *Climacteric*. 1998;**1**(4): 264–70.

45. Avis NE, Brambilla D, McKinlay SM, *et al.* A longitudinal analysis of the association between menopause and depression. Results from the Massachusetts Women's Health Study. *Ann Epidemiol*. 1994;**4**(3):214–20.

46. Freeman EW, Sammel MD, Liu L, Gracia, *et al.* Hormones and menopausal status as predictors of depression in women in transition to menopause. *Arch Gen Psychiatry*. 2004;**61**(1):62–70.

47. Schmidt PJ, Haq N, Rubinow DR. A longitudinal evaluation of the relationship between reproductive status and mood in perimenopausal women. *Am J Psychiatry*. 2004;**161**(12):2238–44.

48. Harlow BL, Wise LA, Otto MW, *et al.* Depression and its influence on reproductive endocrine and menstrual cycle markers associated with perimenopause: the Harvard Study of Moods and Cycles. *Arch Gen Psychiatry*. 2003;**60**(1):29–36.

49. Klaiber EL, Broverman DM, Vogel W, *et al.* Estrogen therapy for severe persistent depressions in women. *Arch Gen Psychiatry*. 1979;**36**(5):550–4.

50. Amsterdam J, Garcia-Espana F, Fawcett J, *et al.* Fluoxetine efficacy in menopausal women with and without estrogen replacement. *J Affect Disord*. 1999;**55**(1):11–7.

51. Shapira B, Oppenheim G, Zohar J, *et al.* Lack of efficacy of estrogen supplementation to imipramine in resistant female depressives. *Biol Psychiatry*. 1985;**20**(5):576–9.

52. Pearce J, Hawton K, Blake F. Psychological and sexual symptoms associated with the menopause and the effects of hormone replacement therapy. *Br J Psychiatry*. 1995;**167**(2):163–73.

53. Miller KJ. The other side of estrogen replacement therapy: outcome study results of mood improvement in estrogen users and nonusers. *Curr Psychiatry Rep*. 2003;**5**(6):439–44.

54. Zweifel JE, O'Brien WH. A meta-analysis of the effect of hormone replacement therapy upon depressed mood. *Psychoneuroendocrinology*. 1997;**22** (3):189–212. Erratum in: *Psychoneuroendocrinology*. 1997;**22**(8):655.

55. Schmidt PJ, Nieman L, Danaceau MA, *et al.* Estrogen replacement in perimenopause-related depression: a preliminary report. *Am J Obstet Gynecol*. 2000; **183**(2):414–20.

56. Soares CN, Almeida OP, Joffe H, *et al.* Efficacy of estradiol for the treatment of depressive disorders in perimenopausal women: a double-blind, randomized, placebo-controlled trial. *Arch Gen Psychiatry*. 2001;**58** (6):529–34.

57. Canada SA, Hofkamp M, Gall EP, *et al.* Estrogen replacement therapy, subsyndromal depression, and orthostatic blood pressure regulation. *Behav Med*. 2003;**29**(3):101–6.

58. Cohen LS, Soares CN, Poitras JR, *et al.* Short-term use of estradiol for depression in perimenopausal and postmenopausal women: a preliminary report. *Am J Psychiatry*. 2003;**160**(8):1519–22.

59. Altshuler LL. The use of SSRIs in depressive disorders specific to women. *J Clin Psychiatry*. 2002;**63**(Suppl 7):3–8.

60. Halbreich U, Rojansky N, Palter S, *et al*. Estrogen augments serotonergic activity in postmenopausal women. *Biol Psychiatry*. 1995;**37**(7):434–41.

61. Grigoriadis S, Kennedy SH, Bagby RM. A comparison of antidepressant response in younger and older women. *J Clin Psychopharmacol*. 2003;**23**(4): 405–7.

62. Kornstein SG, Schatzberg AF, Thase ME, *et al*. Gender differences in treatment response to sertraline versus imipramine in chronic depression. *Am J Psychiatry*. 2000;**157**(9):1445–52.

63. Oppenheim G. A case of rapid mood cycling with estrogen: implications for therapy. *J Clin Psychiatry*. 1984;**45**(1):34–5.

64. Young RC, Moline M, Kleyman F. Hormone replacement therapy and late-life mania. *Am J Geriatr Psychiatry*. 1997;**5**(2):179–81.

65. Schneider LS, Small GW, Hamilton SH, *et al*. Estrogen replacement and response to fluoxetine in a multicenter geriatric depression trial. Fluoxetine Collaborative Study Group. *Am J Geriatr Psychiatry*. 1997;**5**(2):97–106.

66. Schneider LS, Small GW, Clary CM. Estrogen replacement therapy and antidepressant response to sertraline in older depressed women. *Am J Geriatr Psychiatry*. 2001;**9**(4):393–9.

67. Rasgon NL, Altshuler LL, Fairbanks LA, *et al*. Estrogen replacement therapy in the treatment of major depressive disorder in perimenopausal women. *J Clin Psychiatry*. 2002;**63**(Suppl 7):45–8.

68. Rasgon NL, Dunkin J, Fairbanks L, *et al*. Estrogen and response to sertraline in postmenopausal women with major depressive disorder: a pilot study. *J Psychiatr Res*. 2007;**41**(3/4):338–43.

Chapter 13

Different forms of soy processing may determine the positive or negative impact on cognitive function of Indonesian elderly

Eef Hogervorst, Linda Kushandy, Wita Angrianni, Yudarini, Sabarinah, Theresia Ninuk, Vita Priantina Dewi, Amina Yesufu, Tony Sadjimim, Philip Kreager, and Tri Budi W. Rahardjo

Editors' introduction

Hogervorst and colleagues review the complex topic of soy effects on cognition and risk of dementia. In an attempt to address one aspect of this complexity, they conducted a comparative analysis of fermented (e.g., tempe) versus non-fermented (e.g., tofu) forms. Results of their analyses indicate that high intake of tofu was associated with lower cognitive function and an increased risk for dementia, particularly in those participants who were older than 68 years of age. These findings are consistent with previous analyses of hormone therapy and tofu consumption. They also found a complex association with genistein levels. Relatively younger participants (52–68 years of age) appeared to have optimal genistein levels relating to optimal memory function, whereas persons older than 68 years of age with high genistein levels exhibited lower cognitive performance and an increased risk of dementia. These results are reminiscent of the window of opportunity theory (Chapters 4 and 5) or the healthy cell bias theory (Chapter 6). Higher folate levels within tempe (which contains high phytoestrogen levels) may be a mediating factor for its reported protective effects. Further studies to determine the interaction between serum phytoestrogens and folate levels and their relationship to dementia risk are suggested.

Introduction

Natural estrogenic substances, such as phytoestrogens, have received increasing attention over the past years, e.g., as a safer alternative to estrogen treatment for menopausal complaints or as general food supplements to enhance health. Accordingly, their consumption has steadily increased over the last decades in the West [1]. One class of phytoestrogens is the isoflavones, of which genistein is the most potent, followed by daidzein and glycitein. These micronutrients are abundant in soy products, such as tempe and tofu [2, 3]. Lignans are another form of phytoestrogens and are most abundant in flax seeds [3]. This chapter will mainly discuss associations of isoflavones with cognitive function in the elderly.

Biological plausibility of protective effects of phytoestrogens on the brain

It is not entirely clear what effect phytoestrogens could have on the aging brain. Phytoestrogens have long been thought to reduce the risk for cardiovascular disease [2]. Age-related cognitive decline and pathological cognitive aging, such as Alzheimer's disease (AD, the most common type of dementia) share many risk factors with cardiovascular disease [4–6], perhaps allowing phytoestrogens to exert protection on the brain through these mechanisms. On the other hand, in Japan, where phytoestrogen consumption is on average three times higher than in the West, the prevalence of vascular dementia was found to be higher, while that of AD was lower than in Western cohorts [3, 7]. This could suggest other than vascular protective mechanisms. Differences between cohorts and difficulty in accurate diagnostics of different types of dementias cross-culturally may hamper true comparisons.

Phytoestrogens can exert estrogenic effects and act via estrogen receptors as they are chemically similar to estrogens [3]. Numerous animal and in vitro cell studies have shown that estrogens can exert potential

Hormones, Cognition and Dementia: State of the Art and Emergent Therapeutic Strategies, ed. Eef Hogervorst, Victor W. Henderson, Robert B. Gibbs, and Roberta Diaz Brinton. Published by Cambridge University Press.
© Cambridge University Press 2009.

protective effects on the aging brain and act on almost all mechanisms implicated in cognitive decline and AD (see for reviews: [8, 9]). One of these mechanisms would be through the capacity of estrogen-like compounds to act as antioxidants [8]. Oxidative stress has been implicated in cognitive ageing and AD. Several studies found that phytoestrogens could exert antioxidant effects in cortical [10] and hippocampal neuron cultures, e.g., after these had been exposed to toxic substances, such as kainic acid [11], glutamate, or beta-amyloid [12].

Phytoestrogens did not, however, have the same potent neurotrophic effects as estrogens in some experimental paradigms [12]. In addition, when estrogen levels are elevated, phytoestrogens can actually exert antagonistic estrogenic properties through their weak binding to the estrogen receptor and thus act as a partial agonist/antagonist [13, 14].

Treatment trials and observational studies of phytoestrogens in women and men

Relatively small randomized controlled trials (RCTs) of phytoestrogens in elderly women to maintain cognitive function have rendered inconclusive results, similar to the effects of treatment with estrogens [4, 15]. In a recent collaboration RCT with Dr. L. Dye at Leeds University, we found that a two-month cross-over 100 mg/day phytoestrogen treatment improved memory functions, but decreased visual sensitivity in postmenopausal women younger than 65 years of age (Dye, in preparation). In a series of other RCTs, we found that 100 mg phytoestrogens given once as a primer treatment improved procedural memory in young women [75]. A recent excellent and extensive review of this literature investigating phytoestrogen RCTs [3] concluded that of seven studies of postmenopausal women (not including Howes et al., 2004 [20]), four studies showed beneficial effects of soy supplementation. These were mainly on executive function in postmenopausal women who were younger than 66 years of age [16–18], and in one with a mixed age-group (average age 61 years, range 55–74: [19]). Effects on memory were also seen in these studies, but these were not always consistently on the same tests and/or function between studies, e.g., sometimes only short-term [16], long-term episodic memory [17], or only semantic memory [19] was improved after treatment.

This is very similar to the heterogeneity found in studies investigating effects of estrogen treatment on cognitive function [15]. Studies that included postmenopausal women of an older average age (of 60 [20], 64 [21], and 67 years of age [22]) all found no effects of soy on cognitive function.

These findings may substantiate the "age-dependent" and "window of opportunity" hypotheses (see discussion). Briefly, these hypotheses relate to sensitivity of the brain to estrogenic effects, which may be reduced in women who are too far removed from the age of menopause to benefit from estrogen's protective effects (see Chapters 4 and 5). On the other hand, a study with postmenopausal women of a younger age group (48–65 years) also found no significant effects of different types of soy treatment on cognitive function [23]. It was argued [3] that there was a large spread in age since menopause (1–35 years) between women in this particular study, which could have interfered with the effectiveness of soy treatment. This would be in line with the "window of opportunity" hypothesis.

The review concluded that differences in treatment compositions; age and age since menopause; habitual dietary soy intake (e.g., relating to sensitivity to soy)[1]; and the inter-individual differences in the production of equol (a metabolite from daidzein, which has very strong estrogenic effects) could all be responsible for inconsistent findings between studies [3].

In line with the window of time or age-dependent argument, an observational follow-up study (the Honolulu Asia Aging Study) found that elderly (>71 years of age) men and their wives who had reported to consume tofu more than twice a week in midlife had a higher risk of dementia, more brain atrophy, and lower cognitive function in later life than those who consumed less tofu [24]. The Kame project [25] also found negative associations of high tofu consumption (more than three times a week) with cognitive decline over a two-year period in Japanese American elderly. In stratified analyses this remained significant only for women who were hormone replacement users, but not for those who were not hormone users, elderly

---

[1] For example the study by Ho et al. [22] was conducted in Chinese women who consumed soy on a regular basis and who may not have been sensitive to the amount given in the intervention.

men, or those who consumed moderate (twice a week) to low amounts of tofu. These data suggest that there may be optimal levels of phytoestrogens, perhaps interacting with age, sex, and estrogen levels. The Study of Women's Health Across the Nation (SWAN) [26] of 195 Japanese and 185 Chinese women between 42 and 52 years of age found no association between genistein intake (as calculated from Food Frequency Questionnaires, or FFQ) and cognitive function (memory, processing speed, and executive function). The authors surmised that the effects might only be present in women who are in low-estrogen (postmenopausal) states. However, the cognitive tests used (e.g., context memory rather than word lists using free recall) may not have had sufficient resolution to show relatively small associations with soy intake tertiles. A Dutch study of n = 301 women aged 60–75 years also did not find any associations of dietary isoflavones (assessed using FFQ) and memory, processing speed, or executive function, although high lignan intake was associated with better processing speed and executive function [27]. In this cohort average consumption was much lower than that of the other cohorts (the median intake was 15 mg/day in the highest quartile, compared to 60 mg/day minimum in other cohorts) and therefore may not have had the detrimental effects as described in the cohorts of participants who had Asian diets [24, 25]. Asian diets have been calculated to be three-fold higher in isoflavone content than most Western diets. In traditional Asian diets more soy (a rich source of isoflavones) [3] is eaten than in Western diets [28, 29]. In Western diets phytoestrogen intake is predominantly in the form of lignans [27] and second-generation soy foods with very low levels of isoflavones [30].

Phytoestrogen levels were not actually measured in the studies described and self reports may not be reliable indicators of intake. Notwithstanding, data could be in line with the thesis that (phyto)estrogens may have optimal levels to maintain cognitive function in the middle aged, but not in the old (>65 years of age), in whom high consumption could be related to negative consequences for cognitive function. This negative effect is hypothesized on the basis of the age-dependent hypothesis of estrogens and the limited observational data. To our knowledge, no study has investigated associations of actual phytoestrogen levels and cognitive function in elderly men and women.

Why investigate dementia and phytoestrogen intake in Indonesia?

The Indonesian traditional diet contains high levels of phytoestrogens, in the form of soy products such as tempe (fermented whole soybean) and tofu or tahoe (soybean curd). Currently in Indonesia 8% (17 million) of the population is over 60 years old. This figure is expected to double by 2025 [31]. Age is a major risk factor for developing AD [32]. By 2050, 70% of older people will live in developing countries, such as Indonesia, who are burdened by few resources and a combination of non-communicable and communicable diseases [33]. This leads to increased dependence, a higher risk of primary and secondary dementias, and lower productivity. This will have important consequences as many older people still contribute to family finances in Indonesia as was shown in the Aging in Indonesia study [34]. Affordable preventive measures are thus of utmost importance. Dementia prevalence in Indonesia is at present unknown. In India, dementia prevalence is estimated at 5% of people aged over 60 years old [35]. Due to the similar demographic pyramid structure and similar life expectancy, similar dementia prevalence is expected in Indonesia.

In the present study we aimed to investigate the association between salivary phytoestrogen (using linear and non-linear terms) and cognitive function on Java. Low levels of education and the female gender are also important risk factors for AD [32] so in all analyses, sex, age, and education were taken along as covariates as well as in secondary analyses: socioeconomic status, site, and intake of other foods.

Methods

Participants

This cross-sectional feasibility study was carried out between April and June 2006 among mainly Javanese elderly men (n = 109) and women (n = 188) between 56 and 90 years of age, residing either in urban Central and South Jakarta (n = 188) or in rural Borobudur Yogyakarta (n = 109) on Java, Indonesia. In the rural Borobudur site (Central Java, a two-hour drive from Yogyakarta), all Javanese elderly covered by the Borobudur Community Heath Center were tested at the local health center, while two elderly with limited mobility were visited at home. For Central and South Jakarta (North-West Java), a convenience sample was included, who were either attending the local community health centers or lived in a care home in the area (n = 49). Those living in Jakarta comprised a mixed ethnic group (47% Javanese, 17% Sundanese, and others). Ethnic diversity, age, education, and socioeconomic status (those in rural areas were slightly older and less educated with 72% working as farmers or laborers) reflected the 2000 Indonesian demographic census. Governmental and local permits, ethical approval, and informed consent had all been obtained prior to the study onset. The present analyses only include the initial n = 297 participants who were tested between April and June 2006. Data on the full cohort (n = 719) of food intake relating to memory performance are published in [36].

Assessments

All participants had been informed of the study and after giving consent they were contacted to arrange a test-session with their carer present. Testing was done by trained research assistants between 8 and 11 am to avoid circadian interference and the effects of heat. Participants gave a saliva sample and were surveyed for demographic characteristics and nutritional intake (based on the Food Frequency Questionnaires [37] all corroborated by a carer). Questions about dietary intake included intake of tempe, tofu, and other genistein containing foods, as well as questions about intake of rice, fruit (whole or as juice), orange or red vegetables, green vegetables, or fish, which have all previously been found to lower dementia risk [e.g., 38]. These were calculated as intake per week (i.e., once a month = 0.25/week, 3 times a day = 21/week, etc.).

Participants were tested for cognitive function using the Hopkins Verbal Learning Test (HVLT, [39]) and Mini-Mental State Examination (MMSE, [40]) to assess global cognitive function. Some test items were slightly changed to adapt to local knowledge after a pilot study, in a similar way as the Hindi version used in India [41]. The HVLT is a word learning test measuring episodic memory, which consists of twelve words from three low-frequency categories (for version A: "human shelter," "animals," and "precious stones"). These words were all repeated three times to obtain a total immediate recall measure. After 30 minutes a delayed recall was obtained as a memory assessment. Memory is one of the first functions to show a decline in dementia, and this test was found to be sensitive to different forms – and the

early stages – of dementia [39, 42–44]. Verbal memory was also hypothesized to be most sensitive to estrogenic effects [15, 45]. Distribution of performance on both cognitive tests was similar to that of a comparable group of elderly from Oxfordshire. Back-translation was done successfully for tests and questionnaires, which were all well tolerated.

Dementia risk was assessed using a validated algorithm developed on the basis of data from the Oxford Project to Investigate Memory and Ageing, which had 91% sensitivity and 98% specificity using a cut-off of 24.5 for the translated MMSE [40] and 14.5 for the HVLT memory test for cases and 19.5 for controls [44]. In addition, for actual dementia estimates within the sample, performance on the Instrumental Activities of Daily Life had to be below 9, indicating impairment in functional capacity [46]. Confirmation by a carer using the Dementia Questionnaire [47] was also included. These questionnaires both validated the progressive cognitive and the functional impairment not attributable to other morbidity indicative of dementia [48].

In the total cohort dementia was estimated to occur in between 4% and 6% of participants over 60 years of age, confirming earlier estimates. A higher percentage of participants were suspected to have dementia in rural sites (9% in Borobudur and 6% in Cintegah) versus only 2% of the younger and better educated participants in Jakarta. Age and education explained most of the variance in test performance between sites and are the most important risk factors for dementia [32]. For the current analyses only the cognitive algorithm was used to identify those at possible dementia/ cognitive impairment risk and controls.

Genistein (the most potent phytoestrogen), daidizein, and glycitein levels were assayed in a university laboratory in Bogor using reversed-phase high-performance liquid chromatography (HPLC) (see for detail, [49]). The HPLC method has various advantages over other analytical instruments in its sensitivity and selectivity when dealing with very low levels of phytoestrogen [50]. Various studies comparing different methods of assessing phytoestrogen levels in bodily fluids have been published (for a review see [51]). The HPLC coulometric array detection method has been compared with a gas chromatography–mass spectrometry (GC-MS) technique and has been found to be "a practical, affordable means of phytoestrogen determination suitable for metabolic, pharmacokinetic and tissue distribution studies" [50]. Furthermore, it has the advantages of having simple sample preparation, higher sensitivity and specificity than the ultraviolet or diode array detection HPLC methods, and a wide analytical range [52]. The coulometric array method is thus suited to this study as it eliminates the need for sample re-extraction because large peaks of high concentrations do not saturate the detector [53]. In the present analyses only data on genistein are reported.

Results
Demographic characteristics and overall soy intake

The average age of participants was 70 ± 8 years. Thirty percent of participants had received no formal education, while 19% had received more than primary education. Only 7% of the cohort reported poor health. Most consumed soy products on a daily basis and only 2.4% of the cohort ate no tempe or tofu at all. Average consumption of both foods was ten times a week, but there was significant spread in the data reflected in the distribution of genistein levels (Fig. 13.1). Soy consumption was analyzed using median splits (44% of the cohort consumed the soy products more than once daily) or in continuous format.

Analyses pertaining to reported soy intake

High tempe consumption (more than once daily) was associated with better memory (delayed recall HVLT beta = 0.23, 95% CI = 0.31 to 2.82), while tofu was independently associated with worse memory (beta = −0.34, %95 CI = −3.65 to −1.12). Age and education also had a significant association, but there was no gender difference in performance.

There was a lower risk of possible dementia with high tempe consumption (OR = 0.10, 95% CI = 0.01 to 0.72) and an independent ten-fold higher risk with high tofu consumption (OR = 10.17, 95% CI = 1.3 to 78.2). All analyses were controlled for age, sex (which was non-significant), and education.

Controlling for intake of other foods (rice, fish, vegetables, etc.), ethnicity, socioeconomic status, or district did not alter results and also suggested that results were not explained by other factors and general deprivation.

Analyses stratified for median age (at 68 years) showed that negative associations of high tofu intake remained significant in those participants over 68 years of age, but not in those younger than 68 years of age. This would be in line with the age dependent/healthy cell hypothesis of estrogenic effects on the brain.

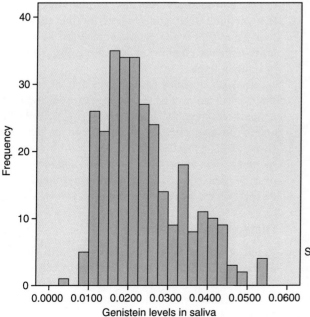

Fig. 13.1 Distribution of unmodified genistein levels (in ppm) in the cohort.

Mean = 0.023876 ppm
Std. dev. = 0.0101037 ppm
N = 297

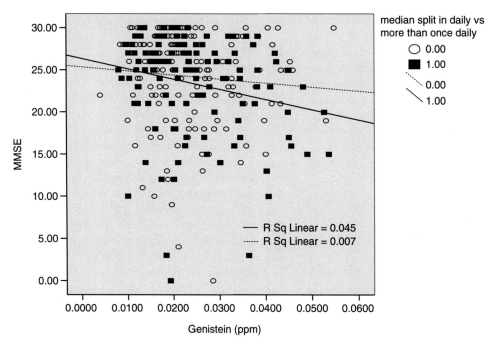

Fig. 13.2 Tofu intake (median split "0" once daily or less, "1" more than once a day), genistein levels (in ppm) and Mini-Mental State Examination (MMSE) performance in the cohort.

Analyses pertaining to genistein levels

Genistein levels were higher (p < 0.05) in possible dementia cases (N = 89, 0.027 ± 0.01) than in controls (N = 81, 0.024 ± 0.01). There was a trend for genistein levels to be associated with lower MMSE scores (p = 0.08) in analyses adjusted for age, sex, and education (Fig. 13.2). The curvilinear term (genistein squared) did not have a significant contribution when entered in these analyses. In age-stratified analyses (again using the median age of 68 years) controlled for age, sex, and education, the MMSE had a trend significant negative association with genistein when included as a linear term, but only for those participants who were 68 years and older (beta = −0.16, p = 0.055).

There was no overall association of genistein when entered as a linear term with memory performance (HVLT delayed recall) in linear regression analyses (p = 0.17) controlled for age, sex, and education. However, when the curvilinear term was also entered, both terms became significant, suggesting optimal levels of genistein associated with optimal memory function (Table 13.1). In age-stratified analyses these results remained significant for those participants younger than 68 years of age, but not for those who were 68 years of age and older.

In analyses stratified for sex, for women there was a significant negative linear association of genistein with MMSE performance (beta = −14, p = 0.05), while for men trends were seen in the same direction (but also including p = 0.10 for the curvilinear term). For memory function, similar trends were seen in both men and women for the curvilinear term (p = 0.07) while genistein included as a linear term remained significant indicating the possibility of optimal levels.

Analyses stratified for both age and sex indicated that for women over 68 years of age (n = 98) there was a significant negative linear (beta = −1.05, p = 0.02) and a positive curvilinear association of genistein (beta = 0.85, p = 0.05) with MMSE performance. For memory these associations were also found for men over 68 years of age and for women younger than 68 years of age, but not for women 68 years and older.

Discussion

Results reported herein are consistent with findings of the Honolulu-Asia Aging Study (HAAS) and the Kame studies [24, 25], in that high tofu consumption was associated with worse cognitive function and a higher risk of possible dementia. Tempe may offset

Table 13.1 Analyses (pertaining to men and women) of phytoestrogen levels with memory function.

Model	Unstandardized coefficients		Standardized coefficients		
	B	Std. error	Beta	t	sig.
(Constant)	7.088	2.215	–	3.200	0.002
Genistein squared	−3060.043	1510.089	−0.516	−2.026	0.044
Genistein (ppm) as a linear term	188.795	88.061	0.550	2.144	0.033
How old are you (age at your last birthday)?	−0.120	0.022	−0.289	−5.380	0.000
What was the highest education level you graduated from?	0.973	0.120	0.468	8.124	0.000
Sex	0.563	0.388	0.079	1.451	0.148

Note: Dependent variable: delayed recall, adjusted R squared = 30%.

this effect, but it had no significant associations with cognition by itself. Genistein levels had an optimal level relationship with memory performance particularly in women younger than 68 years of age and in older men. In line with the data on tofu, in older participants there was a trend negative association for genistein with global cognitive function. In analyses stratified for sex, associations were strongest in women, but there were fewer men in this cohort and power issues could have explained these results.

There are several limitations to this study. First, self report may not be a reliable reflection of intake, particularly in those with dementia because of the very nature of their morbidity [54]. Carers, when present (in 40% of possible cases and controls), also substantiated the information given by participants, which hopefully increased validity of this measure. However, if this was an issue, *low* but not high tofu consumption would have been associated with lower global cognitive function. In addition, other longitudinal cohorts found similar associations, which strengthen the possibility of accuracy of the finding. Importantly, genistein was associated with cognitive and memory performance. Analyses of genistein levels also reflected the results of the analyses pertaining to tofu intake. On the other hand, correlations between phytoestrogen levels and weekly total tofu intake (r = 0.12, p < 0.001 daidzein, r = 0.09, p < 0.05, glycitein, and r = 0.08, p = 0.07 for genistein) were weak. As people may or may not have eaten soy on testing days, these data are perhaps not surprising. It is thus unclear whether we investigated short (levels) or long-term effects of soy intake. Our follow-up

study will investigate consistency in dietary intake and the long-term effects of this on cognitive change. It should be noted that the genistein assay used may have not been optimal. Measuring phytoestrogen in saliva is in its early stages. We are further investigating reliability and validity of the method described versus blood standards and GC-MS to further substantiate the data.

It could also be argued that the cognitive tests used may not have been cross-culturally applicable. However, similar distributions were seen in test performance as in Oxfordshire and in general tests were well tolerated and had been adapted to local knowledge after a pilot. Back-translations were all satisfactory. Results reported were also independent of education and socioeconomic status, despite there being a large spread in these variables within the cohort. On the other hand, soy products are an economical form of protein, which is widely used in developing countries as a food source. Low socioeconomic status is an independent risk factor for AD [55] and it may be the case that the association between soy intake and cognition merely reflects degree of poverty as an underlying confounder. As stated, results found were independent of socioeconomic status, but more in-depth research of socioeconomic status using more appropriate measures than job and house ownership will be included in the follow-up to assess these influences in depth. There were no formal objective measures of health and it is unclear whether health-related factors may have mediated the associations found. Also, no formal clinical assessment of dementia was conducted. Future follow-up studies should be able to rectify these issues.

The Kame project suggested that the use of hormones determined whether tofu consumption had a negative association with cognition in women. In this study, no data on the use of hormone replacement were collected. However, some of the women in this study were younger than 60 years of age and may still have had intact menstrual function with fluctuating high levels of estrogens, which could affect phytoestrogens' effect on the brain [56]. Subsequent in-depth follow-up will enable us to investigate whether serum and salivary endogenous estrogens interact with phytoestrogen intake. However, in the present study, negative associations of tofu were most apparent in those *over* 68 years of age and were thus not expected to be explained through their antagonistic effect on endogenous estrogens. The findings of possible optimal genistein levels for memory function in women younger than 68 years of age could explain why no linear associations were found in the SWAN study.

Data from the current study could be consistent with data on estrogens described in this book. Similar to phytoestrogens, on the basis of cell and animal studies, observational data of estrogen users and small human treatment studies, estrogens were hailed as the most promising treatment for dementia in the nineties [4, 15]. However, results of recent large randomized controlled trials of elderly healthy women [4] and women with AD [57] indicated that estrogen treatment actually increased the risk for AD and could not prevent cognitive decline in women over 65 years of age. The Oxford Project to Investigate Memory and Ageing (OPTIMA) was one of the first studies to report that high estrogen levels were an independent risk factor for AD in women over 65 years of age [58]. Others have since reported similar associations [59, 60]. Women with higher total estradiol levels were also found to have smaller hippocampal volumes and poorer memory performance [61], both early markers of AD [62]. According to meta-analyses, a lack of assay sensitivity and/or accidental inclusion of hormone users may have to led to earlier reports of *lower* levels of estrogens in women with AD [63]. It is unclear why women with AD would have higher levels of estrogens and why increasing estrogen levels would put some women at risk for dementia. It is possible that certain genetic polymorphisms associated with sex steroid metabolism and synthesis play a role in this (see Chapter 15).

As described in this book, one hypothesis is that there are no effects of estrogens in those women who are too far removed from the age of menopause. A "window of opportunity" (see Chapters 4 and 5) may exist for estrogens to exert positive effects on the brains of women who have only relatively recently undergone menopause [8, 64]. This hypothesis, however, would not explain potential negative effects of estrogens. Another hypothesis is that estrogens have negative effects on cognitive function in older women (>65 years of age), the "age-dependent" hypothesis [65], which could be related to findings that cells undergoing pathological changes (which are more prevalent in older brains) respond negatively to estrogens (see Chapter 6).

A third hypothesis is that optimal sex steroid levels exist for optimal cognitive functions ("curvilinear associations"), which may be different for women and men [65–67]. This hypothesis may be complementary to the earlier hypotheses, when these optimal curves move to the left with age due to lower sensitivity and/or higher risk for adverse effects of sex steroids in the older brain. However, in contrast to women, men with AD were found to have lower levels of sex steroids than controls [58, 59, 68, 69]. Others reported that men over the age of 74 years who had high levels of free estradiol had increased risk of brain lacunes and cognitive decline [67, 70]. On the other hand, experimental studies have shown that in healthy men aged 50 to 90 conversion of testosterone into estradiol is required for positive effects of testosterone on verbal memory functions [71]. Associations of estrogens with cognitive performance in elderly men are perhaps not well understood [66]. Optimal levels and the degree of pathology experienced could potentially explain differences in findings between studies. However, in the present study (as in the HAAS) men older than 68 years of age, similar to women, seemed to be negatively affected by high genistein levels.

A strength of the present study was that several foods and different types of soy foods were investigated simultaneously. The fermented soy product tempe (which may protect against dementia and memory impairment) contains twice the level of the estrogen-like genistein of tofu [72]. Consistent with the findings of optimal levels of genistein for those participants who were younger than 68 years of age and negative associations of genistein with cognitive function in those over 68 years of age, tempe no longer had a positive significant contribution to the age-stratified analyses in those over 68 years of age. Power issues in this small sample could be responsible for this.

If power issues were related to no longer finding significant positive associations of tempe in stratified analyses, an alternative hypothesis for the protective effect of tempe in the overall analyses could be the following. Fermentation increases the folate content of tempe to 5.2-fold higher levels than those found in boiled soybean, which is the basis of tofu. This may be due to *de novo* formation of folate by molds in the fermentation process [73]. Folate has protective effects on brain function and could reduce dementia risk [74]. In earlier analyses of an Oxford-based cohort, we found that (a) elderly women with high serum estrogen levels were at risk for dementia, (b) those women with high estrogen levels and high folate levels did not fall below the cut-off score for dementia on the MMSE [63]. It is unclear how folate or other factors could protect against high levels of phytoestrogens.

In summary, in this chapter, similar to results in estrogen studies, high intake of tofu and genistein levels were both associated with lower cognitive function and an increased risk for dementia particularly in those participants who were older than 68 years of age. Results for tofu may reflect those of earlier longitudinal cohort studies. For those younger than 68 years of age, optimal genistein levels seemed to be present for optimal memory function. These data could tie in with those of the window of opportunity theory (Chapters 4 and 5) or the healthy cell bias theory (Chapter 6). Future studies to determine the interaction between serum phytoestrogens and folate levels and their relationship to dementia risk are warranted.

Acknowledgments

This pilot study was funded by the Alzheimer's Research Trust (ART/PPG2006A/2), which is committed to supporting research into varied forms of dementia. We would like to thank the following investigators from the University of Indonesia, Jakarta, who made substantial contributions to this study: Sabarinah Prasetyo, MD MSc; Purwaningtyastuti, MD PhD; Linda Kusdany, DDS PhD; Sudijanto Kamso, MD PhD; Siti Setiati, MD PhD; Wita Anggraini, DDS PhD. None of the authors or co-workers has any conflict of interest.

Disclosure

All authors had full access to all of the data in the study and take responsibility for the integrity of the data and the accuracy of the data analysis. None of the authors has any potential conflicts of interest, including financial interests and relationships and affiliations relevant to the subject of their manuscript.

References

1. FDA. Soy: health claims for soy protein, questions about other components, 2000. Available at: http://www.fda.gov/fdac/features/2000/300_soy.html. Accessed 2008.

2. Kris-Etherton PM, Hecker KD, Bonanome A, *et al.* Bioactive compounds in foods: their role in the prevention of cardiovascular disease and cancer. *Am J Med.* 2002;**113**(Suppl 9B):71S–88S.

3. Zhao L, Brinton RD. WHI and WHIMS follow-up and human studies of soy isoflavones on cognition. *Expert Rev Neurother.* 2007;7(11):1549–64.

4. Hogervorst E. The short-lived effects of hormone therapy on cognitive function. In Rasgun NL, ed. *Effects of Estrogen on Brain Function.* Baltimore, MD: John Hopkins University Press, 2006, pp. 46–78.

5. Hogervorst E, Ribeiro HM, Molyneux A, Budge M, Smith AD. Plasma homocysteine levels, cerebrovascular risk factors, and cerebral white matter changes (leukoaraiosis) in patients with Alzheimer disease. *Arch Neurol.* 2002;**59**(5):787–93.

6. Budge MM, de Jager C, Hogervorst E, Smith AD, Oxford Project to Investigate Memory and Ageing (OPTIMA). Total plasma homocysteine, age, systolic blood pressure, and cognitive performance in older people. *J Am Geriatr Soc.* 2002;**50**(12):2014–18.

7. Zaccai J, Ince P, Brayne C. Population-based neuropathological studies of dementia: design, methods and areas of investigation – a systematic review. *BMC Neurol.* 2006;**6**:2.

8. Gibbs RB. Preclinical data relating to estrogen's effects on cognitive performance. In Rasgon NL, ed. *Effects of Estrogen on Brain Function.* Baltimore, MD: John Hopkins University Press, 2006, pp. 9–45.

9. Henderson VW. Hormone therapy and Alzheimer's disease: benefit or harm? *Expert Opin Pharmacother.* 2004;**5**(2):389–406.

10. Sonee M, Sum T, Wang C, Mukherjee SK. The soy isoflavone, genistein, protects human cortical neuronal cells from oxidative stress. *Neurotoxicology.* 2004;**25**(5):885–91.

11. Azcoitia I, Moreno A, Carrero P, Palacios S, Garcia-Segura LM. Neuroprotective effects of soy phytoestrogens in the rat brain. *Gynecol Endocrinol.* 2006;**22**(2):63–9.

12. Zhao L, Chen Q, Diaz Brinton R. Neuroprotective and neurotrophic efficacy of phytoestrogens in cultured

hippocampal neurons. *Exp Biol Med.* 2002;**227**(7): 509–19.

13. Fitzpatrick LA. Soy isoflavones: hope or hype? *Maturitas.* 2003;**44**(Suppl 1):S21–9.

14. Grodstein F, Mayeux R, Stampfer MJ. Tofu and cognitive function: food for thought. *J Am Coll Nutr.* 2000;**19**(2):207–9.

15. Hogervorst E, Williams J, Budge M, Riedel W, Jolles J. The nature of the effect of female gonadal hormone replacement therapy on cognitive function in post-menopausal women: a meta-analysis. *Neuroscience.* 2000;**101**(3):485–512.

16. File SE, Hartley DE, Elsabagh S, Duffy R, Wiseman H. Cognitive improvement after 6 weeks of soy supplements in postmenopausal women is limited to frontal lobe function. *Menopause.* 2005;**12**(2):193–201.

17. Duffy R, Wiseman H, File SE. Improved cognitive function in postmenopausal women after 12 weeks of consumption of a soya extract containing isoflavones. *Pharmacol Biochem Behav.* 2003;**75**(3):721–9.

18. Casini ML, Marelli G, Papaleo E, *et al.* Psychological assessment of the effects of treatment with phytoestrogens on postmenopausal women: a randomized, double-blind, crossover, placebo-controlled study. *Fertil Steril.* 2006;**85**(4):972–8.

19. Kritz-Silverstein D, Von Muhlen D, Barrett-Connor E, Bressel MA. Isoflavones and cognitive function in older women: the SOy and Postmenopausal Health In Aging (SOPHIA) Study. *Menopause.* 2003;**10**(3):196–202.

20. Howes JB, Bray K, Lorenz L, Smerdely P, Howes LG. The effects of dietary supplementation with isoflavones from red clover on cognitive function in postmenopausal women. *Climacteric.* 2004;**7**(1):70–7.

21. Kreijkamp-Kaspers S, Kok L, Grobbee DE, *et al.* Effect of soy protein containing isoflavones on cognitive function, bone mineral density, and plasma lipids in postmenopausal women: a randomized controlled trial. *JAMA.* 2004;**292**(1):65–74.

22. Ho SC, Chan AS, Ho YP, *et al.* Effects of soy isoflavone supplementation on cognitive function in Chinese postmenopausal women: a double-blind, randomized, controlled trial. *Menopause.* 2007;**14**(3 Pt 1):489–99.

23. Fournier LR, Ryan Borchers TA, Robison LM, *et al.* The effects of soy milk and isoflavone supplements on cognitive performance in healthy, postmenopausal women. *J Nutr Health Aging.* 2007;**11**(2):155–64.

24. White LR, Petrovitch H, Ross GW, *et al.* Brain aging and midlife tofu consumption. *J Am Coll Nutr.* 2000;**19**(2):242–55.

25. Rice MM, Graves AB, McCurry SM, *et al.* Tofu consumption and cognition in older Japanese American men and women. *J Nutr.* 2000;**130**(3):676S.

26. Huang MH, Luetters C, Buckwalter GJ, *et al.* Dietary genistein intake and cognitive performance in a multiethnic cohort of midlife women. *Menopause.* 2006;**13**(4):621–30.

27. Kreijkamp-Kaspers S, Kok L, Grobbee DE, *et al.* Dietary phytoestrogen intake and cognitive function in older women. *J Gerontol A Biol Sci Med Sci.* 2007;**62**(5):556–62.

28. Wu AH, Ziegler RG, Nomura AM, *et al.* Soy intake and risk of breast cancer in Asians and Asian Americans. *Am J Clin Nutr.* 1998;**68**(6 Suppl):1437S–1443S.

29. Mulligan AA, Welch AA, McTaggart AA, Bhaniani A, Bingham SA. Intakes and sources of soya foods and isoflavones in a UK population cohort study (EPIC-Norfolk). *Eur J Clin Nutr.* 2007;**61**(2):248–54.

30. Murkies AL, Wilcox G, Davis SR. Clinical review 92: Phytoestrogens. *J Clin Endocrinol Metab.* 1998;**83**(2):297–303.

31. Wibowo S, Boedhi-Darmojo R, Kreager P, *et al. Indonesia's Elderly: Problem and Potential.* Indonesia: University of Indonesia Center for Health Research and University of Oxford, Oxford Institute of Aging, 2004.

32. Launer LJ, Andersen K, Dewey ME, *et al.* Rates and risk factors for dementia and Alzheimer's disease: results from EURODEM pooled analyses. EURODEM Incidence Research Group and Work Groups. European Studies of Dementia. *Neurology.* 1999;**52**(1):78–84.

33. Kalache A, Aboderin I, Hoskins I. Compression of morbidity and active ageing: key priorities for public health policy in the 21st century. *Bull World Health Organ.* 2002;**80**(3):243–4.

34. Kreager P. Migration, social structure and old-age support networks: a comparison of three Indonesian communities. *Ageing Soc.* 2006;**26**:37–60.

35. Biswas A, Chakraborty D, Dutt A, Roy T. Dementia in India – a critical appraisal. *J Indian Med Assoc.* 2005;**103**(3):154–8.

36. Hogervorst E, Sadjimim T, Yesufu A, Kreager P, Rahardjo TB. High tofu intake is associated with worse memory in elderly Indonesian men and women. *Dement Geriatr Cogn Disord.* 2008;**26**(1):50–7.

37. Frankenfeld CL, Lampe JW, Shannon J, *et al.* Frequency of soy food consumption and serum isoflavone concentrations among Chinese women in Shanghai. *Public Health Nutr.* 2004;**7**(6):765–72.

38. Barberger-Gateau P, Raffaitin C, Letenneur L, *et al.* Dietary patterns and risk of dementia: the Three-City cohort study. *Neurology.* 2007;**69**(20):1921–30.

39. Brandt J. The Hopkins Verbal Learning Test: development of a new memory test with six equivalent forms. *Clin Neuropsychol.* 1991;**5**:125–42.

40. Folstein MF, Folstein SE, McHugh PR. 'Mini-mental State': a practical method for grading the cognitive state of patients for the clinician. *J Psychiat Res.* 1975;**12**:189–98.

41. Ganguli M, Ratcliff G, Chandra V, *et al.* A Hindi version of the MMSE: the development of a cognitive screening instrument for a largely illiterate rural elderly population in India. *Int J Geriatr Psychiatry.* 1995;**10**:367–77.

42. Schrijnemaekers AM, de Jager CA, Hogervorst E, Budge MM. Cases with mild cognitive impairment and Alzheimer's disease fail to benefit from repeated exposure to episodic memory tests as compared with controls. *J Clin Exp Neuropsychol.* 2006;**28**(3):438–55.

43. De Jager CA, Hogervorst E, Combrinck M, Budge MM. Sensitivity and specificity of neuropsychological tests for mild cognitive impairment, vascular cognitive impairment and Alzheimer's disease. *Psychol Med.* 2003;**33**(6):1039–50.

44. Hogervorst E, Combrinck M, Lapuerta P, *et al.* The Hopkins Verbal Learning Test and screening for dementia. *Dement Geriatr Cogn Disord.* 2002;**13**(1):13–20.

45. Sherwin BB. Estrogen and/or androgen replacement therapy and cognitive functioning in surgically menopausal women. *Psychoneuroendocrinology.* 1988;**13**(4):345–57.

46. Lawton MP, Brody EM. Assessment of older people: self-maintaining and instrumental activities of daily living. *Gerontologist.* 1969;**9**(3):179–86.

47. Ellis RJ, Jan K, Kawas C, *et al.* Diagnostic validity of the dementia questionnaire for Alzheimer disease. *Arch Neurol.* 1998;**55**(3):360–5.

48. American Psychiatric Association. *Diagnostic and Statistical Manual of Mental Disorders*, 4th edn. American Psychiatric Association, 1994.

49. Griffith AP, Collison MW. Improved methods for the extraction and analysis of isoflavones from soy-containing foods and nutritional supplements by reversed-phase high-performance liquid chromatography and liquid chromatography-mass spectrometry. *J Chromatogr A.* 2001;**913**(1/2):397–413.

50. Gamache PH, Acworth IN. Analysis of phytoestrogens and polyphenols in plasma, tissue, and urine using HPLC with coulometric array detection. *Proc Soc Exp Biol Med.* 1998;**217**(3):274–80.

51. Wu Q, Wang M, Simon JE. Analytical methods to determine phytoestrogenic compounds. *J Chromatogr B Analyt Technol Biomed Life Sci.* 2004;**812**(1/2):325–55.

52. Wilkinson AP, Wahala K, Williamson G. Identification and quantification of polyphenol phytoestrogens in foods and human biological fluids. *J Chromatogr B Analyt Technol Biomed Life Sci.* 2002; **777**(1/2):93–109.

53. Laboratorytalk. Determination of xenoestrogens. 2003. Available at: http://www.laboratorytalk.com/news/esa/esa134.html. Accessed June 30, 2008.

54. Petitti DB, Buckwalter JG, Crooks VC, Chiu V. Prevalence of dementia in users of hormone replacement therapy as defined by prescription data. *J Gerontol A Biol Sci Med Sci.* 2002;**57**(8):M532–8.

55. Karp A, Kareholt I, Qiu C, *et al.* Relation of education and occupation-based socioeconomic status to incident Alzheimer's disease. *Am J Epidemiol.* 2004;**159**(2):175–83.

56. Chen WH, Lin CC, Chen TS, Misra TK, Liu CY. Capillary electrochromatographic analysis of aliphatic mono- and polycarboxylic acids. *Electrophoresis.* 2003;**24**(6):970–7.

57. Hogervorst E, Yaffe K, Richards M, Huppert FA. Hormone replacement therapy for cognitive function in postmenopausal women with dementia. *Cochrane Database Syst Rev.* 2009;**21**(1): CD003799. Review.

58. Hogervorst E, Combrinck M, Dowsett M, Smith AD. Methodological and conceptual difficulties in assessing the association between sex hormone levels and Alzheimer's disease. The Graylyn Conference on Women's Health. Poster Women's Cognitive Health, Graylyn International Conference Centre of Wake Forest University, Winston-Salem, North Carolina, Nov 8–10, 2001. (Won best poster award.)

59. Paoletti AM, Lello S, Fratta S, *et al.* Psychological effect of the oral contraceptive formulation containing 3 mg of drospirenone plus 30 microg of ethinyl estradiol. *Fertil Steril.* 2004;**81**(3):645–51.

60. Cunningham CJ, Sinnott M, Denihan A, *et al.* Endogenous sex hormone levels in postmenopausal women with Alzheimer's disease. *J Clin Endocrinol Metab.* 2001;**86**(3):1099–103.

61. den Heijer T, Geerlings MI, Hofman A, *et al.* Higher estrogen levels are not associated with larger hippocampi and better memory performance. *Arch Neurol.* 2003;**60**(2):213–20.

62. Smith AD, Jobst KA. Use of structural imaging to study the progression of Alzheimer's disease. *Br Med Bull.* 1996;**52**(3):575–86.

63. Hogervorst E, Williams J, Combrinck M, Smith AD. Measuring serum estradiol in women with Alzheimer's disease: the importance of the sensitivity of the assay method. *Eur J Endocrinol.* 2003;**148**:67–72.

64. Henderson VW. Only a matter of time? Hormone therapy and cognition. *Menopause.* 2005;**12**(1):1–3.

65. Hogervorst E, Bandelow S, Moffat SD. Increasing testosterone levels and effects on cognitive functions in elderly men and women: a review. *Curr Drug Targets CNS Neurol Disord.* 2005;**4**(5):531–40.

66. Hogervorst E, De Jager C, Budge M, Smith AD. Serum levels of estradiol and testosterone and performance in different cognitive domains in healthy elderly men and women. *Psychoneuroendocrinology.* 2004;**29**(3):405–21.

67. Muller M, Aleman A, Grobbee DE, de Haan EH, van der Schouw YT. Endogenous sex hormone levels and cognitive function in aging men: is there an optimal level? *Neurology.* 2005;**64**(5):866–71.

68. Hogervorst E, Combrinck M, Smith AD. Testosterone and gonadotropin levels in men with dementia. *Neuro Endocrinol Lett.* 2003;**24**(3/4):203–8.

69. Moffat SD, Zonderman AB, Metter EJ, *et al.* Free testosterone and risk for Alzheimer disease in older men. *Neurology.* 2004;**62**(2):188–93.

70. Irie F, Strozyk D, Peila R, *et al.* Brain lesions on MRI and endogenous sex hormones in elderly men. *Neurobiol Aging* 2006;**27**(8):1137–44.

71. Cherrier MM, Matsumoto AM, Amory JK, *et al.* The role of aromatization in testosterone supplementation: effects on cognition in older men. *Neurology.* 2005;**64**(2):290–6.

72. Wang H, Murphy PA. Isoflavone content in commercial soybean products. *J Agric Food Chem.* 1994;**42**:1666–73.

73. Ginting E, Arcot J. High-performance liquid chromatographic determination of naturally occurring folates during tempe preparation. *J Agric Food Chem.* 2004;**52**(26):7752–8.

74. Smith AD. Homocysteine, B vitamins, and cognitive deficit in the elderly. *Am J Clin Nutr.* 2002;**75**(5):785–6.

75. Yesufu A, Rahardjo T, Bandelow S, Hogervorst E. Soy, tofu and brain function in the elderly. In Martin C ed., *The Handbook of Behavior, Diet and Nutrition.* London: Karger, 2010.

Hypothalamus-pituitary-adrenal axis activity in aging women: its impact on the brain and the potential influence of estradiol

Oliver T. Wolf

Editors' introduction

Acute and chronic stress have well documented effects on memory consolidation and retrieval. As we age, the ability of the brain to cope with stress is often diminished, even as the presence of physical and emotional stressors increase. In this chapter, Wolf summarizes the latest evidence pertaining to effects of stress hormones, particularly cortisol, on memory, as well as evidence that activity of the hypothalamus-pituitary-adrenal (HPA) axis increases with age. Indications that women in particular are likely to experience chronically elevated levels of cortisol with advanced age is discussed, as well as the possibility that estrogens provide neuroprotection from chronically elevated stress hormones. Based on these data, the author proposes that the loss of estrogens may contribute significantly to increased HPA activity in postmenopausal women, and confer greater susceptibility to the negative effects of chronically elevated stress hormones on memory.

Introduction

Multiple endocrine changes occur during aging and these alterations not only influence processes in the periphery, but also impact on the aging brain. In the present chapter the focus is going to be on the HPA axis, a system which mostly is known for its important involvement in the stress response. While the acute stress response is important for the re-establishment of homeostasis, chronic stress or chronic alterations of the stress hormone system can compromise brain functioning. Here recent findings on this topic will be summarized with a focus on cognition and dementia in aging women. In this context the influence of the female sex steroid estradiol on the HPA axis and brain

effects mediated via the HPA will be discussed. In addition, a few other lines for the development of preventive interventions or treatment strategies against stress-associated brain dysfunction are touched upon.

The neuroendocrine stress response

A commonly used working definition states that stress occurs when a person perceives a real or anticipated challenge to his or her internal or external balance (homeostasis) [1, 2]. Thus when events do not turn out as expected stress occurs [3]. A *stressor* is the specific event that induces stress. Stressors can be physical or psychological in nature. In addition, a stressor can be acute (an upcoming job interview) or chronic (work overload, inadequate housing conditions, marital problems, etc.). Especially in humans, the subjective evaluation of the stressor as well as the evaluation of available coping resources is crucial in determining the impact of a stressor on the individual [4]. What might be an exciting challenge for one person could be perceived as a major threat by another.

Interaction with a stressor leads to a cascade of neuroendocrine responses designed to facilitate adaptation. The hypothalamus-pituitary-adrenal (HPA) axis and the sympathetic nervous system are of special relevance in this respect. Sympathetic nervous system activity leads to rapid release of (nor)epinephrine from the adrenal medulla, which constitutes the first response wave. The HPA response is somewhat slower and is conceptualized as a second response wave. Hypothalamus-pituitary-adrenal activity is increased when the paraventricular nucleus of the hypothalamus receives excitatory input from other brain regions [1]. Corticotrophin-releasing hormone (CRH) and vasopressin reach the pituitary through

Hormones, Cognition and Dementia: State of the Art and Emergent Therapeutic Strategies, ed. Eef Hogervorst, Victor W. Henderson, Robert B. Gibbs, and Roberta Diaz Brinton. Published by Cambridge University Press.
© Cambridge University Press 2009.

the portal blood system, where they initiate the secretion of adrenocorticotropic hormone (ACTH) in the bloodstream. In response to ACTH the adrenal glands secrete glucocorticoids (GCs). In most laboratory rodents (rats and mice) corticosterone dominates, whereas in humans cortisol is the main adrenal GC. Only a small fraction (5–10%) of the released cortisol levels is available as free "unbound" cortisol. The rest is bound onto cortisol binding globulin or albumin. It is believed that only the free fraction is biologically active [5].

After stress the negative feedback of cortisol leads to a decreased HPA activation and thus GC levels return to baseline values within hours [1, 6]. In situations of chronic stress, permanent alterations of the HPA axis (hyper- but also hypoactivity) can occur [2].

As lipophilic steroid hormones, GCs enter the brain where they initiate multiple effects in several target regions. Of interest for the present review is the fact that GCs influence brain regions that are important for memory (e.g., the amygdala, the hippocampus, and the prefrontal cortex). These effects are mediated through the two receptors for the hormone: the mineralocorticoid receptor (MR) and the glucocorticoid receptor (GR). These receptors differ in their affinity for cortisol (with the MR having a much higher affinity) and in their localization throughout the brain. In addition, GCs can exert rapid non-genomic effects by influencing ion channels or neurotransmitter receptors at the membrane level [1, 7].

Acute stress and memory

Stress exerts complex effects on several forms of learning and memory [8, 9]. This chapter will only focus on declarative long-term memory, which refers to the explicit storage of facts and events that can later be intentionally retrieved [10]. This type of memory is tested in human studies with word lists, paired associates, or short stories. In daily life it corresponds to remembering items from your grocery list, or recalling the phone number of a person you have recently met. Long-term memory can be further divided into different memory phases, namely acquisition (or initial learning), consolidation (or storage), and retrieval (or recall). An intact medial temporal lobe (hippocampus and surrounding cortical structures) is essential for the successful completion (acquisition and consolidation) of a declarative long-term memory task. The role of the hippocampus in memory retrieval is debated. For intentional retrieval the prefrontal cortex is very important [10].

The literature regarding the effects of stress on declarative memory has been confusing, with groups reporting enhancing as well as impairing effects; however, it has become more and more apparent that this is largely due to the fact that the different memory phases are influenced by GCs in an opposing fashion [11].

The stress-associated rise in GCs enhances memory consolidation, and this aspect represents the adaptive and beneficial effect of stress on memory. In rodents, making a memory task more stressful leads to superior consolidation of the task. In humans cortisol treatment as well as post-learning stress causes enhanced memory consolidation, especially for emotionally arousing material. Elevated glucocorticoid levels potentiate the enhancing effect of emotional arousal on memory consolidation [8, 9, 11]. A stressful episode is thus remembered better than a non-stressful episode; this could help the individual to avoid a similar threatening event in the future.

Roozendaal and McGaugh used site-specific injections of GC receptor and adrenergic receptor agonists and antagonists, as well as selective lesions, to shown that GCs interact with noradrenergic activity in the basolateral amygdala, thereby influencing memory processes in other brain regions (e.g., the hippocampus for spatial long-term memory or the prefrontal cortex for working memory [11]).

Although the enhanced memory consolidation is adaptive and beneficial, the process appears to occur at the cost of impaired retrieval. In animals, as well as humans, acute stress or GC treatment at the time of retrieval leads to impaired retrieval of previously learned information [11]. In humans exposure to a brief laboratory stressor as well as the pharmacological administration of a single dose of cortisol reliably leads to impaired memory retrieval [8, 9]. Thus, in a stressful situation we are less able to remember the name of a certain medication, the phone number of a friend, or the description of the location of a new store in our neighborhood. In line with these laboratory studies, there are observational studies showing that self-reported stress is associated with memory problems in older adults [12].

Roozendaal and colleagues have summarized their findings on stress and long-term memory as indicative that stress puts the brain into a "consolidation mode," which is accompanied by impaired retrieval [11]. Taken together, studies in animals and humans converge on the idea that acute stress or elevated GCs at the time of initial learning (acquisition) enhance memory consolidation, while acute stress at the time of recall impair memory retrieval.

Effects of chronic stress on brain structure and memory

Animal research has provided insight into the structural alterations in the brain caused by chronic stress. In the hippocampus chronic stress leads to retraction of dendrites (dendritic atrophy; [7, 13]) and similar effects occur in the medial prefrontal cortex (mPFC) [14]. This atrophy is reversible after stress termination, demonstrating substantial neuroplasticity [15, 16]. In addition stress leads to reduced neurogenesis in the dentate gyrus and the mPFC [7, 17]. Even though the function of these newborn neurons is disputed, an impairment of memory and learning resulting from reduced neurogenesis is likely [17]. At the behavioral level impaired performance in hippocampal dependent spatial memory tasks can be observed [7, 18, 19].

In contrast to the hippocampus, the amygdala becomes hypertrophic in conditions of chronic stress [20]. Increases in dendritic arborization and spine density take place. Moreover activity of the corticotropin-releasing factor (CRF) system in the amygdala, which is involved in anxiety, is enhanced [21]. Behaviorally chronically stressed animals show enhanced fear conditioning [22]. Under chronic stress the brain seems to shift from a cognitive rational mode to a more affective (fearful) and automated response style [9].

Interestingly there is evidence that the negative effect of chronic stress on spatial memory might occur only in male rats, and not in female rats [23]. In line with these findings stress-induced dendritic atrophy in the hippocampus was observed in male rats, but not in female rats [24]. Similarly, acute stress impairs spatial memory only in males [25]; however, female rodents are more impaired by stress than their male counterparts with regard to other memory domains (e.g., working (short-term) memory or classical (Pavlovian) eyelid conditioning; [26, 27]). Thus, sex differences in how stress influences memory are task specific, which most likely translates to different sensitivities of specific brain regions to stress [9].

In humans, exposure to chronic stress (e.g., shift workers, airplane personnel, and soldiers) is associated with cognitive deficits in several domains (e.g., working memory and declarative memory) [28, 29].

These observed deficits might in part reflect elevated GC levels in situations of chronic stress. This conclusion would be in line with experimental studies administering GCs for days to weeks and observing cognitive impairments (e.g., [30]). Further evidence comes from studies with patients receiving GC therapy [31]. Whether the negative effects on memory reflect acute or chronic effects and whether they are reversible is currently unknown [8, 9]. A recent study suggests that at least the negative effects of the GC on memory retrieval are rapidly reversible and only reflect the acute impact of the daily medication [32].

Data from patients with Cushing's disease (hyper-adrenocorticism) point in the same direction. Cognitive impairments and hippocampal volume reductions [33] have been reported. Hippocampal atrophy might be reversible once successful treatment has occurred [34]. This would be in line with the remaining plasticity of this structure observed in animal studies.

The HPA axis in aging

Aging leads to alterations of the HPA axis, even though there is substantial variability among individuals. Several studies observed that basal activity increases [35]. This effect is especially prominent during the nadir phase, late evening and the first half of the night, when older subjects have higher levels of cortisol. In addition negative feedback of the HPA axis is less efficient. Thus after exogenous cortisol administration, in the dexamethasone suppression test or in the combined Dex/CRH test, older subjects display higher ACTH and cortisol levels [35, 36]. These alterations lead to a higher exposure to endogenous cortisol with aging. These changes might reflect age-associated diseases, stress exposure over the lifespan, genetic vulnerabilities, the long-term consequences of early adversity, or a combination of the above [13].

There is evidence that the HPA alterations during aging are more pronounced in women. This has been reported in studies measuring cortisol levels over the course of the day (e.g., [35]) as well as in studies using pharmacological or psychological challenges in order to investigate changes in the responsivity or the feedback of the HPA axis (e.g., [37]). Of relevance for the present chapter are findings from a meta-analysis containing 26 studies. Otte and co-workers reported that the age-associated increase in cortisol response to pharmacological or psychological challenges was three times larger in women than in men [36].

Memory in old age: influences of the HPA axis

Animal studies have repeatedly documented that memory impairment in aging is associated with enhanced HPA activity. For example in one study by Issa and colleagues older memory-impaired rats had elevated basal corticosterone levels as well as a more pronounced and longer lasting HPA stress response when compared to young rats. In contrast, older animals that showed no evidence of decreasing memory functioning were characterized by HPA axis activity similar to young animals [38]. Findings along this line have been reported by other laboratories.

In older otherwise healthy humans, observational studies have reported associations between elevated cortisol levels and declarative memory impairments. This has been reported in cross-sectional studies [39, 40], in studies using cortisol levels for the prediction of future cognitive decline [41–43], as well as in longitudinal studies [44, 45]. In some studies these associations were specific to hippocampal-based declarative memory, while in other studies rising cortisol levels were associated also with more global measures of cognitive functioning (also including working memory or attention). It has to be kept in mind that, obviously, none of these human studies allow a clear cause-and-effect interpretation, but instead represent observed associations.

The neuroanatomical correlate of these hormone performance associations in humans remains to be established. Here, the possible association between rising cortisol levels and atrophy of the hippocampus or the prefrontal cortex (measured with magnetic resonance imaging) is insufficiently understood. While several small studies detected a negative correlation between cortisol levels and hippocampal volumes in older healthy subjects [44, 46] a larger study detected associations between cortisol levels and cognition, but failed to find any associations between cortisol and regional brain volumes [40].

There is evidence that patients with Alzheimer's dementia (AD) show signs of HPA hyperactivity when compared to healthy older control subjects [47, 48]. This could just reflect the damage to HPA feedback centers in the brain, but might also be causally involved in disease progression [49].

Recent work in transgenic mice has documented that HPA hyperactivity can negatively influence amyloid metabolism as well as tau phosphorylation [50, 51]. In human AD patients a placebo-controlled randomized double-blind trial revealed that treatment with the synthetic glucocorticoid prednisone for one year resulted in an exaggerated memory loss [52]. Supporting the notion that glucocorticoids can increase AD pathology comes from another study. Here a genetic susceptibility for AD could be linked to the gene encoding 11 beta hydroxysteroid dehydrogenase type 1 (11bHSD1), an enzyme that influences local GC metabolism in the brain [53]. Finally, a large epidemiological study found that subjects who reported a high level of stress susceptibility had a substantially greater dementia risk [54].

Taken together, there is emerging evidence from multiple sources to suggest that chronically elevated cortisol levels can contribute directly as well as indirectly to cognitive decline in older women and men.

Stress, aging, and memory: a role for estrogens?

When discussing the potential role of estrogens in the context of age-associated HPA alterations and their impact on the brain two potential mechanisms can be distinguished. On the one hand, estrogens might be able to prevent the age-associated HPA hyperactivity, on the other hand, estrogens might be able to prevent elevated cortisol levels from impairing brain functions by antagonizing some of the GC effects in the brain. Those two potential mechanisms will be discussed below.

As mentioned above, there is evidence that cortisol levels increase with age more in women than in men [35, 36]. Moreover, recent evidence suggests that basal urinary cortisol levels increase temporarily during the menopausal transition [55]. In this context, questions have been raised about the potential role of estrogens in preventing age-associated HPA hyperactivity in women. As of today, the empirical situation is unsatisfying. Evidence from a few small studies will be summarized below.

Estradiol and basal HPA activity in older women

Studies investigating the effects of estrogens on basal cortisol levels have led to mixed findings. It is important to consider the fact that treatment with oral estrogens leads to an increase in cortisol binding globulin via its impact on the liver. Thus more cortisol can be bound. As a compensatory response cortisol production is increased leading to higher levels of total serum cortisol. In contrast, the biologically active free fraction of the hormone appears to remain relatively stable [56, 57]. These alterations (increase in cortisol binding globulin and total cortisol) do not occur in response to transdermal estradiol treatment [56, 57].

Our group recently conducted a placebo controlled randomized study (six months' treatment length) with older menopausal women to test the effects of oral estradiol treatment or a combination of oral estradiol together with oral progesterone on memory and mood [58]. In addition, salivary cortisol levels were measured throughout the day. In line with the studies mentioned above no effect of the gonadal hormones on free salivary cortisol levels were obtained.

However, since all of these studies tested only a small number of subjects and often investigated only a relatively brief treatment period, more evidence-based information on this important topic is needed.

Estradiol and HPA response to challenge in aging women

A few studies have investigated the effects of estrogenic treatment on the HPA response to a challenge in menopausal women. In a small observational study (N = 28) it was observed that women on postmenopausal estrogenic therapy had basal cortisol levels comparable to those of young women. In contrast, older women not taking hormone treatment had elevated levels of cortisol. More importantly, women on hormone treatment showed a less pronounced cortisol stress response to a laboratory stressor [59]. In contrast, Burleson and co-workers failed to find differences in the HPA response to a psychological stressor between women not taking hormones (N = 25), women on estrogenic treatment (N = 16), and women taking estrogens together with a progestin (N = 14).

Randomized treatment studies might be better suited to uncover a causal influence of estradiol on HPA reactivity in older women. In one small (N = 12) study, transdermal estradiol treatment for eight weeks resulted in a reduced HPA response (ACTH and cortisol) to a psychological stressor [60]. Similarly, Lindheim and colleagues observed that transdermal estradiol given for six weeks, when compared to placebo, led to a blunted HPA response to a psychological stressor [61]. Interestingly, a follow-up study demonstrated that the addition of medroxy-progesterone acetate (MPA) abolished the favorable effects of

estradiol on the HPA response to stress [62]. A separate study with 28 subjects, however, found that transdermal estradiol treatment had no effect on the HPA response to psychosocial stress [37].

In the latter study an additional pharmacological challenge test was employed. In the combined Dex/CRH test older women treated with placebo showed evidence for an exaggerated HPA response compared to younger women, which is in agreement with other studies on this topic [36]. In contrast, participants treated with estradiol for two weeks showed a response pattern that was highly similar to the response pattern of a young control group [37]. Thus this study provides initial evidence for a beneficial effect of estradiol treatment in postmenopausal women on their HPA response to a pharmacological challenge. Additional evidence for a reduced HPA reactivity after estradiol treatment comes from a study that tested the stimulatory influence of an endotoxin on the HPA response. Here transdermal estradiol treatment again led to a blunted ACTH as well as cortisol response to this immunological challenge [63].

Taken together, while the existing literature is suggestive of a beneficial effect of estradiol on the HPA stress response to a challenge [64] more research is needed before any firm conclusions can be drawn. In addition, the possible impact of progesterone has not received the attention needed.

Influence of estradiol on the impact of GCs in the brain

Another potential beneficial effect of estradiol could be a direct protective effect within brain regions sensitive to GC-induced damage. For example, stress in laboratory rodents leads to memory impairments and dendritic atrophy within the hippocampus in male rats only [24]. Female rats appear to be protected, and there is evidence that this is due, in part, to their higher estradiol levels [13, 23]. In older animals these sex differences are no longer present [65].

Note that glucocorticoids can exacerbate free radical toxicity and this effect might be of importance for the pathogenesis of AD. In contrast, estradiol is able to protect neurons from free radical induced stress and thus may block some of the deleterious effects of GCs in the brain [66].

In summary, there is initial evidence from several lines of research that estradiol might prevent age-associated HPA hyperactivity, and may also be able to reduce the negative impact of chronic stress on some parts of the brain. Having said this, current empirical evidence is not solid enough to allow clinical recommendations for the practitioner. Hopefully, HPA reactivity measures will be included in future trials of estrogenic therapy in order to fill this empirical gap.

Other intervention strategies

While the potential of estradiol as a stress-protective agent remains to be further explored, several other potentially beneficial intervention strategies should be mentioned briefly. These concern physiological states in which HPA hyperactivity is often observed. Chronic stress due to work overload has been associated with increased HPA axis activity in several studies [1, 2]. Here, psychological intervention – such as social competence training, relaxation techniques, social support, or active leisure activities (exercise) – should be recommended [67].

Several psychiatric disorders are associated with HPA hyperactivity, most notably major depression [7, 68]. In this situation, antidepressant treatments or psychotherapeutic interventions are indicated. Clinicians need to be sensitive to mood alterations in their age-advanced patients. The clinical relevance of this is highlighted by the fact that depression in older adults is associated with a higher dementia risk [69].

Another condition often associated with increased HPA activity is the metabolic syndrome and type 2 diabetes. The prevalence of both conditions increases substantially with age [70]. There are close links between the stress system and the glucoregulatory system. Several authors have suggested that chronic stress facilitates the occurrence of the metabolic syndrome by influencing visceral fat deposition, impairing insulin sensitivity, or by changing eating habits towards unhealthier (comfort) food [71, 72]. Alternatively, the negative impact of glucose intolerance on the brain might lead to HPA hyperactivity and in turn elevated cortisol levels [70]. Against the metabolic syndrome and type 2 diabetes, lifestyle modifications (e.g., diet and exercise) are often successful if started early enough. If lifestyle changes alone are not sufficient to prevent or treat type 2 diabetes, several pharmacological approaches are currently available [67]. Such interventions are important, since the metabolic syndrome and, even more so, type 2 diabetes is associated with memory impairment, hippocampal atrophy, and an increased dementia risk [70].

In addition to the somewhat indirect approaches mentioned above, there is very promising initial evidence that drugs aimed at influencing local GC concentrations within the brain might be effective agents for the prevention of cortisol-induced memory decline in aging. Local steroid concentrations are, in part, determined by the activity of the enzyme 11 beta hydroxysteroid dehydrogenase type 1 (11bHSD1), which regenerates active GCs from their inactive 11-keto derivatives. Thus, the enzyme increases tissue levels of corticosterone and cortisol. Removal of this enzyme in transgenic mice results in lower intrahippocampal corticosterone levels and reduces GC-associated cognitive decline during aging [73, 74]. In humans, two small, pharmacological, placebo-controlled crossover intervention studies in older subjects or age-advanced patients with type 2 diabetes showed that 11bHSD1 inhibition with the drug carbenoxolone was able to improve some aspects of memory [75]. More research is needed in order to establish the benefits and potential harm of this interesting intervention strategy.

Summary and conclusions

This chapter has highlighted how stress acutely enhances memory consolidation but impairs memory retrieval. In contrast, chronic stress is associated mostly with memory dysfunctions. Activity of the HPA axis increases with aging, and these alterations are more pronounced in women. Thus, the aging female brain is exposed to elevated levels of cortisol. Several studies suggest that this increase is associated with memory impairments. Animal studies and preliminary small-scale experimental studies in humans suggest that pharmacological or behavioral interventions will in the future be able to protect aging women in a more targeted fashion from the negative impact of chronically elevated stress hormone levels. The potential role of estrogens in this context remains to be established.

References

1. De Kloet ER, Joels M, Holsboer F. Stress and the brain: from adaptation to disease. *Nat Rev Neurosci.* 2005; 6:463–75.

2. McEwen BS. Protective and damaging effects of stress mediators. *New Engl J Med.* 1998;**338**(3):171–9.

3. Ursin H, Eriksen HR. The cognitive activation theory of stress. *Psychoneuroendocrinology.* 2004;**29**(5):567–92.

4. Lazarus RS. Coping theory and research: past, present, and future. *Psychosom Med.* 1993;**55**(3):234–47.

5. Mendel CM. The free hormone hypothesis: a physiologically based mathematical model. *Endocr Rev.* 1989;**10**(3):232–74.

6. Dickerson SS, Kemeny ME. Acute stressors and cortisol responses: a theoretical integration and synthesis of laboratory research. *Psychol Bull.* 2004; **130**(3):355–91.

7. Herbert J, Goodyer IM, Grossman AB, *et al.* Do corticosteroids damage the brain? *J Neuroendocrinol.* 2006;**18**(6):393–411.

8. Wolf OT. Effects of stress hormones on the structure and function of the human brain. *Expert Rev Endocrinol Metabol.* 2006;**1**(5):623–32.

9. Wolf OT. The influence of stress hormones on emotional memory: relevance for psychopathology. *Acta Psychol. (Amst)* 2008;**127**(3):513–31.

10. LaBar KS, Cabeza R. Cognitive neuroscience of emotional memory. *Nat Rev Neurosci.* 2006;**7**(1):54–64.

11. Roozendaal B, Okuda S, de Quervain DJ, McGaugh JL. Glucocorticoids interact with emotion-induced noradrenergic activation in influencing different memory functions. *Neuroscience.* 2006;**138**:901–10.

12. Neupert SD, Almeida DM, Mroczek DK, Spiro A, III. Daily stressors and memory failures in a naturalistic setting: findings from the VA Normative Aging Study. *Psychol Aging.* 2006;**21**(2):424–9.

13. McEwen BS. Sex, stress and the hippocampus: allostasis, allostatic load and the aging process. *Neurobiol Aging.* 2002;**23**(5):921–39.

14. Radley JJ, Morrison JH. Repeated stress and structural plasticity in the brain. *Ageing Res Rev.* 2005;**4**(2):271–87.

15. McEwen BS. Mood disorders and allostatic load. *Biol Psychiatry.* 2003;**54**(3):200–7.

16. Radley JJ, Rocher AB, Janssen WG, *et al.* Reversibility of apical dendritic retraction in the rat medial prefrontal cortex following repeated stress. *Exp Neurol.* 2005;**196**:199–203.

17. Gould E, Tanapat P, Rydel T, Hastings N. Regulation of hippocampal neurogenesis in adulthood. *Biol Psychiatry.* 2000;**48**(8):715–20.

18. Bodnoff SR, Humphreys AG, Lehman JC, *et al.* Enduring effects of chronic corticosterone treatment on spatial learning, synaptic plasticity, and hippocampal neuropathology in young and mid-aged rats. *J Neurosci.* 1995;**15**(1 Pt 1):61–9.

19. Conrad CD, Galea LA, Kuroda Y, McEwen BS. Chronic stress impairs rat spatial memory on the Y-maze, and this effect is blocked by tianeptine pretreatment. *Behav Neurosci.* 1996;**110**(6):1321–34.

20. Sapolsky RM. Stress and plasticity in the limbic system. *Neurochem Res.* 2003;**28**(11):1735–42.

21. Schulkin J, Gold PW, McEwen BS. Induction of corticotropin-releasing hormone gene expression by glucocorticoids: implication for understanding the states of fear and anxiety and allostatic load. *Psychoneuroendocrinology.* 1998;**23**(3):219–43.

22. Conrad CD, LeDoux JE, Magarinos AM, McEwen BS. Repeated restraint stress facilitates fear conditioning independently of causing hippocampal CA3 dendritic atrophy. *Behav Neurosci.* 1999;**113**(5):902–13.

23. Luine V. Sex differences in chronic stress effects on memory in rats. *Stress.* 2002;**5**(3):205–16.

24. Galea LA, McEwen BS, Tanapat P, *et al.* Sex differences in dendritic atrophy of CA3 pyramidal neurons in response to chronic restraint stress. *Neuroscience.* 1997;**81**(3):689–97.

25. Conrad CD, Jackson JL, Wieczorek L, *et al.* Acute stress impairs spatial memory in male but not female rats: influence of estrous cycle. *Pharmacol Biochem Behav.* 2004;**78**(3):569–79.

26. Shansky RM, Rubinow K, Brennan A, Arnsten AF. The effects of sex and hormonal status on restraint-stress-induced working memory impairment. *Behav Brain Funct.* 2006;**2**:8.

27. Shors TJ. Learning during stressful times. *Learn Mem.* 2004;**11**(2):137–44.

28. Cho K. Chronic 'jet lag' produces temporal lobe atrophy and spatial cognitive deficits. *Nat Neurosci.* 2001;**4**(6):567–8.

29. Morgan CA, III, Doran A, Steffian G, Hazlett G, Southwick SM. Stress-induced deficits in working memory and visuo-constructive abilities in Special Operations soldiers. *Biol Psychiatry.* 2006;**60**(7):722–9.

30. Newcomer JW, Selke G, Melson AK, *et al.* Decreased memory performance in healthy humans induced by stress-level cortisol treatment. *Arch Gen Psychiatry.* 1999;**56**(6):527–33.

31. Wolkowitz OM, Reus VI, Canick J, Levin B, Lupien S. Glucocorticoid medication, memory and steroid psychosis in medical illness. *Ann N Y Acad Sci.* 1997;**823**:81–96.

32. Coluccia D, Wolf OT, Kollias S, *et al.* Glucocorticoid therapy-induced memory deficits: acute versus chronic effects. *J Neurosci.* 2008;**28**(13):3474–8.

33. Starkman MN, Gebarski SS, Berent S, Schteingart DE. Hippocampal formation volume, memory dysfunction, and cortisol levels in patients with Cushing's syndrome. *Biol Psychiatry.* 1992;**32** (9):756–65.

34. Starkman MN, Giordani B, Gebarski SS, *et al.* Decrease in cortisol reverses human hippocampal atrophy

following treatment of Cushing's disease. *Biol Psychiatry*. 1999;**46**(12):1595–602.

35. Van Cauter E, Leproult R, Kupfer DJ. Effects of gender and age on the levels and circadian rhythmicity of plasma cortisol. *J Clin Endocrinol Metab*. 1996;**81**(7):2468–73.

36. Otte C, Hart S, Neylan TC, *et al*. A meta-analysis of cortisol response to challenge in human aging: importance of gender. *Psychoneuroendocrinology*. 2005;**30**(1):80–91.

37. Kudielka BM, Schmidt-Reinwald AK, Hellhammer DH, Kirschbaum C. Psychological and endocrine responses to psychosocial stress and dexamethasone/corticotropin-releasing hormone in healthy postmenopausal women and young controls: the impact of age and a two-week estradiol treatment. *Neuroendocrinology*. 1999;**70**(6):422–30.

38. Issa AM, Rowe W, Gauthier S, Meaney MJ. Hypothalamic-pituitary-adrenal activity in aged, cognitively impaired and cognitively unimpaired rats. *J Neurosci*. 1990;**10**(10):3247–54.

39. Lee BK, Glass TA, McAtee MJ, *et al*. Associations of salivary cortisol with cognitive function in the Baltimore memory study. *Arch Gen Psychiatry*. 2007;**64**(7):810–8.

40. MacLullich AM, Deary IJ, Starr JM, *et al*. Plasma cortisol levels, brain volumes and cognition in healthy elderly men. *Psychoneuroendocrinology*. 2005;**30**(5):505–15.

41. Greendale GA, Kritz-Silverstein D, Seeman T, Barrett-Connor E. Higher basal cortisol predicts verbal memory loss in postmenopausal women: Rancho Bernardo Study. *J Am Geriatr Soc*. 2000;**48**(12):1655–8.

42. Li G, Cherrier MM, Tsuang DW, *et al*. Salivary cortisol and memory function in human aging. *Neurobiol Aging*. 2006;**27**(11):1705–14.

43. Karlamangla AS, Singer BH, Chodosh J, McEwen BS, Seeman TE. Urinary cortisol excretion as a predictor of incident cognitive impairment. *Neurobiol Aging*. 2005;**26**(Suppl 1):80–4.

44. Lupien SJ, de Leon M, De Santi S, *et al*. Cortisol levels during human aging predict hippocampal atrophy and memory deficits. *Nat Neurosci*. 1998;**1**(1):69–73.

45. Seeman TE, McEwen BS, Singer BH, Albert MS, Rowe JW. Increase in urinary cortisol excretion and memory declines: MacArthur studies of successful aging. *J Clin Endocrinol Metab*. 1997;**82**(8):2458–65.

46. Wolf OT, Convit A, de Leon MJ, Caraos C, Quadri SF. Basal hypothalamo-pituitary-adrenal axis activity and corticotropin feedback in young and older men: relationship to magnetic resonance imaging derived hippocampus and cingulate gyrus volumes. *Neuroendocrinology*. 2002;**75**:241–9.

47. de Leon MJ, McRae T, Tsai JR, *et al*. Abnormal cortisol response in Alzheimer's disease linked to hippocampal atrophy. *Lancet*. 1988;**2**(8607):391–2.

48. O'Brien JT, Ames D, Schweitzer I, Mastwyk M, Colman P. Enhanced adrenal sensitivity to adrenocorticotrophic hormone (ACTH) is evidence of HPA axis hyperactivity in Alzheimer's disease. *Psychol Med*. 1996;**26**(1):7–14.

49. Csernansky JG, Dong H, Fagan AM, *et al*. Plasma cortisol and progression of dementia in subjects with Alzheimer-type dementia. *Am J Psychiatry*. 2006;**163**(12):2164–9.

50. Kang JE, Cirrito JR, Dong H, Csernansky JG, Holtzman DM. Acute stress increases interstitial fluid amyloid-beta via corticotropin-releasing factor and neuronal activity. *Proc Natl Acad Sci USA*. 2007;**104**(25):10673–8.

51. Rissman RA, Lee KF, Vale W, Sawchenko PE. Corticotropin-releasing factor receptors differentially regulate stress-induced tau phosphorylation. *J Neurosci*. 2007;**27**(24):6552–62.

52. Aisen PS, Davis KL, Berg JD, *et al*. A randomized controlled trial of prednisone in Alzheimer's disease. Alzheimer's Disease Cooperative Study. *Neurology*. 2000;**54**(3):588–93.

53. de Quervain DJ, Poirier R, Wollmer MA, *et al*. Glucocorticoid-related genetic susceptibility for Alzheimer's disease. *Hum Mol Genet*. 2004;**13**(1):47–52.

54. Wilson RS, Evans DA, Bienias JL, *et al*. Proneness to psychological distress is associated with risk of Alzheimer's disease. *Neurology*. 2003;**61**(11):1479–85.

55. Woods NF, Carr MC, Tao EY, Taylor HJ, Mitchell ES. Increased urinary cortisol levels during the menopause transition. *Menopause*. 2006;**13**(2):212–21.

56. Qureshi AC, Bahri A, Breen LA, *et al*. The influence of the route of oestrogen administration on serum levels of cortisol-binding globulin and total cortisol. *Clin Endocrinol. (Oxf)* 2007;**66**(5):632–5.

57. Shifren JL, Desindes S, McIlwain M, Doros G, Mazer NA. A randomized, open-label, crossover study comparing the effects of oral versus transdermal estrogen therapy on serum androgens, thyroid hormones, and adrenal hormones in naturally menopausal women. *Menopause*. 2007;**14**(6):985–94.

58. Wolf OT, Heinrich AB, Hanstein B, Kirschbaum C. Estradiol or estradiol/progesterone treatment in older women: no strong effects on cognition. *Neurobiol Aging*. 2005;**26**:1029–32.

59. Patacchioli FR, Simeoni S, Monnazzi P, *et al*. Menopause, mild psychological stress and salivary cortisol: influence of long-term hormone replacement therapy (HRT). *Maturitas*. 2006;**55**(2):150–5.

60. Komesaroff PA, Esler MD, Sudhir K. Estrogen supplementation attenuates glucocorticoid and catecholamine responses to mental stress in perimenopausal women. *J Clin Endocrinol Metab.* 1999;**84**(2):606–10.

61. Lindheim SR, Legro RS, Bernstein L, *et al.* Behavioral stress responses in premenopausal and postmenopausal women and the effects of estrogen. *Am J Obstet Gynecol.* 1992;**167**(6):1831–6.

62. Lindheim SR, Legro RS, Morris RS, *et al.* The effect of progestins on behavioral stress responses in postmenopausal women. *J Soc Gynecol Investig.* 1994;**1**(1):79–83.

63. Puder JJ, Freda PU, Goland RS, Wardlaw SL. Estrogen modulates the hypothalamic-pituitary-adrenal and inflammatory cytokine responses to endotoxin in women. *J Clin Endocrinol Metab.* 2001;**86**(6):2403–8.

64. Kajantie E, Phillips DI. The effects of sex and hormonal status on the physiological response to acute psychosocial stress. *Psychoneuroendocrinology.* 2006;**31**(2):151–78.

65. Bowman RE, MacLusky NJ, Diaz SE, Zrull MC, Luine VN. Aged rats: sex differences and responses to chronic stress. *Brain Res.* 2006;**1126**:156–66.

66. Behl C, Moosmann B, Manthey D, Heck S. The female sex hormone oestrogen as neuroprotectant: activities at various levels. *Novartis Found Symp.* 2000;**230**:221–34.

67. Wolf OT. Stress, memory and aging: relevance for the peri- and postmenopausal women. *Menopause Management* 2007;**16**:22–30.

68. Ising M, Kunzel HE, Binder EB, *et al.* The combined dexamethasone/CRH test as a potential surrogate marker in depression. *Prog Neuropsychopharmacol Biol Psychiatry.* 2005;**29**(6):1085–93.

69. Wilson RS, Barnes LL, Mendes De Leon CF, *et al.* Depressive symptoms, cognitive decline, and risk of AD in older persons. *Neurology.* 2002;**59**(3):364–70.

70. Convit A. Links between cognitive impairment in insulin resistance: an explanatory model. *Neurobiol Aging.* 2005;**26**(Suppl. 1):31–5.

71. Dallman MF, Pecoraro N, Akana SF, *et al.* Chronic stress and obesity: a new view of "comfort food". *Proc Natl Acad Sci USA.* 2003;**100**(20):11696–701.

72. Rosmond R. Stress induced disturbances of the HPA axis: a pathway to Type 2 diabetes? *Med Sci Monit.* 2003;**9**(2):RA35–RA39.

73. Seckl JR, Walker BR. 11beta-hydroxysteroid dehydrogenase type 1 as a modulator of glucocorticoid action: from metabolism to memory. *Trends Endocrinol Metab.* 2004;**15**(9):418–24.

74. Yau JL, Noble J, Kenyon CJ, *et al.* Lack of tissue glucocorticoid reactivation in 11beta-hydroxysteroid dehydrogenase type 1 knockout mice ameliorates age-related learning impairments. *Proc Natl Acad Sci USA.* 2001;**98**(8):4716–21.

75. Sandeep TC, Yau JL, MacLullich AM, *et al.* 11β-Hydroxysteroid dehydrogenase inhibition improves cognitive function in healthy elderly men and type 2 diabetics. *Proc Natl Acad Sci USA.* 2004; **101**:6734–9.

15

Possible genetic polymorphisms related to sex steroid metabolism and dementia in women

Eef Hogervorst, Stephan Bandelow, and Chris Talbot

Editors' introduction

This chapter explains why two meta-analyses of treatment studies only found time-limited positive effects of estradiol in both women with and without dementia. The findings in women with dementia do not substantiate the "window of opportunity" theory. Negative effects of longer term treatment (>1year) have also been reported in both women with and without dementia.

The meta-analyses reported that the most substantial effects of estradiol on cognition were seen in women who had undergone surgical menopause. Another large observational study found an increased risk for dementia when women had undergone surgical menopause. This chapter attempts to explain these findings by speculating that some women who are more at risk for medical indications for surgical menopause have particular genotypes implicated in sex steroid metabolism and synthesis. These genotypes expose these women to high estradiol levels. This may explain why these women show such strong responses to undergoing surgical menopause, as this induces a very sharp decline in their previously high estradiol levels. If these women also have genetic polymorphisms that predispose them to high levels of toxic estrogenic metabolites (such as catecholestrogens) this could lead to DNA damage. In the first instance that could lead to medical indications for surgical menopause, such as ovarian or endometrial cancer, endometriosis, cysts, etc. If these women are given estrogens at a later time in their lives, they might also be more susceptible to dementia, which has previously also been associated with DNA damage. The brain is apparently less able to compensate for this type of damage in later life, which could explain the more substantial negative effects on cognition and dementia risk found in the older women. Future genetic screening for these polymorphisms might allow more targeted treatment for those women who are not genetically at risk.

Biological plausibility versus WHIMS

As discussed in previous chapters, there is abundant evidence from animal and cell culture studies to suggest that sex steroids, such as estrogens (Es) and testosterone (T), could protect the aging brain. In the nineties, sex steroids were hailed as one of the most promising lines of treatment for Alzheimer's disease (AD), the most prevalent type of dementia, which seemed to be substantiated by observational studies and small treatment trials [1, 2]. However, at the turn of the century several larger and better controlled trials showed that estrogen treatment did not improve cognitive function in women with dementia [3, 4] and even seemed to worsen dementia symptoms in some cases [5]. The Women's Health Initiative Memory Study (WHIMS, see Chapter 1) indicated a doubled risk for AD in women who had been allocated to conjugated equine estrogens (CEE) treatment, particularly when this was combined with medroxy-progesterone acetate (MPA [6, 7], see also Chapter 1). Cognitive function did not show the same improvement over time in women treated with estrogens compared to those women who had been given placebo [8, 9]. In addition, the WHIMS confirmed earlier reported increased risks with hormone treatment (HT) for dangerous adverse events, such as cardiovascular disease, breast cancer, etc. [6]. Results of the WHIMS have had a significant impact, as 66% of women were estimated to have stopped taking conjugated equine estrogens (Premarin®) with MPA (33% for Premarin® alone) in the year after publication, between 2002 and 2003 [10].

Hormones, Cognition and Dementia: State of the Art and Emergent Therapeutic Strategies, ed. Eef Hogervorst, Victor W. Henderson, Robert B. Gibbs, and Roberta Diaz Brinton. Published by Cambridge University Press.

Age and the window of opportunity theory in animal and human studies

Women in the HT studies who showed negative effects on cognitive function mentioned above, were all over 65 years of age, which led to the "window of opportunity" theory (see Chapter 4). Although explained in more detail in the other chapters, briefly, this theory states that estrogens should be given close to the onset of menopause to be effective in protecting the brain. Animal studies using surgically induced menopausal female rodents support this theory. Work by Gibbs (see Chapter 5) and others showed that oophorectomized female rats showed a decline in cognitive function. This could be reversed using estradiol treatment. However, if the interval between induced menopause and hormone treatment was too long, positive effects on cognitive function and brain function were no longer detected.

The "window of opportunity" theory also seems to apply to humans (see Chapter 4). An observational study [11] indicated that postmenopausal women who were relatively close to the age of menopause (50–63 years of age) showed a positive association between treatment with estrogens and cognitive function. However, this was not found to be the case for the older women of this cohort. Another much cited observational study [12] also reported that former, but not current, estrogen treatment users (of an average age of 74.5 years) were protected against dementia. This may suggest that older users of estrogens and/or those women who are far removed from their age at menopause are not protected against dementia when they take estrogens.

The effect of oophorectomy in humans and animals

In line with the animal studies, a number of relatively small studies [13, 14] of the effect of surgical menopause on women showed a substantial decline in cognitive function in the months after oophorectomy. A recent observational study presented by the Mayo Clinic team in Minnesota [15] reported that having undergone surgical menopause overall also increased the risk of dementia or cognitive impairment by 45%. For women who had undergone bilateral oophorectomy, but only received hormone treatment up to the age of 46, this risk was increased by 79%. However, when women were treated with estrogens up to the natural age of menopause there was no increased risk of dementia. Another earlier observational study found an association between better cognitive function and estrogen use, but only in surgically menopausal women who were younger than 58 years of age. No associations were reported between estrogen use and cognition in older surgically menopausal women and were also not found in younger and older naturally menopausal women [16].

The current consensus is that undergoing natural menopause is not necessarily associated with an abrupt loss of cognitive function (see Chapter 4). On the other hand, this may be the case when women are subjected to a surgical menopause, particularly when this is performed at a relatively young age. These data all substantiate the "window of opportunity" theory.

Similar to animal studies, the effect of estradiol treatment after surgical menopause on cognitive function in humans is substantial. A Cochrane meta-analysis was updated in 2006 [2]. Over 15 trials of 566 postmenopausal women were included. Of these, six studies did not have adequate data for analyses. Despite inclusion of the large WHIMS data in these updated meta-analyses, the positive effects of 10 mg estradiol bolus injections intramuscularly monthly in relatively young surgically menopausal women on the paired associate learning test immediate recall ($z = 2.40$, $p < 0.05$, chi-square test $= 1.12$, $p = 0.29$, SMD $= 1.02$, 95% CI $= 0.19$–1.85), on a test of abstract reasoning ($z = 10.45$, $p < 0.0001$, WMD $= 6.80$, 95% CI $= 5.52$–8.08), and a test of speed and accuracy ($z = 9.16$, $p < 0.0001$, WMD $= 6.00$, 95% CI $= 4.72$–7.28) remained significant. However, there was no evidence of an effect on other verbal or visuo(spatial) memory, mental rotations, speed, or accuracy measures. There was also little evidence that Premarin®, the most widely prescribed hormone treatment, had positive effects on cognitive function in women without dementia.

It was thus concluded that a very high dose of bolus estradiol given intramuscularly was beneficial for women without dementia who had recently undergone surgical menopause [2]. It should be noted that recalculation of standard deviations (SD) of the mean difference based on error bars or given means and SDs of before and after treatment (which was necessary when this had not been given in the study results), raised concerns regarding the possibility of false negative findings in the meta-analysis. Some results reported to be significant by the authors could, for instance, not be replicated in the Cochrane meta-analysis using the calculated SD of the mean difference. Calculating SD from data and comparing these to existing data gave up to a factor 2 difference, especially in the smaller studies. Independent of this potential confound, however, these data from the meta-analysis reflect the fact that the magnitude of the effect size was most impressive in surgical menopausal women, and suggests that women who undergo surgical menopause may respond more dramatically to a loss of hormones than those who experience natural menopause. However, the positive effects of estradiol on cognition in surgically menopausal women were only significant for up to two to three months of treatment.

Short-lived effects of estradiol in surgically menopausal women, but also in women with dementia: data that contrast with the "window of opportunity" theory

Similar short-lived positive effects of estrogen treatment in women with dementia contrast with the "window of opportunity" theory. Another recently updated Cochrane meta-analysis of women with dementia (Hogervorst et al., 2009 [52], abstract shown in Text box 1) also showed that estradiol could exert significant positive effects on cognition in women with dementia, most of whom would be at least 65 years of age. This positive effect was again only observed to occur for a few months (see Text box 1). Given an average age of menopause onset around 51 years of age and the age of late onset AD after age 65 years, this would put women who are afflicted with dementia at least 14 years beyond the age of menopause. These data thus do not substantiate the "window of opportunity" theory.

In summary, positive effects of transdermal estradiol were detected in women with dementia up to two months of treatment (see also Chapter 8). Importantly, an early trial in 1954 of institutionalized women with probable dementia already reported that some cognitive functions declined after 18 months of treatment with an estradiol bolus injection [17]. We found similar effects in an unblinded study using an oral estradiol and a progestagen in women without dementia who had severe menopausal complaints after a year of

treatment (data not published of the study mentioned in [25]). Furthermore, an observational study reported that surgically menopausal women who had an estradiol implant for ten years had worse cognitive function than untreated surgically menopausal women [26]. It is unclear whether initial benefits of treatment on cognitive function had been seen or were reported in these women. In WHIMS, the first negative effects were also already seen after one year, but earlier measurements had, to our knowledge, not been carried out. Some authors have argued that the type of estrogens administered (see Chapter 7) affects the outcome of the study. Indeed, meta-analysis in women without dementia did not reveal strong effects of CEEs, but small effects of this type of treatment have been seen in women with dementia. Basic science data also seem to suggest that CEEs do have the propensity to have positive effects on brain function (see Chapter 6).

On the basis of this limited information, longer term ($>$ 6 months) treatment with estrogens (either estradiol or CEEs) using current regimens may not be indicated in protecting women against dementia and may even worsen cognitive function in the longer term in some women. This begs the questions (i) why there would be initial positive short-lived effects of estrogens, and (ii) why these might subsequently reverse into negative effects on brain function.

High levels of estrogens are a risk factor for dementia

Rocca et al. [15] speculated that there may be another reason for finding an association between surgical menopause and dementia. For instance, they proposed a genetic predisposition that could increase the risk for both outcomes independently. We propose that there are genetic factors resulting in a common factor that relates to both outcomes (see also [1, 27]) and which may explain the association found between surgical menopause and dementia.

The OPTIMA data showing higher estradiol levels in AD female cases when compared to controls ([33] see Text box 2) were later replicated in several other cohorts [34, 35]. In a recent longitudinal study where none of the participants had dementia at baseline, high estradiol levels ($>$ 10 pg/mL) were also associated with a 75% increase in risk for all cause dementia (and 94% for AD but not VaD). No associations were found for testosterone (or for men and dementia with sex steroid levels) [36]. In another longitudinal study,

Text box 1 Cochrane meta-analyses of women with dementia

Nine double-blind placebo-controlled trials of postmenopausal women with dementia were identified using Cochrane search strategies up to November 2007 with a PubMed update in May 2008 (for keywords used see [52]). In two trials [17, 18] there was insufficient information about the randomization procedure. In accordance with the Cochrane guidelines, these studies were excluded from analysis. For the current meta-analysis, a total of 7 trials including 351 women with AD were analyzed.

Subjects: screening and selection

The total number of participants randomized in the trials varied from 14 to 120. In total, 351 women with dementia were included (266 had completed the studies) with an average of 38 participants per study. Drop-outs were described in four studies (but not in [19] and [20]; although their data suggested that no drop-out had occurred). 21/176 of treated women (11%) dropped out compared with 13/131 of placebo users (10%) for a wide variety of reasons, but mostly these seemed unrelated to the use of active medication.

Most studies required very rigorous health screening [3–5, 21, 22]. One study [19] had less rigorous criteria (age <70, depression, non-AD dementia syndromes) and was a preliminary analysis on 20 subjects, which was published in a general article on estrogen and hormonal replacement therapy. No follow-up of these data (or a more detailed description of the study) has been reported to our knowledge. Power analyses had been carried out by two studies [3, 5] but were not mentioned in the smaller studies [19, 22, 23] while Wang et al. [4] also failed to mention a power analysis but would (on the basis of the calculations of the first two studies) have had numbers (N = 50) to obtain sufficient power for comparisons.

Subjects: dementia assessment

All studies reported inclusion of people with dementia of the Alzheimer's type (DAT) or Alzheimer's disease (AD). Most studies employed the NINCDS/ADRDA criteria for probable AD (but see [19], where no criteria were given) and participants were in general considered to have mild to moderate dementia (MMSE between 10 and 28).

Subjects: age and other confounding factors

Mean age of the women with AD was 75 years, but some studies had a wide age-range ([5]: range 56–91) and had thus included early and late onset AD. In one study only early age-onset AD patients (<63 years of age) were included with mild AD [20]. Age, education, and depression were usually not controlled for in the analyses. Some studies included only women who had undergone natural menopause [21] while others included mixed groups of surgically and naturally menopausal women (e.g., [3, 5, 22]) or did not provide data on this.

Design

All studies used a parallel-groups design. Duration of treatment varied from 8 weeks to 12 months, with an average of 4.4 months. We did not include the 5 weeks treatment time point of Asthana et al. [21] as the authors pointed out that data may not have been reliable, since 2 (of 12) participants had been tested elsewhere.

Cognitive assessments

Not all studies used similar cognitive tests, which made comparisons difficult. One of the problems in two otherwise well designed studies [4, 5] was that no common test of verbal memory was used. Verbal memory has been thought likely to be the most sensitive cognitive function to the effects of estrogens [24].

Different types of treatment and estradiol levels

Four RCTs prescribed Premarin® (conjugated equine estrogens, or CEE, produced by Wyeth). Of these, three used the 1.25 mg/day dosage [3–5] and two employed the lower dosage of 0.625 mg/day [5, 19]. One study [19] also added a progestagen to the estrogen to prevent endometrial hyperplasia. In another study [20] a Chinese estrogenic compound was used (Beimeili) containing conjugated oestrogen, which was manufactured by Wyeth-Ayerst in the USA (which also produces CEE) and that was thought to probably be similar to CEE. Unfortunately, little information could be found about this product, which seems to be marketed mainly in China. Two studies used transdermal estradiol [22, 23]. Compliance checks were done using pill counts [3] or serum estrogen checks [4, 5, 22, 23]. Some studies [19, 20] gave no data on compliance checks.

Text box 1   (cont.)

Statistics
Some studies reported separate within-group comparisons for participants in treatment and placebo groups [19, 20], which can result in chance accumulation and a risk of the type I error. Five studies had performed "completers" analyses ([3, 5, 19, 20, 23] but data not shown) and three had performed "intention-to-treat" analyses [4, 5, 22].

Methodological quality of included studies
Three studies described their randomization procedures in detail [3, 5, 22] and received a Cochrane quality rating of A. In these studies an external person had performed the allocation. The other studies reported having "randomly assigned treatments" but did not describe the randomization procedures in detail, and in accordance with Cochrane collaboration standards received a quality rating of B. For two studies no randomization procedure was reported and these were not included in the analyses [17, 18].

Results
Seven studies thus met inclusion criteria and had performed adequate or intermediate allocation procedures. These studies had all been published in peer-reviewed journals.

Analyses showed that there was a limited positive effect of low dose conjugated equine estrogens (CEE, 0.625 mg once a day) but not of the higher dosage (1.25 mg of CEE once a day) on the Mini-Mental Status Examination (MMSE) after two months (WMD = 1.28, 95% CI = 0.26 to 2.30, z = 2.45, p < 0.01). The effect disappeared after 3, 6 and 12 months of treatment. This effect was also small (it disappeared after correction for multiple testing) and was probably not clinically relevant, as there was only a difference of 1 point on average on the MMSE, in comparison with the placebo users (the scale range is 0–30). There were also short-term (1 and 4 months, respectively) effects of 1.25 mg of CEE on tests of concentration and executive function, namely the Trail Making Test-B (WMD = −40.90, 95% CI − 79.29 to −2.51, z = 2.09, p < 0.05) and Digit Span backward (WMD = 0.67, 95% CI = −0.01 to 1.34, z = 1.94, p < 0.05). Both effects also disappeared after corrections for multiple testing. With regard to memory, only cued delayed recall of a word list was positively affected by two months of transdermal estradiol (E_2) (WMD = 6.50, 95% CI = 4.04 to 8.96, z = 5.19, p < 0.0001). No treatment effects were seen on other word lists, or on the Paragraph Recall or Paired Associate Learning test. In addition, no effects were seen on visual memory, language functions, most speeded tests, clinical rating scales, or depression scales. Controls had better performance on the delayed recall of the Paragraph Test (overall WMD = −0.45, 95% CI = −0.79 to −0.11, z = 2.60, p < 0.01) after one month than CEE users. However, there was a trend for reversal of this effect after four months. Controls were better on the Finger Tapping test after 12 months of placebo (WMD = −3.90, 95% CI = −7.85 to 0.05, z = 1.93, p < 0.05) and clinicians gave controls a better score on a dementia rating scale (CDR, overall WMD = 0.35, 95% CI = 0.01 to 0.69, z = 1.99, p < 0.05). Positive findings in favor of treatment or placebo could have been random effects caused by multiple analyses. However, after correction for multiple testing, the short-term positive treatment effect of transdermal estradiol on memory up to two months remained, but also the positive effects of placebo over active treatment were not altered by corrections.

Text box 2   Levels of estradiol in women with dementia

In contrast to the accepted paradigm that estrogens should protect against AD and that estrogen levels would thus be lower in women with AD, sufficiently sensitive assays (3 pmol/L) indicated that women with AD (n = 66) actually had slightly, but significantly, higher levels of estradiol than controls (n = 62) of the Oxford Project to Investigate Memory and Ageing (OPTIMA). Diagnoses of cases and controls in OPTIMA were performed during consensus meetings also using computerized systems to improve validity and inter-rater reliability of the diagnoses [28]. In the analyses of estradiol levels, 37 of the NINCDS/ADRDA AD cases [29] also fulfilled the Consortium to Establish a Registry for Alzheimer's Disease (CERAD) histopathological criteria for probable or definite AD [30]. All participants had undergone a full medical examination, which included blood sampling, brain scans (CT or MRI and SPECT) and cognitive assessment using the Cambridge Examination for Mental Disorders of the Elderly (CAMDEX [31]). None of the participants had active systemic morbidity or was institutionalized. None of the women used medication that could have interfered with hormone levels, such as antipsychotics or other hormone treatment, etc. This study was thus carefully controlled and had also controlled for any other factors that could affect sex steroid metabolism, such

Text box 2 (*cont.*)

as smoking, body mass index, use of alcohol, morbidity, etc. Non-fasting blood serum samples had been obtained between 10:00 and 12:00 hours and had then been stored at $-70°C$ for an average of 2.3 ± 2.1 years. For total estradiol, two assays were used. For the first technique, duplicate serum samples were extracted with ether. Total estradiol was then assessed by radio-immunoassay using a highly specific polyclonal rabbit-derived anti-human estradiol antiserum. The lower limit or sensitivity of this assay was 3 pmol/L. The validity of this assay when compared with other commercial assays (such as DPC C-A-C) was good ($r > 0.99$). The second total estradiol assay was the commercial Bayer Immuno 1 assay (Bayer©, Bayer Corporation, 511 Benedict Avenue, Tarrytown, NY 10591–5097 USA). The lower detection limit for this commercial assay was 37 pmol/L. However, expected values for postmenopausal women are between 0 to 172 pmol/L. Consequently, when using this technique, 80% of the data for the women of this particular age group were found to be missing in OPTIMA. The between assay correlation (between the sensitive ether extraction immuno-assay, "x", and less sensitive Bayer, "y", immuno-assay) was $r = 0.90$, $p < 0.005$ ($n = 157$) and the overall regression equation was $y = 0.81x + 1.13$. Using meta-analysis over several other studies, which had reported estradiol levels in AD cases and controls, low estradiol assay sensitivity and/or the accidental inclusion of control women using estrogen treatment were the most likely causes for other and earlier reports of *lower* estradiol levels in women with AD [32].

women with higher total estradiol levels had smaller hippocampal volumes and poorer memory performance, both indicative of an increased risk for AD [37]. Interesting with regard to this, were data presented at the Alzheimer's Association meeting in 2006 by Voyager Pharmaceuticals (and discussed in Chapter 26), which indicated that leuprolide acetate (which lowers gonadotropin levels such as luteinizing hormone, but thus also (indirectly) estrogens levels) improved cognitive function in women with AD. Data on men were not revealed. It could be proposed that the reduction of high levels of estrogens actually led to improvement in these women rather than (or as well as) the reduction in neurotoxic high levels of luteinizing hormone (see Chapter 26).

Genetics of sex steroid metabolism underlying both dementia pathology and medical indications for surgical menopause

It is currently unclear why women with AD would have higher levels of estrogens and why increasing estrogens levels for a longer period of time would put some women at risk for AD. It could be hypothesized that for some women, increasing levels of estrogens for a longer period of time is associated with higher risks for dementia. We propose that genetic polymorphisms related to estrogens synthesis and metabolism may be responsible for this.

It could be hypothesized that women at risk for AD have particular genetic profiles associated with

sex steroid metabolism and synthesis, which could result in high levels of toxic estrogenic metabolites. These toxic metabolites may be implicated in both AD [27] and also in morbidity that can be a clinical indication for surgical menopause. This hypothesis may thus be an alternative explanation to why Rocca *et al.* [15] found an increased AD risk in women who had undergone surgical menopause. High levels of estrogens and their toxic end products have been implicated in endometriosis, cysts, endometrioid ovarian cancer, and endometrial carcinoma, all often indications to induce surgical menopause in women [38]. Women with cancers had been excluded from the Mayo Clinic cohort study, but endometriosis and cysts had been the main indications for oophorectomy in this study [15].

The focus could be on genetic polymorphisms in the following candidate genes described in Text box 3 that are involved in sex steroid synthesis and catabolism (Fig. 15.1) and that have already been implicated in morbidity sensitive to high levels of estrogens, such as endometrial and breast cancer [39–41] and possibly also in AD. A potential common underlying mechanism, that would need to be further explored, could be DNA damage. DNA damage has been associated with these polymorphisms (e.g., of CYP19 and COMT) in endometrial cancer [39] and might also be a potential pathological factor in AD [42].

We would thus hypothesize that the discussed genotypes CYP17 (A2), CYP1A1 (m1), CYP1B1 (Val432), CYP19 (A6 or 8 r allele), and COMT (met) are more frequent in women with AD than in controls. These genotypes are associated with high levels of toxic

Text box 3 Genetic polymorphisms in candidate genes possibly related to AD and endometrial cancer

CYP17 variants: A1/A2 (5′ UTR SNP that creates/deletes an SP1 element)

  enzyme: cytochrome P450c17a. Sex steroid synthesis. The A2 allele (enhanced promoter activity) increases the amount of enzyme produced, which may result in higher levels of estradiol [43].

CYP1A1 variants: m1 (non-coding), m2 (iso462/val462)

  enzyme: P450(CYP)1A1. Sex steroid catalysis. The m1 variant is associated with higher levels of 2-hydroxycate-cholestrogen (which is a potentially toxic reactive estrogenic metabolite) that can cause oxidative stress and DNA damage which has been implicated in cancer [44].

CYP1B1 variants: valine432/leucine432

  enzyme: cytochrome P450(CYP)1B1. Sex steroid catalysis. Produces 4-hydroxy-estradiol, another reactive catecholestrogen metabolite (see CYP1A1 above). The Val432 allele variant has higher efficiency for the conversion of estradiol into the toxic 4-hydroxy-estradiol leading to high levels of the toxic metabolite [45, 46].

COMT variants: val108,158/met

  enzyme: catechol-o-methyltransferase inactivates reactive estrogenic metabolites. The 'met' allele polymorphism results in higher levels of the metabolites, which could lead to accumulation of toxic end products [46]. Women with genotypes CYP17 A2, CYP1A1 m1, CYP1B1 Val432, and COMT met may thus produce very high levels of toxic estrogenic metabolites, which may put them at risk for AD. COMT genotyping was carried out on OPTIMA participants with no differences between cases and controls [47], but analyses were yet not stratified for sex (see below).

CYP19 has a long allele variant that produces higher levels of aromatase (see Fig. 15.1), an enzyme that converts testosterone into estradiol. Aromatase is encoded by the CYP19 gene located at 15q21.1. Subjects with the CYP 19 (aromatase) polymorphism with the long allele variant (A6 or 8 r allele) have higher estrogen levels and lower androgen levels. CYP19 data are currently under investigation in OPTIMA.

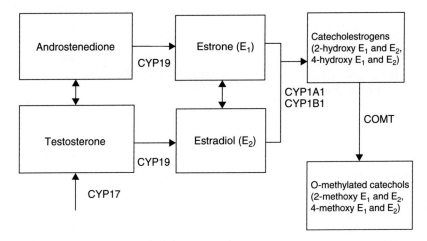

Fig. 15.1 Genetic polymorphisms associated with sex steroid metabolism and synthesis. (Based on Tworoger *et al.*, *Cancer Epidemiol Biomarkers Prev* 2004; 13(1): 94.)

estrogenic metabolites and subsequent DNA damage, which could be implicated in an increased risk for AD, as well as for morbidity associated with the necessity of inducing surgical menopause.

This model could potentially explain the duration of treatment effect. DNA damage to cells may take longer to become apparent, i.e., until this process eventually overrules the initial positive and short-lived effects of estrogens (dendritic sprouting, cerebral blood flow, neurotransmitter effects, etc., as described in earlier chapters). It might also explain why negative effects of treatment may be worse in women over age 65 years, who perhaps have fewer compensatory and protective mechanisms against DNA damage. Lastly, the model could tentatively explain why surgically menopausal women are so much more affected by a drop in estradiol levels, as they have been exposed to much higher estradiol levels throughout their life.

An earlier study [48] found no difference in CYP17, CYP1A1, and COMT polymorphism frequencies between AD cases and controls, but their sample was small (n = 66 AD, n = 86 controls) and their analyses were not stratified for sex. However, 69% of AD cases had at least one CYP17 A2 allele (vs. 58.4% of controls, p = 0.06), which would have been predicted on the basis of our model. Power analyses indicated that the sample should have been n = 111 for both samples using a 50% beta error level (www.dssresearch.com/toolkit/sscalc/size_p2.asp). Similarly, Nicholl et al. [49] found no difference in CYP1A1 polymorphisms in analyses not stratified for sex, but also only had 23 AD cases. For CYP1A1 and COMT polymorphisms, power analyses on the basis of the data from Wang [48] would indicate that 700 to 800 participants would have been necessary to reach significance in these analyses. In addition, associations of AD with COMT polymorphisms may be modified by presence of psychosis in AD [50], which should thus be controlled for in statistical analyses.

In sum, previous studies into these polymorphisms were all too small to allow stratification for sex. This is important as associations between sex steroids and brain function are hypothesized to be different for men and women (see Chapter 18).[1]

---

[1] Briefly, in contrast to findings in women, we and others found *lower* levels of both T and E_2 in men with AD [34, 53, 54]. Rosario [55] reported lower levels of T (but not of E_2) in the brains of men with AD, also in those in the very early, non-detectable stages of AD with early brain pathological – but non-clinical – symptoms. Men who had not yet developed AD, but who did have the APOE epsilon 4 genotype (a genetic risk factor for AD) also already had lower levels of T [56]. Having an APOE epsilon 4 genotype was hypothesized to contribute to cognitive decline in transgenic mice by reducing the number of androgen receptors (AR) in the brain [57]. Lehmann et al. [58] reported that in OPTIMA men with AD were more likely to carry short androgen receptor (AR) CAG repeat alleles (≤20 CAG repeats) than controls. The combination of the short AR allele variant and low T levels increased the risk for AD (OR = 4.2, 95% CI = 1.4–13) in men, but not women. While this polymorphism is associated with increased AR sensitivity, Krithivas et al. [59] also found that age-related decline in T was faster in men with short CAG repeat lengths. This would tie in with our earlier observation that men with AD seem to exhibit accelerated age-related endocrinological changes with earlier decreases in T and thyroid stimulating hormone (TSH) and earlier increases in sex hormone binding globulin (SHBG) and gonadotropin levels than age-matched controls [60]. Different mechanisms and genetic polymorphisms are thus hypothesized to explain associations between sex hormones and dementia in men and women (see Chapter 18).

Pending research outcomes using large data bases stratified for sex, genetic screening could be a useful future tool in determining risks for women who would like to use hormones to reduce perimenopausal complaints. This is an important topic to further investigate as many of the women, after initial discontinuation of treatment, restarted using hormone treatment [51]. This may not be surprising as HT has been shown to be the most effective treatment for menopausal complaints. Analyzing risks and benefits for the individual with menopausal symptoms is a primary concern for future clinicians.

References

1. Hogervorst E. The short-lived effect of hormone therapy on cognition function. In Rasgon N, ed. *The Effects of Estrogen on Brain Function*. Baltimore: Johns Hopkins Press, 2006, pp. 46–78.

2. Yesufu A, Bandelow S, Hogervorst E. Meta-analyses of the effect of hormone treatment on cognitive function in postmenopausal women. *Women's Health*. 2007; 3(2):173–95.

3. Henderson VW, Paganini-Hill A, Miller BL, et al. Estrogen for Alzheimer's disease in women. *Neurology*. 2000;54(January 2):295–301.

4. Wang PN, Liao SQ, Liu RS, et al. Effects of estrogen on cognition, mood, and cerebral blood flow in AD. *Neurology*. 2000;54(January 1):2061–66.

5. Mulnard RA, Cotman CW, Kawas C. et al. Estrogen replacement therapy for treatment of mild to moderate Alzheimer's disease. *JAMA*. 2000;283:1007–15.

6. Shumaker SA, Legault C, Rapp SR, et al. Estrogen plus progestin and the incidence of dementia and mild cognitive impairment in postmenopausal women. *JAMA*. 2003;289:2651–62.

7. Shumaker SA, Legault C, Kuller L, et al. Conjugated equine estrogens and incidence of probable dementia and mild cognitive impairment in postmenopausal women: the Women's Health Initiative Memory Study. *JAMA*. 2004;291(24):2947–58.

8. Rapp SR, Espeland MA, Shumaker SA, et al. Effect of estrogen plus progestin on global cognitive function in postmenopausal women: the Women's Health Initiative Memory Study: a randomized controlled trial. *JAMA*. 2003;289(20):2663–72.

9. Espeland MA, Rapp SR, Shumaker SA, et al. Conjugated equine estrogens and global cognitive function in postmenopausal women: the Women's Health Initiative Memory Study. *JAMA*. 2004;291(24):2959–68.

10. Hersh AL, Stefanick ML, Stafford RS. National use of postmenopausal hormone therapy. *JAMA*. 2004; **291**(1):47–53.

11. Henderson VW, Benke KS, Green RC, *et al.* Postmenopausal hormone therapy and Alzheimer's disease risk: interaction with age. *JNNP*. 2005;**76** (1):103–5.

12. Zandi PP, Carlson MC, Plassman BL, *et al.* Hormone replacement therapy and incidence of Alzheimer disease in older women the Cache County Study. *JAMA*. 2002;**288**(17):2123–9.

13. Sherwin BB. Estrogen and/or androgen replacement therapy and cognitive functioning in surgically menopausal women. *Psychoneuroendocrinology*. 1988;**13**:345–57.

14. Nappi RE, Sinforiani E, Mauri M, *et al.* Memory functioning at menopause impact of age in ovariectomized women. *Gynecol Obstet Invest*. 1999;**47**:29–36.

15. Rocca WA, Bower JH, Maraganore DM, *et al.* Increased risk of cognitive impairment or dementia in women who underwent oophorectomy before menopause. *Neurology*. 2007;**69**(11): 1074–83.

16. Szklo M, Cerhan J, Diez-Roux AV, *et al.* Estrogen replacement therapy and cognitive functioning in the artherosclerotic risk in communities (ARIC) study. *Am J Epidemiol*. 1996;**144**:1048–57.

17. Caldwell BM. An evaluation of psychological effects of sex hormone administration in aged women II. Results of therapy after 18 months. *J Gerontol*. 1954;**9**(2):168–74.

18. Honjo H, Ogino Y, Tanaka K, *et al.* An effect of conjugated estrogen to cognitive impairment in women with senile dementia-Alzheimer's type: a placebo-controlled double-blind study. *J Jpn Menopause Soc*. 1993;**1**:161–71.

19. Birge SJ. The role of estrogen in the treatment of Alzheimer's disease. *Neurology*. 1997;**48**:S36–S41.

20. Zhang YX, Luo G, Guo ZJ, Wang LQ, Zhou CL. Quantitative evaluation of the intervention of estrogen on Alzheimer's disease. *Chin J Clin Rehab*. 2006; **10**(30):37–91.

21. Asthana S, Craft S, Baker LD, *et al.* Cognitive and neuroedocrine response to transdermal estrogen in postmenopausal women with AD: results of a placebo-controlled, double-blind pilot study. *Psychoneuroendocrinology*. 1999;**24**:657–77.

22. Asthana S, Baker LD, Craft S, *et al.* High-dose estradiol improves cognition for women with AD: results of a randomized study. *Neurology*. 2001;**57**(4):605–12.

23. Asthana S, Craft S, Baker LD, *et al.* Transdermal estrogen improves memory in women with Alzheimer's Disease. *Soc Neurosci Abstr*. 1996;**22**: A200.

24. Hogervorst E, Williams J, Budge M, Riedel W, Jolles J. The nature of the effect of female gonadal hormone replacement therapy on cognitive function in post-menopausal women: a meta-analysis. *Neuroscience*. 2000;**101**(3):485–512.

25. Hogervorst E, Boshuisen M, Riedel WJ, Willekes C, Jolles J. The effect of hormone replacement therapy on cognitive function in elderly women. *Psychoneuroendocrinology*. 1999;**24**:43–68.

26. File SE, Heard JE, Rymer J. Trough oestradiol levels associated with cognitive impairment in post-menopausal women after 10 years of oestradiol implants. *Psychopharmacology (Berl)*. 2002;**161** (1):107–12.

27. Hogervorst E, Bandelow S. Should surgically menopausal women be treated with estrogens to decrease the risk for dementia? Invited Editorial. *Neurology*. 2007;**69**(11):1070–1.

28. Hogervorst E, Bandelow S, Combrinck M, Irani M, Smith AD. The validity and reliability of 6 sets of clinical criteria to classify Alzheimer's disease and vascular dementia in post-mortem confirmed cases: added value of a decision-tree approach. *Dementia*. 2003;**16**(3):170–80.

29. McKhann G, Drachmann D, Folstein M, *et al.* Clinical diagnosis of Alzheimer's disease: report of the NINCDS-ADRDA work group under the auspices of Department of Health and Human Services Task Force on Alzheimer's Disease. *Neurology*. 1984;**34**:939–44.

30. Mirra SS, Heyman A, McKeel D, *et al.* The Consortium to Establish a Registry for Alzheimer's Disease (CERAD). II. Standardization of the neuropathologic assessment of Alzheimer's disease. *Neurology*. 1991;**41**:479–86.

31. Roth M, Huppert FA, Tym E, Mountjoy CQ. *CAMDEX: The Cambridge Examination for Mental Disorders of the Elderly*. Cambridge: Cambridge University Press, 1988.

32. Hogervorst E, Williams J, Combrinck M, Smith AD. Measuring serum oestradiol in women with Alzheimer's disease: the importance of the sensitivity of the assay method. *Eur J Endocrinol*. 2003;**148**(1):67–72.

33. Hogervorst E, Barnetson L, Williams J, *et al.* Women with dementia of Alzheimer's type have higher levels of estradiol than healthy controls: prize winning poster. Paper presented at the 5th Annual Graylyn Conference on Women's Health, 1999; Winston-Salem.

34. Paoletti AM, Congia S, Lello S, *et al.* Low androgenization index in elderly women and elderly

men with Alzheimer's disease. *Neurology.* 2004;
62(2):301–3.

35. Cunningham CJ, Sinnott M, Denihan A, *et al.*
Endogenous sex hormone levels in postmenopausal
women with AD. *J Clin Endocrinol Metab.* 2001;
86(3):1099–103.

36. Ravaglia G, Forti P, Maiolo F, *et al.* Endogenous sex
hormones as risk factors for dementia in elderly men
and women. *J Gerontol A Biol Sci Med Sci.* 2007;
62(9):1035–41.

37. Den Heijer T, Geerlings MI, Hofman A, *et al.*
Higher estrogen levels are not associated with larger
hippocampi and better memory performance. *Arch
Neurol.* 2003;**60**(2):213–20.

38. Rees M. Gynaecological oncology perspective on
management of the menopause. *Eur J Surg Oncol.*
2006;**32**(8):892–7.

39. Berstein L, Zimarina T, Imyanitov E, *et al.* Hormonal
imbalance in two types of endometrial cancer and
genetic polymorphism of steroidogenic enzymes.
Maturitas. 2006;**54**(4):352–5.

40. Szyllo K, Smolarz B, Romanowicz-Makowska H,
Kulig A. The polymorphisms of the CYP17 and CYP19
genes in endometrial cancer patients. *Pol J Pathol.*
2006;**57**(1):35–40.

41. Aban M, Arslan M, Tok E, *et al.* CYP17 genetic
polymorphism in patients with endometrial hyperplasia
and cancer. *Int J Gynecol Cancer.* 2006;**16**(1):448–51.

42. Kruman R, Wersto F, Cardozo-Pelaez L, *et al.* Cycle
activation linked to neuronal cell death initiated by
DNA damage. *Neuron.* 2004;**41**(4):549–61.

43. Sharp L. CYP17 gene polymorphisms. A HuGE review.
Am J Epid. 2004;**160**(8):729–40.

44. Huang CS, Chern HD, Chang KJ, *et al.* Breast cancer
risk associated with genotype polymorphism of the
estrogen-metabolizing genes CYP17, CYP1A1, and
COMT: a multigenic study on cancer susceptibility.
Cancer Res. 1999;**59**(19):4870–5.

45. Cecchin E. Lack of association of CYP1B1*3
polymorphism and ovarian cancer. *Int J Biol Markers.*
2004;**19**(2):160–3.

46. Tworoger SS, Chubak J, Aiello EJ, *et al.* Association of
CYP17, CYP19, CYP1B1, and COMT polymorphisms
with serum and urinary sex hormone concentrations
in postmenopausal women. *Cancer Epidemiol
Biomarkers Prev.* 2004;**13**(1):94–101.

47. Turnbridge EM, Harrison PJ, Warden DR, *et al.*
Polymorphisms in the catechol-O-methyltransferase
(COMT) gene influence plasma total homocysteine
levels. *Am J Med Genet B Neuropsychiatr Genet.*
2008;**147B**(6): 996–9.

48. Wang PN. Estrogen-metabolizing gene COMT
polymorphism synergistic APOE epsilon4 allele
increases the risk of Alzheimer disease. *Dementia.*
2005;**19**(2/3):120–5.

49. Nicholl DJ, Bennett P, Hiller L, *et al.* A study of five
candidate genes in Parkinson's disease and related
neurodegenerative disorders. *Neurology.* 1999;**53**(7):
1415–21.

50. Borroni B, Agosti C, Archetti S, *et al.* COMT
polymorphism is associated with risk for psychosis
in AD. *Neurosci Lett.* 2004;**370**(2/3):127–9.

51. Wegienka G, Havstad S, Kelsey JL. Menopausal
hormone therapy in a health maintenance organization
before and after WHI hormone trials termination.
J Women's Health. 2006;**15**(4):369–78.

52. Hogervorst E, Yaffe K, Richards M, Huppert FA.
Hormone replacement therapy to maintain
cognitive function in women with dementia. *Cochrane
Database Syst Rev.* 2009;**21**(1):CD003799. Review.

53. Hogervorst E, Williams JW, Budge M, Barnetson L,
Smith AD. Serum total testosterone is lower in men
with Alzheimer's disease. *Neuro Endocrinol Lett.*
2001;**22**(3):163–8.

54. Moffat SD, Zonderman AB, Metter EJ, *et al.* Free
testosterone and risk for Alzheimer disease in older
men. *Neurology.* 2004;**62**(2):188–93.

55. Rosario ER, Chang L, Stanczyk FZ, Pike CJ.
Age-related testosterone depletion and the development
of Alzheimer disease. *JAMA.* 2004;**292**(12):1431–2.

56. Hogervorst E, Lehmann DJ, Warden DR, McBroom J,
Smith AD. Apolipoprotein E ε4 and testosterone
interact in the risk of Alzheimer's disease in men.
Int J Geriatr Psychiatry. 2002;**17**(16):938–40.

57. Raber J, Bongers G, Le Fevour A, Buttini M, Mucke L.
Androgens protect against apolipoprotein E4-induced
cognitive deficits. *Neurosci.* 2002;**22**(12):5204–9.

58. Lehmann DJ, Hogervorst E, Warden DR, *et al.*
The androgen receptor CAG repeat and serum
testosterone in the risk of Alzheimer's disease in
men. *J Neurol Neurosurg Psychiatry.* 2004;**75**(1):163–4.

59. Krithivas K, Yurgalevitch SM, Mohr BA, *et al.*
Evidence that the CAG repeat in the androgen
receptor gene is associated with the age-related decline
in serum androgen levels in men. *J Endocrinol.* 1999;
162(1):137–42.

60. Hogervorst E, Bandelow S, Moffat SD. Increasing
testosterone levels and effects on cognitive function
in elderly men and women: a review. *Curr
Drug Targets CNS Neurol Disord.* 2005;**4**(5):
531–40.

Chapter 6

Genetics related to sex steroids: implications for Alzheimer's disease

Chris Talbot

Editors' introduction

In this chapter, Chris Talbot discusses the evidence for involvement of genetic factors related to sex steroids in Alzheimer's disease (AD). He addresses the limitations of studies carried out including their small cohort sizes, a lack of stratification for sex, and a lack of consideration of other factors that might modify genetic risk such as age and prior hormone use. He concludes that currently the best evidence for genetic associations for AD with sex hormone genes are for the ERα and Aromatase genes in the estrogen metabolism pathway and DAPK1 for the estrogen responsive genes. However, given that genes in the sex hormone metabolism pathways operate in a coordinated fashion and that therefore epistatic interactions are likely, there is a need to analyze data on multiple SNPs in multiple genes simultaneously. Furthermore, since endogenous and exogenous hormones regulate the expression of the pathway genes, it may be crucial to measure circulating sex hormone metabolites and include these as co-factors in the analysis. Novel statistical techniques allowing higher order interactions used on combinations of large cohorts will hopefully render data that will allow future clinicians to take into account genetic profiles in deciding on an optimal hormone treatment plan.

Genetics of Alzheimer's disease

The heritability of Alzheimer's disease (AD) has been estimated by a large twin study to be 58% [1]. This is supported by the observation that having a first degree relative with AD raises an individual's risk six-fold [2]. Some families have been observed to segregate AD in a Mendelian fashion, predominantly for cases of the disease arising before 65 years of age

(early-onset AD or EOAD). Since the first AD gene was discovered in 1991 there has been a very large amount of effort put in to identify the causative disease genes. This work has led to the finding that mutations in the APP, PS1, and PS2 genes account for the majority of familial early-onset cases, but less than 2% of all AD cases. It has long been thought that most of the remaining genetic variance for AD consists of common alleles that affect risk by a small amount, in line with the common disease/common variant hypothesis. In addition, there are thought to be some remaining Mendelian loci in familial AD.

An early success was the finding that alleles of the APOE gene could be reproducibly shown to affect disease risk and lower the age at onset. There has been disagreement, however, about how much of the heritability of late-onset AD is accounted for by the APOE locus. One analysis concluded that APOE explains 7% to 9% of variation in age at onset and presented modeling that suggested that there may be four or more genetic effects of the same size or greater [3]. This, though, appears to be contradicted by the findings of the whole-genome association studies for AD (see below).

Ongoing genetic AD studies

A number of linkage studies have identified genetic loci, with the AlzGene database listing 20 loci with at least two suggestive p values. The most studied loci are on chromosomes 9, 10, and 12, but there has been a lack of success in unambiguously identifying the causative genes. This may be because there are several causative genes in the loci or the mutations are rare.

Following on from the APOE association there have been a plethora of candidate gene association

---

Hormones, Cognition and Dementia: State of the Art and Emergent Therapeutic Strategies, ed. Eef Hogervorst, Victor W. Henderson, Robert B. Gibbs, and Roberta Diaz Brinton. Published by Cambridge University Press.
© Cambridge University Press 2009.

studies. The AlzGene database of the Alzheimer Research Forum keeps an up-to-date list of these. As of June 2009, they report 1196 studies on 579 genes [4]. Of these AlzGene calculates that 32 genes show positive association on meta-analysis across at least four studies, with APOE being the strongest association. These studies are now being supplemented with whole-genome association approaches, enabled by advances in genotyping technology.

Coon *et al.* detected a genetic effect near APOE with a p value of 5×10^{-34} but no other significant results at all [5]. A later study by the same group stratified the cohorts by APOE genotype and identified the GAB2 gene as being associated in those bearing the APOE risk allele [6]. Grupe *et al.* showed similar results with SNPs near APOE the only ones to show study-wide significance, though variation in the GALP gene showed suggestive association [7]. Li *et al.* again showed APOE as the strongest genetic effect with some evidence for GOLPH2 as well as in some intergenic regions [8]. Thus these studies clearly suggest that there are no common genetic effects anywhere near the size of APOE, and by identifying different genes as runner-ups emphasizing the difficulty of finding any further consistent genetic associations.

An important caveat is that although these studies used many thousands of cases and controls, the huge degree of multiple testing still means that they are not powered to be able to detect genetic effects after controlling for sex, age at onset of AD, APOE genotype, and other factors such as history of hormone treatment. One possible explanation for the paucity of success so far in association studies is that the common disease–common variant (CDCV)[1] hypothesis does not hold for AD, apart from the case of APOE. The remaining genetic variance in AD might be accounted for by a number of mechanisms including: rare mutations with incomplete penetrance or recessive inheritance; common variants only affecting a subset of the population, e.g., women who have had hormone treatment; or epistatic interactions between multiple loci. All of these would be very hard to detect with current whole genome analyses (WGA) studies, but might be amenable to a more targeted approach.

---

[1] This assumes that complex diseases are influenced by genetic variants (single-nucleotide polymorphisms, SNPs) that are relatively common in human populations.

Association studies in estrogen related genes

Estrogen receptors

Association studies with other disease

Genetic variation in the estrogen receptor genes has been tested for associations with a range of diseases and conditions, many of which have differences in risk according to sex, including: obesity, cancer, osteoarthritis, endometriosis, type 2 diabetes, bone mineral density, cardiovascular disease, and neurological diseases (reviewed in [9]). In many of these diseases there are conflicting reports on association, with both positive and negative studies. The likely complications are those common to complex disease genetics including ethnic differences and environmental factors (e.g., hormone treatment use) not being taken into account.

Gene structures and polymorphisms

The ESR1 gene has eight exons and covers nearly 300 kb on chromosome 6. There are no validated non-synonymous coding SNPs or known functional variants. Most studies have concentrated on two SNPs within intron 1 of the gene: rs2234693 (detectable by PvuII cleavage) and rs9340799 (XbaI), but there is an abundance of SNPs across the gene. There is also a TA repeat polymorphism: 1174 bp 5′ of exon 1. The first introns of genes often have important regulatory elements that control gene expression, and for the PvuII polymorphism the T allele has been shown in a luciferase reporter assay to destroy a functional binding site for the B-myb transcription factor [10, 11] and to be associated with reduced postmenopausal estradiol levels [12]. The TA repeat polymorphism has been suggested to be associated with various diseases and to affect expression levels [13]. The latter may be altering its binding to methylated histone 3 (H3K4me3 and H3K27me3) (Genome Institute of Singapore ChIP-PET track at genome.ucsc.edu). An interesting complication is the suggestion that the polymorphisms are associated with increased use of hormone therapy (HT), possibly because women with decreased estrogen response might have more severe menopausal symptoms [14]. If that observation was found to be secure it would imply that any association study using ESR1 that did not take HT use into account would be severely compromised.

The ESR2 gene has 14 exons across about 112 kb of chromosome 14, but only 8 of the exons are coding. There are no non-synonymous coding SNPs and the only synonymous coding SNP is informative in East Asians, but not Europeans or Afro-Americans. There are no reports of SNPs affecting expression of the gene. A recent study did a comprehensive analysis of variation in the gene and concluded that four SNPs could be used to tag the haplotypes in most populations, but that five needed to be used in Africans [15]. There is a CA repeat polymorphism in intron 5 of ESR2 (isoform 1), which has shown associations with androgen levels and several diseases [13].

Association studies with Alzheimer's disease

The first AD association studies with polymorphisms in the ESR1 gene were carried out in 1999. Brandi et al. showed positive associations with the P allele of PvuII and X allele of the XbaI polymorphism, both separately and combined, using 193 Italian AD cases and 202 controls [16]. A similar result was found by Isoe-Wada et al. using 86 Japanese AD cases and 51 controls [17].

Subsequent replication studies have shown eight positive and eight negative results in different cohorts; all using the same two SNPs (see www.alzgene.org). Some of these found a sex-specific effect and others suggest an interaction with the APOE polymorphisms. The largest study up until now used data from a longitudinal cohort of 35,405 Dutch of whom 230 developed AD [18]. This study found no evidence for association with AD risk, although they did find that amygdala size measured by magnetic resonance imaging (MRI) increased in PX bearers. The significance of the latter finding is unclear.

A meta-analysis carried out in 2006 concluded that there was no association in AD cohorts from European-derived populations, but that there was from East Asian cohorts (Chinese and Japanese), with an odds ratio of 1.5 (95% CI 1.1–2.0) for bearing either the P or X allele [19]. As the authors of the meta-analysis concluded, these studies would be more meaningful if they had also controlled for sex, APOE genotype, and age at onset, to which we might add history of hormone treatment. The most recent studies have confirmed the lack of association in European-derived populations, and a Japanese study failed to find association with either SNP [20], which reduces but does not extinguish the effect on meta-analysis: OR 1.3 (95% CI 1.1–1.5) (my calculation).

There has been less work on the ESR2 gene, with four studies to date, all of which suggest some association, but only when controlling for sex or ESR1 genotype. Forsell et al. used the intron 5 CA repeat and found no overall difference between cases and controls, but that allele 5 was protective, but only in men [21]. Lambert et al. used a 3′UTR SNP, rs4986938, finding no effect by itself, but only when combined with ESR1 SNPs [22]. Pirskanen used four intronic SNPs, of which two were associated in women (rs1271573 and rs1256043), but the Lambert SNP, rs4986938, was not [23]. Luckhaus et al. used three 3′UTR SNPs including rs4986938. They found no association for the SNPs considered individually but did in a haplotypic analysis [24]. Combining the data for SNP rs4986938, which is common to three of the studies, gives an insignificant result, OR 0.96 (95% 0.83–1.11), but does not exclude involvement of the locus (my calculation).

Estrogen metabolizing genes
Aromatase

Aromatase is the rate-limiting enzyme in estrogen biosynthesis, converting testosterone to estradiol and androstenedione to estrone. It is a monooxygenase of the cytochrome P450 family. Aromatase is encoded by the CYP19A1 gene, which covers 129 kb on chromosome 15. There is one fairly common non-synonymous coding SNP, rs700519, and two rarer ones. Most of the non-AD studies have focused on a tetranucleotide repeat polymorphism (TTTA) in intron 4, while most AD studies have used multiple SNPs. It has been shown in some studies that subjects with the long allele variant of the polymorphism have higher estrogen levels and lower androgen levels, but other studies have failed to replicate this [25]. In addition, there is a 3 bp TCT insertion/deletion polymorphism upstream by 50 bp of the TTTA repeat, which has been shown in some studies to modulate its effect [26]. There is a reported copy number variation of the CYP19A1 gene, although it occurs in fewer than 1% of people [27].

There have been six studies on the association of CYP19A1 and AD, three finding a positive association and three negative. The first study, in 2004, used nine SNPs across the gene in a large Finnish cohort and found evidence that three of these were associated with disease irrespective of APOE genotype or sex [28]. Two papers using a moderately sized Spanish cohort reported association with SNPs in the gene, but only in combination with others in the BCHE and IL10 genes [29, 30]. Huang and Poduslo used a haplotyping strategy with 18 SNPs across the gene and detected separate haplotypes at the 5′ and 3′ ends of the genes that both affected risk for AD [31]. Two of the WGA studies included SNPs within CYP19A1, with neither finding association in their large cohorts [6, 8]. It is only possible to carry out a meta-analysis on one of the 5′ UTR SNPs, with AlzGene calculating the odds ratio as a non-significant 0.95 (95% CI 0.86–1.04).

Given the importance of the gene, it would be worth genotyping the repeat and insertion polymorphisms in a large cohort and integrating with the SNP data, to achieve a final analysis of whether there is an association with AD.

Catechol o-methyltransferase

Catechol o-methyltransferase (COMT) is involved in one of the main degradative pathways of the catecholamine neurotransmitters as well as inactivating reactive estrogenic metabolites. It is encoded by a small gene covering just 27 kb on chromosome 22. There is only one non-synonymous coding SNP in people of European origin, Met158Val (rs4680). This SNP has been used in numerous genetic studies, with evidence for association with schizophrenia, panic disorder, and bipolar disorder, though it is possible another variation in the gene is also involved [32]. Postmenopausal women not taking HT who had the Met/Met genotype had 28% higher 2-hydroxyestrone levels and 31% higher 16alpha-hydroxyestrone, compared with Val/Val women [33]. There is known to be a segmental duplication that affects the COMT gene and causes a whole gene deletion in 4% of individuals [34].

There is little evidence of an association between alleles of Met158Val and AD, though this may be complicated by the copy number polymorphism. The first two studies published found no evidence of association for risk of AD [35, 36], while two other small studies found marginal evidence after stratification of the cohorts [37, 38]. Given the reported links between COMT and psychiatric disease, it is interesting that Borroni et al. report an association between psychosis in AD and the Val allele, with OR of 2.7 (95% CI 1.6–6.6) [36]. This association has subsequently been replicated, including using other COMT SNPs [39]. The link between estrogen levels and psychosis is further reinforced by the cases of postpartum and perimenopausal psychosis [40, 41]. There

have been some research studies on the therapeutic use of female hormones on psychosis, including in AD, but it is not in regular clinical use [42–44].

CYP17 and CYP1A1

CYP17 and CYP1A1 are other members of the cytochrome P450 family, both of which are involved in key steps in estrogen biosynthesis.

CYP17A1 is a 7 kb gene on chromosome 10, with only one annotated polymorphism that changes an amino acid in 1% of Chinese and sub-Saharan African chromosomes (HapMap data). The most commonly studied polymorphism is an SNP in the 5′ UTR, rs743572, often detected using the MspAI restriction enzyme. The SNP has been reported to affect promoter activity, with each copy of the minor allele (known as A2 allele) halving the mRNA level. The evidence is mixed, however, as to whether the polymorphism affects endogenous hormone levels [45]. There is evidence though that rs743572 is associated with HT use, with A2/A2 homozygotes being only half as likely to be current HT users as compared with women of A1/A1 genotype [46]. If true that would be a potential confounder in studies of postmenopausal women that did not take HT use into account.

CYP1A1 is a 6 kb gene on chromosome 15, which has at least 15 annotated coding SNPs, though all have minor allele frequencies of below 10% except for Ile462Val (rs1048943). Two other SNPs in the 3′ UTR have also been used extensively to test for genetic associations with breast cancer. There is inconsistent evidence as to whether the polymorphisms affect gene expression, protein activity, or metabolite levels [47].

CYP1A1 had been included in a Parkinson's disease association study that included a very small AD cohort, but unsurprisingly found no evidence for association [48]. Wang et al., already mentioned in relation to COMT, also studied polymorphisms in CYP17 and CYP1A1 genes in a Taiwanese AD cohort but found no sign of association [37]. CYP17 is in the chromosome 10 AD linkage region but was not found to be associated in the published chromosome-wide association study [49]. None of these studies was stratified for sex (see previous chapter).

Other estrogen pathway genes

The KEGG pathway for androgen and estrogen metabolism shows that at least 27 separate enzymes control the hormone's biosynthesis and degradation [50].

Many of these enzymes function in multiple metabolic pathways. Each enzyme operates in a carefully controlled network and many are regulated by levels of estrogenic metabolites. Therefore there is every possibility not only that DNA variation in any of the genes could influence levels of hormone in a tissue-specific manner, but that these might operate in a coordinated manner, resulting in epistatic interactions.

Apart from the association studies listed above, most of the other estrogen pathway genes have yet to be considered as candidates for AD. The whole-genome studies of course will have included SNPs in the vicinity of these genes, but are subject to the caveats noted above.

Estrogen responsive genes

The genes we have so far considered are those that directly affect estrogen levels and therefore the transcriptional activity of the estrogen receptors. A further way that genetic variation could interact with estrogen functioning and impact on risk for AD is in the estrogen responsive genes.

ERα and ERβ translocate to the nucleus where they bind different subsets of estrogen responsive elements (EREs) in the genome and act as transcription factors. There is sequence variation in the verifiable ERE sequences, which prevents easy computational determination of all functional EREs. There are at least 50 genes that have been shown experimentally to have functional EREs and even more that show estrogen response by an indirect mechanism [51]. Genomics approaches using chromatin immunoprecipitation on microarrays (ChIP-on-chip) have identified at least 3,665 ER binding sites, of which only 4% are in gene promoters, with many lying tens of kilobases upstream of the genes they regulate [52]. Some of the genes thus identified as estrogen responsive by Carroll *et al.* [52] have already been considered as candidates for AD.

Myeloperoxidase (MPO) is a heme-containing protein that is released from leukocytes at sites of inflammation, and is known to activate aromatic amines from tobacco smoke and generate free radicals. The initial association study showed association between an over-expressing promoter allele and risk for AD [53]. Given the estrogen responsiveness it is interesting that the association was sex-specific, with females at increased risk and males having decreased risk. The subsequent eight replication studies gave

mixed results, and the current meta-analysis at AlzGene shows no overall evidence for association (OR = 1.0, 95% CI 0.8–1.3). It must be noted, however, that this does not take sex into account, let alone HT use.

The low density lipoprotein receptor (LDLR) is one of the receptors for APOE, and therefore several SNPs in it have been extensively studied for evidence of association to AD. The original study found no evidence of association to LDLR [54], but two subsequent large studies did show a robust sex-specific effect [55, 56]. Again, the AlzGene meta-analyses are not significant, but do not stratify analyses by sex (exon 13 SNP OR = 1.0, 95% CI 0.9–1.1).

Another estrogen-responsive gene was the aspartyl protease, Cathepsin D, which is thought to modulate APP and tau cleavage. As of July 2008 there were 28 published AD association studies with CTSD, with a near significant meta-analysis for cohorts of European descent (OR = 1.17, 95% CI 0.98–1.41). There is little evidence from the literature for a sex effect.

The last estrogen-responsive gene we shall consider here is Death Associated Protein Kinase 1 (DAPK1). The DAPK1 protein promotes programmed cell death and was identified in a very large study as the disease gene in the chromosome 9 AD linkage region [57]. Two smaller studies have failed to replicate the finding, but the meta-analysis remains significant (rs4878104 OR = 0.88, 95% CI 0.82–0.95). Li *et al.* did not report whether they had analyzed the data stratified for sex.

Gene and hormone treatment interactions

As discussed in other chapters of this book, the WHIMS came to the surprising conclusion that HT increases risk for AD, though it is probably dependent upon the timing of HT after menopause. Genetic variation may also be important, with there being a possibility that exogenous estrogen has different effects on risk, dependent on genotype.

There have been some studies on the interaction between APOE genotype and HT use. Burkhardt *et al.* studied memory performance in a cohort of Australian women with mean age around 65 years of age, and concluded that HT improved cognitive performance, but only in women who did not carry an APOE ε4 allele [58]. A larger family-based study of Latinas from the Caribbean concluded that APOE ε4 risk may be reduced by a history of HT [59]. This conclusion is only partially supported by the data, since the regression analysis suggested that APOE genotype and HT use were independent risk factors. Furthermore, as the authors noted, the HT effect in this study could be caused by the fact that the HT users were younger and had a better education than non-HT users, both factors known to decrease AD risk.

The estrogen receptors and degradative enzymes are obvious candidates for modulating the effect of HT on cognitive performance and risk for AD. Ongoing studies should answer whether there is a genetically defined subgroup of women who would benefit from HT.

Other sex hormone pathways
Androgen genes

The androgen receptor (AR) gene has a CAG repeat polymorphism in exon 1, the expansion of which has been proved to lower gene transcription. Using the OPTIMA cohort Lehmann *et al.* found an increased risk of AD for men with shorter repeat lengths [60]. This finding has been reiterated in a sophisticated grade-of-membership analysis, but has yet to be repeated in a different cohort [61].

Luteinizing hormone

Mark Smith and colleagues have published a series of papers and reviews arguing that the crucial hormone system in AD is luteinizing hormone (LH) [62, 63]. They evince several lines of evidence including raised levels of LH in AD patients, the high concentration of LH receptors in the hippocampus, the detrimental effect of raised LH on AD-model mice, and the beneficial effect of leuprolide acetate, which lowers LH production. To this has recently been added genetic evidence [64].

Luteinizing hormone is a glycoprotein consisting of two protein chains joined by disulfide bonds. The α chain is common to several glycoprotein hormones and is encoded by the CGA gene, while the β chain is specific to LH and is encoded by the LHB gene. There is one main receptor, the luteinizing hormone/choriogonadotropin receptor (LHCGR).

Haasl *et al.* described a study that set out to look for gene–gene interactions between alleles of multiple SNPs in APOE, LHB, and LHCGR [64]. Their results suggested that an allele of an intron 1 SNP in LHCGR

reversed the increased risk of the APOE ε4 allele in males. This study used a small cohort and needs to be replicated.

Conclusions

Genetic association studies in all complex diseases are plagued by the problem of non-replicability of modest risk factors. This is widely thought to be caused by small cohort sizes, no stratification for sex, publication bias, and failure to consider all genetic information such as age, education, and HT use. Beyond the case of APOE there are no unambiguous genetic risk factors for AD, including the sex hormone genes. This may be because there simply are not any other polymorphisms that affect risk for AD to any great extent. The extent of heritability of the disease, however, argues against that notion. An alternative solution is that there are multiple risk factors that only operate in a subset of all AD patients.

Given that sex hormones operate by definition in a sex-specific manner it is plain that all association analyses using pathway genes should take sex into account and stratify analyses for sex. It is likely, though, that it will be necessary to also factor in APOE genotype and other hormone-altering life events such as age at menarche, history of oral contraception, and HT use. Most existing cohorts are of insufficient size to carry out stratified analyses but advanced statistical methods for studying interactions should obviate the need for the reduction in power caused by stratification.

Genes in the sex hormone metabolism pathways operate in a coordinated fashion and therefore epistatic interactions are likely, necessitating the need to analyze data on multiple SNPs in multiple genes simultaneously. The use of multiple genic SNPs allows haplotypic analyses that include the full genetic information. Furthermore, since endogenous and exogenous hormones regulate the expression of the pathway genes it may be crucial to measure circulating sex hormone metabolites and include these as co-factors in the analysis.

The best current evidence for genetic associations with sex hormone genes are for the ERα and aromatase genes in the estrogen metabolism pathway and DAPK1 for the estrogen responsive genes. There are, however, many other genes in the pathways that are yet to be tested, and many of the published studies may have been unable to detect any real genetic effect through not incorporating enough information into the analysis. There is a need for the reanalysis of old data and further large scale studies on well characterized cohorts with measures of circulating hormone levels. One additional possibility would be to study all SNPs that occur genome-wide in ER binding sites, which can be estimated to number around 12,000 (my calculation).

In sum, novel techniques employing multiple interactions simultaneously in combinations of large existing cohorts will hopefully aid clinicians in the future to determine possible AD risk related to sex steroid genetics.

References

1. Gatz M, Reynolds CA, Fratiglioni L, *et al.* Role of genes and environments for explaining Alzheimer disease. *Arch Gen Psychiatry.* 2006;**63**(2):168–74.

2. Mayeux R, Sano M, Chen J, Tatemichi T, Stern Y. Risk of dementia in first-degree relatives of patients with Alzheimer's disease and related disorders. *Arch Neurol.* 1991;**48**(3):269–73.

3. Daw EW, Payami H, Nemens EJ, *et al.* The number of trait loci in late-onset Alzheimer disease. *Am J Hum Genet.* 2000;**66**(1):196–204.

4. Bertram L, McQueen M, Mullin K, Blacker D, Tanzi R. *The AlzGene Database.* Alzheimer Research Forum. 2008 [updated 2008; cited 08/07/08]; Available from: http://www.alzgene.org.

5. Coon KD, Myers AJ, Craig DW, *et al.* A high-density whole-genome association study reveals that APOE is the major susceptibility gene for sporadic late-onset Alzheimer's disease. *J Clin Psychiatry.* 2007; **68**(4):613–18.

6. Reiman EM, Webster JA, Myers AJ, *et al.* GAB2 alleles modify Alzheimer's risk in APOE epsilon4 carriers. *Neuron.* 2007;**54**(5):713–20.

7. Grupe A, Abraham R, Li Y, *et al.* Evidence for novel susceptibility genes for late-onset Alzheimer's disease from a genome-wide association study of putative functional variants. *Hum Mol Genet.* 2007;**16**(8):865–73.

8. Li H, Wetten S, Li L, *et al.* Candidate single-nucleotide polymorphisms from a genomewide association study of Alzheimer disease. *Arch Neurol.* 2008; **65**(1):45–53.

9. Deroo BJ, Korach KS. Estrogen receptors and human disease. *J Clin Invest.* 2006;**116**(3):561–70.

10. Herrington DM, Howard TD, Brosnihan KB, *et al.* Common estrogen receptor polymorphism augments effects of hormone replacement therapy on E-selectin but not C-reactive protein. *Circulation.* 2002;**105** (16):1879–82.

11. Schuit SC, Oei HH, Witteman JC, *et al.* Estrogen receptor alpha gene polymorphisms and risk of myocardial infarction. *JAMA.* 2004;**291**(24):2969–77.

12. Schuit SC, de Jong FH, Stolk L, *et al.* Estrogen receptor alpha gene polymorphisms are associated with estradiol levels in postmenopausal women. *Eur J Endocrinol.* 2005;**153**(2):327–34.

13. McIntyre MH, Kantoff PW, Stampfer MJ, *et al.* Prostate cancer risk and ESR1 TA, ESR2 CA repeat polymorphisms. *Cancer Epidemiol Biomarkers Prev.* 2007;**16**(11):2233–6.

14. Lawlor DA, Timpson N, Ebrahim S, Day IN, Smith GD. The association of oestrogen receptor alpha-haplotypes with cardiovascular risk factors in the British Women's Heart and Health Study. *Eur Heart J.* 2006;**27**(13):1597–604.

15. Cox DG, Bretsky P, Kraft P, *et al.* Haplotypes of the estrogen receptor beta gene and breast cancer risk. *Int J Cancer.* 2008;**122**(2):387–92.

16. Brandi ML, Becherini L, Gennari L, *et al.* Association of the estrogen receptor alpha gene polymorphisms with sporadic Alzheimer's disease. *Biochem Biophys Res Commun.* 1999;**265**(2):335–8.

17. Isoe-Wada K, Maeda M, Yong J, *et al.* Positive association between an estrogen receptor gene polymorphism and Parkinson's disease with dementia. *Eur J Neurol.* 1999;**6**(4):431–5.

18. den Heijer T, Schuit SC, Pols HA, *et al.* Variations in estrogen receptor alpha gene and risk of dementia, and brain volumes on MRI. *Mol Psychiatry.* 2004; **9**(12):1129–35.

19. Luckhaus C, Sand PG. Estrogen Receptor 1 gene (ESR1) variants in Alzheimer's disease. Results of a meta-analysis. *Aging Clin Exp Res.* 2007; **19**(2):165–8.

20. Usui C, Shibata N, Ohnuma T, *et al.* No genetic association between the myeloperoxidase gene-463 polymorphism and estrogen receptor-alpha gene polymorphisms and Japanese sporadic Alzheimer's disease. *Dement Geriatr Cogn Disord.* 2006;**21**(5/6): 296–9.

21. Forsell C, Enmark E, Axelman K, *et al.* Investigations of a CA repeat in the oestrogen receptor beta gene in patients with Alzheimer's disease. *Eur J Hum Genet.* 2001;**9**(10):802–4.

22. Lambert JC, Harris JM, Mann D, *et al.* Are the estrogen receptors involved in Alzheimer's disease? *Neurosci Lett.* 2001;**306**(3):193–7.

23. Pirskanen M, Hiltunen M, Mannermaa A, *et al.* Estrogen receptor beta gene variants are associated

with increased risk of Alzheimer's disease in women. *Eur J Hum Genet.* 2005;**13**(9):1000–6.

24. Luckhaus C, Spiegler C, Ibach B, *et al.* Estrogen receptor beta gene (ESRbeta) 3′-UTR variants in Alzheimer disease. *Alzheimer Dis Assoc Disord.* 2006; **20**(4):322–3.

25. Olson SH, Bandera EV, Orlow I. Variants in estrogen biosynthesis genes, sex steroid hormone levels, and endometrial cancer: a HuGE review. *Am J Epidemiol.* 2007;**165**(3):235–45.

26. Kastelan D, Grubic Z, Kraljevic I, *et al.* Decreased peak bone mass is associated with a 3-bp deletion/insertion of the CYP19 intron 4 polymorphism: preliminary data from the GOOS study. *J Endocrinol Invest.* 2007;**30**(6):465–9.

27. Redon R, Ishikawa S, Fitch KR, *et al.* Global variation in copy number in the human genome. *Nature.* 2006;**444**(7118):444–54.

28. Iivonen S, Corder E, Lehtovirta M, *et al.* Polymorphisms in the CYP19 gene confer increased risk for Alzheimer disease. *Neurology.* 2004;**62**(7): 1170–6.

29. Combarros O, Riancho JA, Infante J, *et al.* Interaction between CYP19 aromatase and butyrylcholinesterase genes increases Alzheimer's disease risk. *Dement Geriatr Cogn Disord.* 2005;**20**(2/3):153–7.

30. Combarros O, Sanchez-Juan P, Riancho JA, *et al.* Aromatase and interleukin-10 genetic variants interactively modulate Alzheimer's disease risk. *J Neural Transm.* 2008;**115**(6):863–7.

31. Huang R, Poduslo SE. CYP19 haplotypes increase risk for Alzheimer's disease. *J Med Genet.* 2006;**43**(8):e42.

32. Mukherjee N, Kidd KK, Pakstis AJ, *et al.* The complex global pattern of genetic variation and linkage disequilibrium at catechol-O-methyltransferase. *Mol Psychiatry.* 2008; doi:10.1038/mp.2008.64.

33. Tworoger SS, Chubak J, Aiello EJ, *et al.* Association of CYP17, CYP19, CYP1B1, and COMT polymorphisms with serum and urinary sex hormone concentrations in postmenopausal women. *Cancer Epidemiol Biomarkers Prev.* 2004;**13**(1):94–101.

34. Locke DP, Sharp AJ, McCarroll SA, *et al.* Linkage disequilibrium and heritability of copy-number polymorphisms within duplicated regions of the human genome. *Am J Hum Genet.* 2006; **79**(2):275–90.

35. Emahazion T, Feuk L, Jobs M, *et al.* SNP association studies in Alzheimer's disease highlight problems for complex disease analysis. *Trends Genet.* 2001;**17**(7):407–13.

36. Borroni B, Agosti C, Archetti S, *et al.* Catechol-O-methyltransferase gene polymorphism is associated with risk of psychosis in Alzheimer disease. *Neurosci Lett.* 2004;**370**(2/3):127–9.

37. Wang PN, Liu HC, Liu TY, *et al.* Estrogen-metabolizing gene COMT polymorphism synergistic APOE epsilon4 allele increases the risk of Alzheimer disease. *Dement Geriatr Cogn Disord.* 2005;**19**(2/3):120–5.

38. Forero DA, Benitez B, Arboleda G, *et al.* Analysis of functional polymorphisms in three synaptic plasticity-related genes (BDNF, COMT AND UCHL1) in Alzheimer's disease in Colombia. *Neurosci Res.* 2006;**55**(3):334–41.

39. Sweet RA, Devlin B, Pollock BG, *et al.* Catechol-O-methyltransferase haplotypes are associated with psychosis in Alzheimer disease. *Mol Psychiatry.* 2005;**10**(11):1026–36.

40. Sit D, Rothschild AJ, Wisner KL. A review of postpartum psychosis. *J Womens Health (Larchmt).* 2006;**15**(4):352–68.

41. Rasgon N, Shelton S, Halbreich U. Perimenopausal mental disorders: epidemiology and phenomenology. *CNS Spectr.* 2005;**10**(6):471–8.

42. Chua WL, de Izquierdo SA, Kulkarni J, Mortimer A. Estrogen for schizophrenia. *Cochrane Database Syst Rev.* 2005(4):CD004719.

43. Kulkarni J, Gurvich C, Gilbert H, *et al.* Hormone modulation: a novel therapeutic approach for women with severe mental illness. *Aust NZ J Psychiatry.* 2008;**42**(1):83–8.

44. Herrmann N, Lanctot KL. Pharmacologic management of neuropsychiatric symptoms of Alzheimer disease. *Can J Psychiatry.* 2007;**52**(10):630–46.

45. Sharp L, Cardy AH, Cotton SC, Little J. CYP17 gene polymorphisms: prevalence and associations with hormone levels and related factors. A HuGE review. *Am J Epidemiol.* 2004;**160**(8):729–40.

46. Feigelson HS, McKean-Cowdin R, Pike MC, *et al.* Cytochrome P450c17{{alpha}} gene (CYP17) polymorphism predicts use of hormone replacement therapy. *Cancer Res.* 1999;**59**(16):3908–10.

47. Masson LF, Sharp L, Cotton SC, Little J. Cytochrome P-450 1A1 gene polymorphisms and risk of breast cancer: a HuGE review. *Am J Epidemiol.* 2005; **161**(10):901–15.

48. Nicholl DJ, Bennett P, Hiller L, *et al.* A study of five candidate genes in Parkinson's disease and related neurodegenerative disorders. European Study Group on atypical Parkinsonism. *Neurology.* 1999; **53**(7):1415–21.

49. Grupe A, Li Y, Rowland C, *et al.* A scan of chromosome 10 identifies a novel locus showing

strong association with late-onset Alzheimer disease. *Am J Hum Genet.* 2006;**78**(1):78–88.

50. Kanehisa M, Goto S, Hattori M, *et al.* From genomics to chemical genomics: new developments in KEGG. *Nucleic Acids Res.* 2006;**34**(Database issue):D354–7.

51. O'Lone R, Frith MC, Karlsson EK, Hansen U. Genomic targets of nuclear estrogen receptors. *Mol Endocrinol.* 2004;**18**(8):1859–75.

52. Carroll JS, Meyer CA, Song J, *et al.* Genome-wide analysis of estrogen receptor binding sites. *Nat Genet.* 2006;**38**(11):1289–97.

53. Reynolds WF, Rhees J, Maciejewski D, *et al.* Myeloperoxidase polymorphism is associated with gender specific risk for Alzheimer's disease. *Exp Neurol.* 1999;**155**(1):31–41.

54. Lendon CL, Talbot CJ, Craddock NJ, *et al.* Genetic association studies between dementia of the Alzheimer's type and three receptors for apolipoprotein E in a Caucasian population. *Neurosci Lett.* 1997;**222**(3):187–90.

55. Lamsa R, Helisalmi S, Herukka SK, *et al.* Genetic study evaluating LDLR polymorphisms and Alzheimer's disease. *Neurobiol Aging.* 2008;**29**(6):848–55.

56. Zou F, Gopalraj RK, Lok J, *et al.* Sex-dependent association of a common low-density lipoprotein receptor polymorphism with RNA splicing efficiency in the brain and Alzheimer's disease. *Hum Mol Genet.* 2008;**17**(7):929–35.

57. Li Y, Grupe A, Rowland C, *et al.* DAPK1 variants are associated with Alzheimer's disease and allele-specific expression. *Hum Mol Genet.* 2006;**15**(17):2560–8.

58. Burkhardt MS, Foster JK, Laws SM, *et al.* Oestrogen replacement therapy may improve memory functioning in the absence of APOE epsilon4. *J Alzheimers Dis.* 2004;**6**(3):221–8.

59. Rippon GA, Tang MX, Lee JH, *et al.* Familial Alzheimer disease in Latinos: interaction between APOE, stroke, and estrogen replacement. *Neurology.* 2006;**66**(1):35–40.

60. Lehmann DJ, Butler HT, Warden DR, *et al.* Association of the androgen receptor CAG repeat polymorphism with Alzheimer's disease in men. *Neurosci Lett.* 2003;**340**(2):87–90.

61. Corder EH, Beaumont H. Susceptibility groups for Alzheimer's disease (OPTIMA cohort): integration of gene variants and biochemical factors. *Mech Ageing Dev.* 2007;**128**(1):76–82.

62. Casadesus G, Garrett MR, Webber KM, *et al.* The estrogen myth: potential use of gonadotropin-releasing hormone agonists for the treatment of Alzheimer's disease. *Drugs R D.* 2006;**7**(3):187–93.

63. Webber KM, Perry G, Smith MA, Casadesus G. The contribution of luteinizing hormone to Alzheimer disease pathogenesis. *Clin Med Res.* 2007;**5**(3):177–83.

64. Haasl RJ, Ahmadi MR, Meethal SV, *et al.* A luteinizing hormone receptor intronic variant is significantly associated with decreased risk of Alzheimer's disease in males carrying an apolipoprotein E epsilon4 allele. *BMC Med Genet.* 2008;**9**:37.

Apolipoprotein E, hormone therapy, and neuroprotection

Robert G. Struble and Mary E. McAsey

Editors' introduction

Struble and McAsey propose that apolipoprotein E (APOE) is a pivotal required intermediary in the neuroprotective effects of hormone replacement therapy (HT) not only in dementia but in other chronic neurological diseases. Basic science analyses indicate that 17β-estradiol increases APOE expression, which facilitates neuronal plasticity, neural repair, and could delay progression of several types of neurodegenerative disease. The issue of the APOE4 isoform, which may be a negative regulator of HT outcomes, is considered along with therapeutic implications for either increasing or decreasing its expression. These authors propose that subsequent studies of the impact of HT or selective estrogen receptor modulators on neurological function should include APOE genotyping.

Introduction

The initial finding that a history of HT could decrease the risk for developing clinical dementia [1] led to numerous studies of ovarian hormone effects on brain function. Most epidemiology studies examined the effects of HT in dementia. The intense focus on dementia has largely overshadowed possible roles of neuroprotection by HT in other chronic neurological diseases. Nonetheless, a limited number of studies during the last 15 years suggested that HT's neuroprotective effects were not unique to dementia and occurred in such diverse chronic diseases as multiple sclerosis and Parkinson's disease [2, 3]. Review of this literature suggested that HT was neuroprotective in numerous chronic diseases but that studies of less common diseases may have lacked adequate power to detect an effect.

In spite of the neuroprotective effects of HT in the incidence of dementia, clinical intervention studies generally have been unsuccessful. These negative findings suggested to us that previous clinical trials of HT may have overlooked some critical intermediate variable that could modify the neuroprotective mechanism(s) of HT. Therefore, we searched for a possible intermediary protein that could explain the generalized neuroprotective effects of HT and intervention failures. We propose that apolipoprotein E (APOE) is a candidate intermediate protein. APOE aids in repair and regeneration following damage. It may also function during acute damage, although few studies exist addressing this possibility. A generalized neuroprotective role of APOE could affect the progression of multiple chronic neurological diseases regardless of the etiology of the disease. Moreover, human APOE exists as three isoforms. Studies have suggested an APOE isoform-specific efficacy of HT, which could explain some failures of HT studies. We propose that APOE is a critical intermediary protein for neuroprotection by HT.

Apolipoprotein E

APOE is a 35 kD lipid-associated protein. Lipid binds to the APOE C-terminus and specialized receptors bind the N-terminus. Humans possess three major isoforms of APOE referred to as APOE2, APOE3 and APOE4, which are coded by three alleles, ε2, ε3, and ε4. Variation of these isoforms by one amino acid at two sites modifies the tertiary structure, which in turn, may modify binding affinity to both intracellular and extracellular receptors [4]. The approximate frequencies of ε2, ε3, and ε4 alleles are 0.03, 0.78, and 0.18, respectively showing a Hardy–Weinberg equilibrium.

APOE modifies brain function through specialized receptors. The APOE receptor family range in weight from 130 to 600 kD. Most of these are present in the brain. They include the very low density lipoprotein receptors (VLDLr), the low density lipoprotein receptor (LDLr), the APOE receptor (APOE2r), the lipoprotein receptor related protein (LRP), megalin, and GP330, among others. Importantly, the C-terminus of some of these receptors, including the LRP, has an NPxY motif that, in addition to lipid internalization, modulates numerous intracellular processes. Lipoprotein receptor related protein may be especially important since it has been recognized as a "receptor" for APOE, lactoferrin, α2 macroglobulin, amyloid precursor protein, and the transforming growth factor beta protein, among others. More information about these receptors can be found in an excellent review [5].

If APOE is a critical intermediary for neuroprotection by HT, as we propose, then APOE should meet several criteria. (1) Brain levels of APOE and its receptors must be affected by components of HT including estrogens and/or progestins. (2) Hormone therapy should interact with APOE to influence disease risk or progression. (3) APOE genotype should modify the course of the same diseases affected by HT. (4) Finally, because HT neuroprotection affects multiple diseases, APOE should have a generalized mechanism(s) of action that would not be disease process-specific. Below, we discuss each of these criteria.

Brain APOE is affected by 17β-estradiol (estradiol)

Ovarian hormones affect brain levels of APOE but the mechanisms are complex and the effects may show regional specificity. We showed regionally specific variation in mouse brain APOE levels throughout the estrous cycle [6]. APOE peaked on diestrus and proestrus in hippocampus, cingulate, and frontal cortex with lowest levels on estrus. Olfactory bulb and cerebellum showed an opposite pattern with a peak on estrus. APOE protein in males tended to be slightly less than peak levels in females.

Numerous studies have shown that five to seven days of estradiol replacement increased whole brain APOE mRNA and protein in ovariectomized (OVX) rodents (reviewed in [7]). Estradiol replacement slightly increased neocortical APOE protein (ca. 20%), had a stronger effect in the hippocampus (ca. 40%) and a substantial effect in the olfactory bulb and cerebellum (100%) [6]. We also found that physiological concentrations of 17β-estradiol increased APOE within four hours in adult neocortical cell culture media and this increase was maintained for four days [8]. Hence, APOE is clearly affected by HT.

The receptor specificity of APOE's response to 17β-estradiol replacement is not clear. Previous studies suggested that 17β-estradiol acted through an estrogen receptor (ER) α-like receptor. However, our data and those of others suggested that 17β-estradiol regulation of APOE was more complex than a simple ER response. ERα tends to be more common in cortical regions. ERβ is found in the cerebellum in the absence of ERα. ERβ is the predominant ER in the olfactory bulb [6]. However, regardless of ER subtype, cyclic variation in APOE occurs in these brain regions. The magnitude of APOE increase five to seven days after OVX was greater in the olfactory bulb and cerebellum than in the neocortex or hippocampus suggesting that the absence of ERα did not inhibit a response [6]. As noted above, these structures show few or no immunocytochemically labeled ERα receptors [6]. In contrast, Brinton and co-workers have reported that ERα increased while ERβ decreased APOE expression in hippocampus both in vitro and in vivo (Wang et al., 2006 [51]). These data indicate differential regulation of APOE mRNA and protein expression by estrogen receptor isoforms. Further these data indicate that when ERα and ERβ are co-expressed in the same brain region that their impact on APOE expression can be opposite whereas in the absence of ERα, ERβ can assume a pro-regulatory effect on APOE.

We have also shown that the effects of prolonged 17β-estradiol replacement on APOE and LRP are transient. Replacement of 17β-estradiol by subcutaneous pellets increased APOE, LRP, and synaptophysin at five to seven days after OVX as compared to the OVX-vehicle-treated mice [9, 10]. However, by 14 days of continuous 17β-estradiol, levels of APOE, LRP, and synaptophysin declined to levels comparable to the vehicle-treated mice in all regions, and remained low over the 49 days. Moreover, effects of 17β-estradiol on LRP were brain-region specific. Estradiol replacement increased LRP in the hippocampus, somatosensory cortex, and olfactory bulb, but not the cerebellum [10]. Interestingly, the LDLr was refractory to estradiol replacement showing no changes in any region at any time period. These data suggest that increased APOE and LRP subsequent to 17β-estradiol replacement may not directly modify lipid receptors.

In an unpublished study we treated 16- and 23-week-old mice five days post-OVX with a single dose of 17β-estradiol calculated to elevate serum to proestrus concentration. APOE expression, measured in four brain regions, did not change within 24 hours of estradiol treatment. However, we found increased APOE within 12 hours if the mice had been ovariectomized six weeks prior to 17β-estradiol treatment. Clearly, prolonged absence of ovarian hormones modified the brain response to 17β-estradiol replacement.

We also noted a striking age-specific effect in LRP production when acute replacement was used. Replacement with 17β-estradiol five days post OVX at 16 weeks of age suppressed LRP within hours, but increased LRP if OVX and 17β-estradiol replacement occurred at 23 weeks of age. This observation is important since it would imply that APOE cellular processes mediated by LRP could substantially change as a function of 17β-estradiol-mediated changes in the number of the lipid receptors. Aging in mice, even within this brief time period, has substantial effects.

In sum, these studies show that 17β-estradiol replacement modified brain APOE and LRP, and three major conclusions emerge. First, rapid ER activation followed by rapid APOE protein production probably does not occur. Estradiol replacement after ovariectomy requires between three and seven days to increase APOE, which we feel is probably too protracted for a simple membrane or nuclear receptor-mediated response. Acute responses to a single bolus of 17β-estradiol are only seen two months following ovariectomy.

Second, continuous 17β-estradiol replacement resulted in an acute (five to seven days) increase of APOE (and LRP), but returned within two weeks to the levels observed in ovariectomized, vehicle-treated groups. Continuous 17β-estradiol replacement became non-functional to elevate these proteins. The explanation for this mechanism is not known.

The effects of aging, even within a relatively brief period during the mouse reproductive life (16–23 weeks) could be substantial. The age of OVX clearly interacts with the age of the mouse. Subsequent studies to understand APOE and receptor responses to estradiol replacement as a function of age of intervention are clearly indicated.

Hormone therapy interacts with APOE for disease risk

The literature of the interaction between HT and APOE genotype is limited. Women treated with HT who had an APOE ε4 allele did not show the same degree of neuroprotection from cognitive decline as those with other genotypes [11]. Hormone therapy appeared to improve cognitive function in postmenopausal women who did not have the ε4 allele [12]. Of note, although not directly generic to HT, are parallel observations in males. Higher levels of serum testosterone are associated with better cognitive function unless the APOE ε4 gene is present [13]. Estrogen receptor polymorphisms interacted with APOE4 genotype to increase the risk for developing Alzheimer type dementia suggesting that HT and APOE shared a common mechanism [14]. Hence, neuroprotection by gonadal hormones appears to be moderated by APOE isoforms.

Studies in experimental animals, although limited in number, show a similar interaction. Neuroprotection by 17β-estradiol replacement in an experimental stroke model is absent in mice lacking APOE [15]. An increase rate of synaptogenesis by 17β-estradiol replacement following entorhinal cortex lesion does not occur in the absence of APOE [16]. Finally, we have shown that 17β-estradiol facilitates neurite growth in adult cortical cultures and the dose–response curve for growth facilitation is similar to the curve for 17β-estradiol stimulation of APOE release into the media [8]. Moreover, 17β-estradiol does not stimulate process growth in the absence of APOE or in the presence of APOE4; synergy between 17β-estradiol and APOE showed APOE2 to be more efficacious than APOE3 [8].

Overall, these data suggest that the gonadal hormones, 17β-estradiol and testosterone, probably interact with APOE genotype to modify risk for cognitive decline. Therefore, when designing replacement studies it may be essential to consider the role of the APOE genotype.

APOE genotype modifies the course of numerous chronic neurological diseases

APOE4 is associated with an increased "risk" for numerous chronic neurological diseases, including those modified by HT. Dementia is substantially affected by APOE genotype. Individuals homozygous for ε4 have approximately a 90% risk for dementia by the age of 90 while those homozygous for ε3 had approximately a 30% risk and about 50% of demented patients have at least one ε4 allele [17]. APOE ε2 may lessen the risk but the low frequency of this genotype has made epidemiological risk estimates unreliable. Dementia risk is also modified by polymorphisms of the APOE receptor, LRP [18]. Hence APOE4 is markedly overrepresented in the demented population and polymorphisms of APOE receptors can modify risk for dementia.

The ε2 and ε4 alleles are more frequently associated with Parkinson's disease (PD) than ε3 [19, 20]. Notably, the risk associated with ε4 effect was greater in women than in men, which implicates a role of ovarian hormones in developing PD [21].

Other chronic neurological conditions are also affected by APOE isoform. Dementia following brain trauma is more likely in those with the ε4 genotype [22]. The ε4 genotype is associated with more rapid progression of relapsing–remitting multiple sclerosis [23, 24] and amyotrophic lateral sclerosis [25]. Finally, the progression of temporal lobe epilepsy is more rapid in patients with an APOE4 allele [26]. Hence, the ε4 genotype seems to increase the risk or progression of numerous chronic neurological diseases.

APOE has generalized effects on neuroprotection

APOE clearly has "neuroprotective qualities". Neuroprotection by APOE could involve two mechanisms, either by directly limiting damage from an acute insult or indirectly, by improving recovery from an insult. The latter possibility is supported by more data although few studies have addressed the former.

Only limited data exist on the role of APOE in the acute response to brain damage. Acute damage from stroke is greater in mice lacking APOE (APOE KO) than in controls [15]. Mice with the ε4 allele showed greater damage after stroke than those with ε3 [27].

The role of APOE on stroke risk/outcomes in clinical studies has been equivocal. A meta-analysis of APOE isoform and stroke identified an increased risk associated with having an ε4 allele but also pointed out substantial heterogeneity [28]. In general, death or dependency following stroke (which reflects both stroke severity and recovery) was increased by the presence of an ε4 allele, but this change was significant only for intracerebral or subarachnoid hemorrhages.

Ischemic stroke did not reach significance. These authors emphasize that the numerous variables that are involved in the etiology and outcome measures of strokes require very large sample sizes to identify critical factors.

In contrast to acute protection by APOE, the data on the role of APOE in facilitating repair and regeneration after injury in animal models are compelling. Brain APOE protein and mRNA message expression are substantially increased following injury and remain elevated for weeks after the acute injury during a putative repair period [29, 30]. We have shown that APOE protein in the olfactory bulb doubles after a reversible lesion of the olfactory nerve [29] and is maintained at high levels for about two weeks during the period of axonal regeneration and regrowth. Studies in the hippocampus have reported similar findings for mRNA expression [30]. We have shown that APOE facilitates the rate, but not the endpoint, of olfactory nerve regeneration [31]. Hippocampal synaptogenesis [16] and process growth in culture paradigms [see 8] is increased by APOE. In brief, repair and regeneration (or process growth) is significantly delayed in animals lacking APOE compared to littermates expressing APOE. Also, APOE3 is more effective than APOE4 in supporting process growth. Hence, we think a role in facilitating axonal growth and synaptogenesis may be a critical generalized function for APOE in response to injury.

A final possible mechanism of neuroprotection that combines both direct and indirect effects is suppression of reactive microglia. Reactive microglia are a source of cytokines and reactive oxygen species that are injurious to nearby neurons. Activated microglia produce more of these products and APOE3, but not APOE4, suppresses this increase [32] as does estradiol [33]. In sum, we think the most likely major effects of APOE on general neuroprotection are by facilitating repair and regeneration, and suppressing reactive gliosis.

Relating APOE to clinical observations of neuroprotection by HT

A major goal in this review is to relate neuroprotection by HT to APOE and using this relationship to address controversies in HT. A role of HT in preventing dementia is controversial. Most published observational studies showed that a history of HT decreased the risk for developing dementia [11, 34–36] although a publication bias for positive effects probably exists. In contrast, one prospective study, the Women's Health Initiative Memory Study (WHIMS) of the pharmaceutical preparation of Premarin® alone or PremPro® found no positive effects on cognitive function and in fact, a decline in function when medroxyprogesterone (the progestin component of PremPro®) was included [see 37].

The explanation for the difference in observational studies and the prospective WHIMS may lie in two aspects of the study design. Compliance with daily HT treatment was tightly maintained and the project showed a substantial attrition rate (about 40% in the treatment group). This high attrition rate suggests there might be some bias against compliance. Our rodent data suggest that continuous 17β-estradiol exposure becomes ineffective to modulate either APOE or LRP expression in the brain. In admittedly anecdotal conversations about HT with educated lay audiences, we have found that users admit to taking "HT holidays" when they felt the side effects outweighed the benefits of HT, but reinstated therapy when menopausal symptoms recurred. Perhaps, this self-selected holiday indicated a strategy of spontaneous cycling of HT to maintain positive effects.

Second, the average age of HT initiation in the WHIMS was 64 years. Research has suggested that early (during the perimenopausal period) initiation of HT may be critical for neuroprotection [36]. Our unpublished data have shown a striking difference in response to acute estradiol replacement in 16- vs. 23-week-old mice as discussed above. We have not evaluated more aged mice but our data emphasize that studies in this area should be initiated. The precise effects HT initiated 10 to 15 years after menopause on APOE may be strikingly different when initiated during perimenopause.

Intervention studies with HT in dementia have generally not been successful [38, 39]. To our knowledge, only one study [38] found an improvement and this was with high dose (0.10 mg/day) estradiol patches. However, studies have not reported the APOE genotype of participants. The ε4 genotype appears to limit neuroprotection by HT in human populations [11, 12]. APOE4 protein has also been reported to limit the neuroprotective effects of estradiol replacement in culture paradigms [8]. The ε4 genotype is substantially overrepresented (50%) in the demented population [17]. Including APOE genotype information in these trials might identify a subgroup of individuals that respond differently to

HT. Hence, it is conceivable that a positive effect of hormone replacement in dementia trials may be masked by the high prevalence of women with APOE4. This hypothesis could be tested by examining existing data from these trials and should be performed.

Other chronic diseases show a neuroprotective effect of HT. Hormone therapy has been reported to *slow the progression* [3] or decrease the risk [40] of Parkinson's disease. APOE4 may be a risk factor for females, but not males [21] suggesting an interaction of disease process with ovarian hormones and APOE genotype. Hormone therapy could increase APOE protein, thereby improving repair and delaying clinical symptoms, which may decrease the "risk" of Parkinson's disease.

Hormone therapy may also have a neuroprotective effect in multiple sclerosis (MS). Although a history of HT generally does not reduce the risk for MS, it does affect the progression of the relapsing–remitting variant. A gene for APOE4 appears to accelerate the progression of MS [23, 24] and recovery during the remitting phases may be improved [2, 41]. We speculate that a greater effect of HT to slow the progress of MS might be detected in women not having the ε4 genotype.

In the diseases noted above, HT may delay disease risk and/or progression by regulating APOE. However, there are at least three clinical neurological conditions where APOE isoform affects the disease course, but where HT may not be efficacious: stroke, amyotrophic lateral sclerosis (ALS), and epilepsy.

A history of HT was noted to decrease the risk for stroke and hypertensive damage [34, 42] and estradiol required APOE to be neuroprotective in experimental stroke models [15]. However, the WHI showed increased risk for stroke in those on HT [see 37]. This unclear neuroprotective effect of HT on stroke could represent multiple factors. Hormone therapy improves serum lipid profile and suppresses atherosclerosis but not in those with APOE4 [43, 44]. Hormone therapy may modify peripheral factors predisposing to stroke that function over the long term. Moreover, as our studies have shown, the response of APOE to estradiol replacement in mice is modified by the duration of absence of ovarian hormones and by the duration of continuous replacement. Finally, a receptor for APOE, LRP, exhibits a complicated role in the risk and outcome from stroke. Lipoprotein receptor related protein is able to modulate Ca^{2+} conductance into the cell via the N-methyl D-aspartate receptor [45]. Lipoprotein receptor related protein is also the receptor for the tissue plasminogen activator–inhibitor complex and numerous other acute phase proteins that can affect neuronal function and death [5]. Hence the net effect of HT on neuroprotection from stroke probably involves not only APOE but numerous competing responses involving APOE and receptors. Clarifying the interaction of APOE and HT in stroke risk and recovery would require a large sample and careful parsing as previously proposed [28].

Two other diseases, ALS and epilepsy, show negative effects of a history of HT that may relate to the excitatory effects of estradiol in the brain. The APOE genotype does not modify the risk for ALS, but progression is accelerated in patients with an APOE4 gene [25,46]. However, a history of HT may increase the risk for ALS [47]. In epilepsy, APOE genotype appears to substantially modify disease course; patients with ε4 have a more malignant course [26]. However, HT may increase the risk for seizures [48].

One possible explanation for negative effects of HT is direct stimulation of neuronal activity that may be deleterious in these diseases. Neuronal excitation by 17β-estradiol has been reviewed previously [49]. Perhaps in both of these chronic diseases neuronal stimulation by HT outweighs its advantageous effects of glial stimulation of APOE production.

We suspect that interplay between neurons and glia, which we addressed in a recent review, is a critical factor in HT neuroprotection [7]. We suggested a reciprocal relationship between neuronal and glial activation. In brief, we proposed that a bolus of 17β-estradiol might first have an excitatory effect on neurons, which would, in turn, inhibit glial activation. Glial activation might occur subsequently as neuronal activity declined. Hence, neuronal activation and synaptogenesis could be initiated by estradiol, leading to hyperactivity and possibly excitotoxicity. Although estradiol-stimulated glial production of APOE might be advantageous to support membrane repair and reorganization, the protective effects of HT could be masked by acute toxic effects.

Our working hypothesis for APOE's role in neuroprotection by HT

We propose that chronic neurological diseases are composed of two processes: (a) disease-specific injury and (b) repair and regeneration. Functional decline occurs when repair/regeneration is no longer able to compensate for injury. Based on progression composed of damage and repair, the term "risk" requires qualification (Fig. 17.1). An intervention (such as HT) or genotype factor (such as APOE3) that decreases the

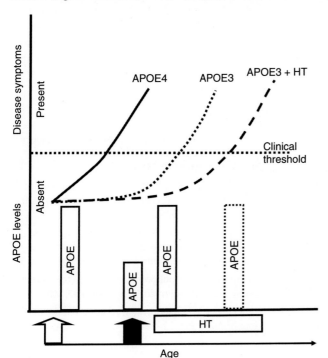

Fig. 17.1 Hypothetical model of disease progression as a function of APOE isoform and HT. All cases develop the initial stages of the disease at approximately the same age (open arrowhead). Those with APOE4 are less able to repair damage. Hence, they display a more rapid progression (solid line) and cross the clinical threshold at an earlier age. Hence women (and men) with APOE4 have an earlier age of onset than those with APOE3 (dotted line) due to poorer repair. At menopause (solid arrowhead) low levels of ovarian hormones may decrease APOE3 and result in a more rapid disease progression that is roughly parallel to the APOE4 isoform. Hormone therapy initiated during the perimenopausal period may increase APOE3 and thereby slow disease progression and conversion to clinical expression. If HT is delayed until well after menopause, the disease course may be too advanced to show protective effects of increased APOE. As illustrated in this model, the curves are fairly parallel after clinical onset. This would predict that HT after clinical expression occurs may not delay disease progression. The effect of women with APOE4 treated with HT is not included since we propose that increasing APOE4 may have no positive effects on repair and plasticity.

progression rate of a disease would result in a later onset of clinical disease expression. This slower progression could be totally independent from the basic etiology of the disease. This situation has been proposed in a study that indicated that the life-time risk of AD was equivalent in those with APOE ε3 or ε4 but age of onset was decreased in the ε4 group. Hence both incidence and prevalence appeared to be increased [see 50].

A similar mechanism may be present in MS. Both HT and APOE3 can suppress microglial activation, decreasing damage in MS [33,34]. Independently, APOE isoform may facilitate axonal regeneration and remyelination by supplying lipids. Hence, HT, acting via APOE might decrease the severity of the relapsing phase and increase the extent of recovery (remitting phase). We would anticipate that this improvement would not be observed in those with the ε4 gene.

One caveat in this scenario is that if degeneration is too advanced, repair may be inadequate to influence the clinical course. Hence, we would not expect demonstrable neuroprotective effects of HT in latter stages of a disease when degeneration has far outstripped neurorepair. We are concerned this might be the case with dementia.

Summary

We propose that a major role of HT in neuroprotection involves increasing apolipoprotein E in the central nervous system. Our data clearly show that 17β-estradiol is able to increase APOE, although the precise mechanism and receptor specificity remains to be fully determined. Increased APOE can facilitate neuronal plasticity and repair, and could slow the progression of numerous chronic neurological diseases. The existence of three APOE isoforms, that display possible differential effects on efficacy of HT, indicate that APOE genotype should be considered in any future investigative studies of HT on neural function.

Two critical issues require further scientific examination regarding the indirect effects of HT on APOE if neuroprotection is a consideration in a woman's choice for clinical application of HT. First, we must determine if APOE4 is either merely inefficient or can counteract the beneficial effects of APOE2 or APOE3 on repair. If APOE4 is merely inefficient then increasing APOE in ε4 heterozygotes may be indicated. Conversely, if APOE4 is injurious, then increasing APOE4 would be contraindicated. To us it is clear that any subsequent studies of HT for neuroprotection should include APOE genotyping.

Second, we must identify the mechanism of action of 17β-estradiol in regulating APOE. Identifying a selective estrogen response modulator (SERM) that could manipulate levels of APOE is indicated. For example, a SERM that could increase APOE but not have systemic effects or increase neuronal excitability might be indicated in epilepsy. Hormone therapy likely has an important role in neuroprotection, but requires a more complex understanding of ovarian hormone function in the intact nervous system. Direct studies of APOE pharmacogenomics may be indicated to develop effective HT therapies specifically designed for neuroprotection.

Acknowledgments

These studies were supported by the Illinois Department of Public Health Alzheimer Disease Fund and the Southern Illinois University School of Medicine Central Research Committee Research Fund. None of the authors has any financial interests related to this work. We wish to sincerely thank Shari Beckman-Randall and Jennifer (Miao) Li for their expert technical assistance; Xiang Xing Cheng, Craig Cady, and Britto Nathan for their contributions to this work; and countless medical and graduate students for their participation in the studies presented herein.

References

1. Paganini-Hill A, Henderson V. Estrogen deficiency and risk of Alzheimer's disease in women. *Am J Epidemiol.* 1994;**140**:256–61.

2. Sicotte NL, Liva SM, Klutch R, *et al.* Treatment of multiple sclerosis with the pregnancy hormone estriol. *Ann Neurol.* 2002;**52**:421–8.

3. Saunders-Pullman R, Gordon-Elliott J, Parides M, *et al.* The effect of estrogen replacement on early Parkinson's disease. *Neurology.* 1999;**52**:1417–21.

4. Weisgraber KH. Apolipoprotein E: structure–function relationships. *Adv Protein Chem.* 1994;**45**:249–302.

5. Herz J, Bock HH. Lipoprotein receptors in the nervous system. *Annu Rev Biochem.* 2002;**71**:405–34.

6. Struble RG, Rosario ER, Kircher ML, *et al.* Regionally specific modulation of brain apolipoprotein E in the

mouse during the estrous cycle and by exogenous 17β estradiol. *Exp Neurol.* 2003;**183**:638–44.

7. Struble RG, Nathan BP, Cady C, Cheng X, McAsey M. Estradiol regulation of astroglia and apolipoprotein E: an important role in neuronal regeneration. *Exp Gerontol.* 2007;**42**:54–63.

8. Nathan BP, Barsukova AG, Shen F, McAsey M, Struble RG. Estrogen facilitates neurite extension via apolipoprotein E in cultured adult mouse cortical neurons. *Endocrinology.* 2004;**145**:3065–73.

9. McAsey ME, Cady C, Jackson LM, *et al.* Time course of response to estradiol replacement in ovariectomized mice: brain apolipoprotein e and synaptophysin transiently increase and glial fibrillary acidic protein is suppressed. *Exper Neurol.* 2006;**197**:197–205.

10. Cheng X, McAsey ME, Li M, *et al.* Estradiol replacement increases the low-density lipoprotein receptor related protein (LRP) in the mouse brain. *Neurosci Lett.* 2007;**417**:50–4.

11. Yaffe K, Haan M, Byers A, Tangen C, Kuller L. Estrogen use, APOE, and cognitive decline: evidence of gene-environment interaction. *Neurology.* 2000;**54**:1949–54.

12. Burkhardt MS, Foster JK, Laws SM, *et al.* Oestrogen replacement therapy may improve memory functioning in the absence of APOE epsilon4. *J Alzheimers Dis.* 2004;**6**:221–8.

13. Hogervorst E, Lehmann DJ, Warden DR, McBroom J, Smith AD. Apolipoprotein E epsilon4 and testosterone interact in the risk of Alzheimer's disease in men. *Int J Geriatr Psychiatry.* 2002;**17**:938–40.

14. Mattila KM, Axelman K, Rinne JO, *et al.* Interaction between estrogen receptor 1 and the epsilon 4 allele of apolipoprotein E increases the risk of familial Alzheimer's disease in women. *Neurosci Lett.* 2000;**282**:45–8.

15. Horsburgh K, Macrae IM, Carswell H. Estrogen is neuroprotective via an apolipoprotein E-dependent mechanism in a mouse model of global ischemia. *J Cereb Blood Flow Metab.* 2002;**22**:1189–95.

16. Stone DJ, Rozovsky I, Morgan TE, Anderson CP, Finch CE Increased synaptic sprouting in response to estrogen via an apolipoprotein E-dependent mechanism: implications for Alzheimer's disease. *J Neurosci.* 1998;**18**:3180–5.

17. Corder EH, Saunders AM, Strittmatter WJ, *et al.* Gene dose of apolipoprotein E type 4 allele and the risk of Alzheimer's disease in late onset families. *Science.* 1993;**261**(5123):921–3.

18. Kolsch H, Ptok U, Mohamed I, *et al.* Association of the C766T polymorphism of the low-density lipoprotein receptor-related protein gene with Alzheimer's disease.

19. Tang G, Xie H, Xu L, *et al.* Genetic study of apolipoprotein E gene, alpha-1 antichymotrypsin gene in sporadic Parkinson disease. *Am J Med Genet.* 2002;**114**:446–9.

20. Zareparsi S, Camicioli R, Sexton G, *et al.* Age at onset of Parkinson disease and apolipoprotein E genotypes. *Am J Med Genet.* 2002;**107**:156–61.

21. Buchanan DD, Silburn PA, Prince JA, Mellick GD. Association of APOE with Parkinson disease age-at-onset in women. *Neurosci Lett.* 2007;**411**:185–8.

22. Jordan BD. Genetic influences on outcome following traumatic brain injury. *Neurochem Res.* 2007;**32**:905–15.

23. Fazekas F, Strasser-Fuchs S, Kollegger H, *et al.* Apolipoprotein E epsilon 4 is associated with rapid progression of multiple sclerosis. *Neurology.* 2001;**57**:853–7.

24. Masterman T, Zhang Z, Hellgren D, *et al.* APOE genotypes and disease severity in multiple sclerosis. *Mult Scler.* 2002;**8**:98–103.

25. Li YJ, Pericak-Vance MA, Haines JL, *et al.* Apolipoprotein E is associated with age at onset of amyotrophic lateral sclerosis. *Neurogenetics.* 2004;**5**:209–13.

26. Briellmann RS, Torn-Broers Y, Busuttil BE, *et al.* APOE epsilon4 genotype is associated with an earlier onset of chronic temporal lobe epilepsy. *Neurology.* 2000;**55**:435–7.

27. Sheng H, Laskowitz DT, Bennett E, *et al.* Apolipoprotein E isoform-specific differences in outcome from focal ischemia in transgenic mice. *J Cereb Blood Flow Metab.* 1998;**18**:361–6.

28. Martínez-González NA, Sudlow CL. Effects of apolipoprotein E genotype on outcome after ischaemic stroke, intracerebral haemorrhage and subarachnoid haemorrhage. *J Neurol Neurosurg Psychiatry.* 2006;**77**:1329–35.

29. Nathan BP, Nisar R, Randall S, *et al.* Apolipoprotein E is upregulated in olfactory bulb glia following peripheral receptor lesion in mice. *Exp Neurol.* 2001;**172**:128–36.

30. Poirier J, Hess M, May PC, Finch CE. Astrocytic apolipoprotein E mRNA and GFAP mRNA in hippocampus after entorhinal cortex lesioning. *Brain Res Mol Brain Res.* 1991;**11**:97–106.

31. Nathan BP, Nisar R, Short J, *et al.* Delayed olfactory nerve regeneration in APOE-deficient mice. *Brain Res.* 2005;**1041**:87–94.

32. Brown CM, Wright E, Colton CAM, *et al.* Apolipoprotein E isoform mediated regulation of

nitric oxide release. *Free Radic Biol Med.* 2002;
32:1071–5.

33. Colton, CA, Brown CM, Vitek MP. Sex steroids, APOE genotype and the innate immune system. *Neurobiol Aging.* 2005;**26**:363–72.

34. Paganini-Hill A, Perez Barreto M. Stroke risk in older men and women: aspirin, estrogen, exercise, vitamins, and other factors. *J Gend Specif Med.* 2001;**4**:18–28.

35. LeBlanc ES, Janowsky J, Chan BK, Nelson HD. Hormone replacement therapy and cognition: systematic review and meta-analysis. *JAMA.* 2001;**285**:1489–99.

36. Henderson VW, Benke KS, Green RC, Cupples LA, Farrer LA. MIRAGE Study Group. Postmenopausal hormone therapy and Alzheimer's disease risk: interaction with age. *J Neurol Neurosurg Psychiatry.* 2005;**76**:103–5.

37. Espeland MA, Rapp SR, Shumaker SA, *et al.* Women's Initiative Memory Study. Conjugated equine estrogens and global cognitive function in postmenopausal women: the Women's Health Initiative Memory Study. *JAMA.* 2004;**291**:2959–68.

38. Asthana S, Baker LD, Craft S, *et al.* High-dose estradiol improves cognition for women with AD: results of a randomized study. *Neurology.* 2001;**57**:605–12.

39. Thal LJ, Thomas RG, Mulnard R, *et al.* Estrogen levels do not correlate with improvement in cognition. *Arch Neurol.* 2003;**60**:209–12.

40. Currie LJ, Harrison MB, Trugman JM, Bennett JP, Wooten GF. Postmenopausal estrogen use affects risk for Parkinson disease. *Arch Neurol.* 2004;**61**:886–8.

41. Holmqvist P, Wallberg M, Hammar M, Landtblom AM, Brynhildsen J. Symptoms of multiple sclerosis in women in relation to sex steroid exposure. *Maturitas.* 2006;**54**:149–53.

42. Simpkins JW, Yang SH, Wen Y, Singh M. Estrogens, progestins, menopause and neurodegeneration:

basic and clinical studies. *Cell Mol Life Sci.* 2005;**62**: 271–80.

43. Lehtimaki T, Dastidar P, Jokela H, *et al.* Effect of long-term hormone replacement therapy on atherosclerosis progression in postmenopausal women relates to functional apolipoprotein e genotype. *J Clin Endocrinol Metab.* 2002;**87**:4147–53.

44. von Muhlen D, Barrett-Connor E, Kritz-Silverstein D. Apolipoprotein E genotype and response of lipid levels to postmenopausal estrogen use. *Atherosclerosis.* 2002;**161**:209–14.

45. Qiu Z, Crutcher KA, Hyman BT, Rebeck GW. APOE isoforms affect neuronal N-methyl-D-aspartate calcium responses and toxicity via receptor-mediated processes. *Neuroscience.* 2003;**122**:291–303.

46. Drory VE, Birnbaum M, Korczyn AD, Chapman J. Association of APOE epsilon4 allele with survival in amyotrophic lateral sclerosis. *J Neurol Sci.* 2001;**190**:17–20.

47. Popat RA, Van Den Eeden SK, Tanner CM, *et al.* Effect of reproductive factors and postmenopausal hormone use on the risk of amyotrophic lateral sclerosis. *Neuroepidemiology.* 2006;**27**:117–21.

48. Harden CL, Pulver MC, Ravdin L, Jacobs AR. The effect of menopause and perimenopause on the course of epilepsy. *Epilepsia.* 1999;**40**:1402–7.

49. Joels M. Steroid hormones and excitability in the mammalian brain. *Front Neuroendocrinol.* 1997;**18**:2–48.

50. Khachaturian AS, Corcoran CD, Mayer LS, *et al.* Apolipoprotein E epsilon4 count affects age at onset of Alzheimer disease, but not lifetime susceptibility: the Cache County Study. *Arch Gen Psychiatry.* 2004;**61**:518–24.

51. Wang JM, Irwin RW, Brinton RD. Activation of estrogen receptor alpha increases and estrogen receptor beta decreases apolipoprotein E expression in hippocampus in vitro and in vivo. *Proc Natl Acad Sci USA.* 2006;**103**:16983–8.

Chapter 8

Testosterone, gonadotropins, and genetic polymorphisms in men with Alzheimer's disease

Eef Hogervorst, Stephan Bandelow, and Donald Lehmann

Editors' introduction

This chapter discusses the possibility that men with Alzheimer's disease (AD) exhibit age-accelerated endocrinological change that increases the risk for AD related pathological processes. This age-accelerated endocrinological change is characterized by an earlier decrease in thyroid stimulating hormone, an earlier increase in sex hormone binding globulin, and a subsequent earlier decrease in free or bioavailable testosterone levels. They also show an earlier increase of gonadotropin levels, which may be an appropriate, if inadequate, response to lower free testosterone levels. However, both these processes (the increase in gonadotropin levels as a response to the lowered levels of free testosterone) have the propensity to negatively affect neuronal health, as subsequent chapters in Section 6 will outline in more detail. This acceleration in age-related endocrinological change may be related to stress and morbidity (which are both known to affect thyroid stimulating hormone) and/or possibly, certain genetic polymorphisms that could predispose to an earlier lowering of free testosterone, which, especially when combined with a decrease of androgen receptors in the brain, leads to a lowered protective environment for the aging brain.

Biological plausibility: testosterone and the brain

As mentioned in more detail in Chapters 25 to 27, there is strong biological plausibility for testosterone to have a positive and protective effect on the brain. Its neuroprotective actions could occur through its conversion into estradiol in the brain or could be direct (e.g., through androgen receptors distributed in the brain). Mechanisms described have been through reduction of oxidative stress [1], of apoptosis [2], and of the accumulation of the toxic β-amyloid [3], all factors that have been deemed important in Alzheimer's disease (AD) pathogenesis. Longitudinal studies found that brain volumes were larger in older men who had high midlife testosterone levels [4] and that cerebral blood flow was better in men who had high testosterone levels at onset of the study, six to ten years before brain scans were performed (see Chapter 21). From this it would follow that testosterone and estradiol might be lower in men with AD, not allowing these patients to benefit from their neuroprotective properties.

Testosterone levels and dementia

One of the first studies to show lower levels of testosterone in post-mortem confirmed men with AD [5] was carried out by the Oxford Project to Investigate Memory and Ageing (OPTIMA). This project was initiated by Professor David Smith, Dr Kim Jobst, and Elizabeth King in 1988 and included at the time of the study more than 800 well characterized dementia cases and controls from the Oxfordshire region. These participants were annually assessed using a medical examination, which included brain scans, blood screening, and history taking, with a full carer's report and a neuropsychological assessment, based on the Cambridge Examination for Mental Disorders of the Elderly (CAMDEX [6]). The study was well controlled. For analyses of the association between levels of sex steroids and AD, all cases with orchidectomy or prostate cancer; those who used medication that could interfere with gonadal steroid function (antipsychotics, hormone medication, etc.); had Cushing's

Hormones, Cognition and Dementia: State of the Art and Emergent Therapeutic Strategies, ed. Eef Hogervorst, Victor W. Henderson, Robert B. Gibbs, and Roberta Diaz Brinton. Published by Cambridge University Press.
© Cambridge University Press 2009.

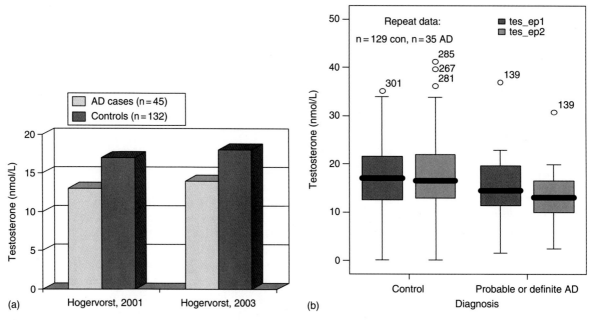

Fig. 18.1 (a) Testosterone levels in men with Alzheimer's disease and controls. (b) Repeat data of testosterone levels over time in men with Alzheimer's disease and controls.

or Addison's disease; or acute systemic or end-stage morbidity were excluded. Blood had been sampled in the morning to avoid the interference of circadian rhythms and had been stored at −70°C. Testosterone and sex hormone binding globulin (SHBG) levels were measured using a DPC Immulite® at the John Radcliffe biochemistry laboratory. Risk for AD (n = 45 vs. 132 controls) was significantly increased with low total testosterone (by 8% for each nmol/L of testosterone less). This was independent of SHBG, age, body mass index (BMI), smoking, alcohol, diabetes mellitus, glucocorticoid- and thyroid-medication use [5]. Results were very similar in another larger OPTIMA cohort (including follow-up data on 35 of the AD cases and 129 controls) whose data were published in 2004 (Fig. 18.1a/b) [7].

The data suggested that total testosterone levels continued to decrease with age in AD cases, but remained relatively unchanged in age-equated controls, although the difference was reversed for free testosterone levels (Fig. 18.2a/b) [7]. These results were further substantiated in the prospective Baltimore Longitudinal Study of Aging (BLSA) [8] and in other cohorts, e.g., [9]. The BLSA data showed that low free testosterone (but not total testosterone) at baseline predicted dementia risk after a follow-up of on average six years in men who did not have dementia at baseline [8]. Further analyses of the data of OPTIMA and BLSA suggested that the relatively younger BLSA cohort was more likely to show larger differences in free testosterone between cases and controls, while greater differences were seen for total testosterone levels between older AD cases and controls, such as those of OPTIMA.

The association of sex hormone binding globulin and pituitary stimulating hormones with dementia and free testosterone levels: the theory of age-accelerated endocrinological change

High sex hormone binding globulin (SHBG) lowers levels of free and bioavailable sex steroids and is increased in response to an older age, wasting, smoking, and lower testosterone levels [10]. In OPTIMA and other cohorts, SHBG levels were independently (of age, BMI, smoking, and testosterone, etc.) higher in cases with AD compared to controls [7, 9, 11]. Subclinical hyperthyroidism (low thyroid stimulating hormone or TSH levels with normal thyroxine levels) is also

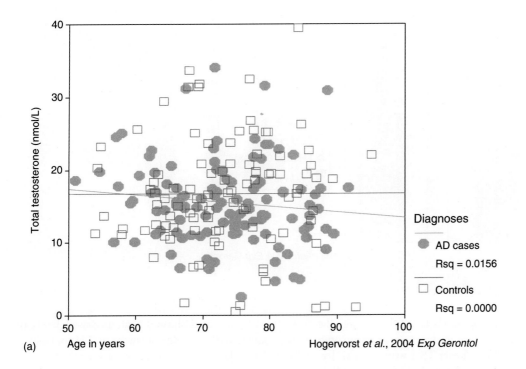

(a)

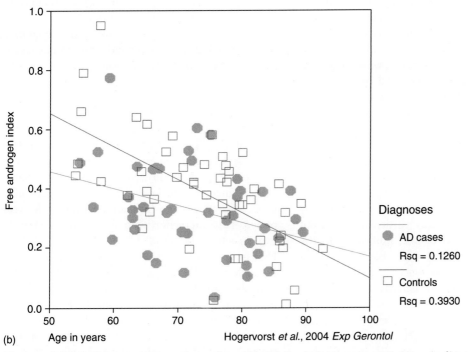

(b)

Fig. 18.2 (a) Levels of total testosterone with age of men with Alzheimer's disease and controls. (b) Levels of bio-available or free testosterone (free androgen index or FAI = TT/SHBG) with age of men with Alzheimer's disease and controls. (See color plate section.)

mIU/L

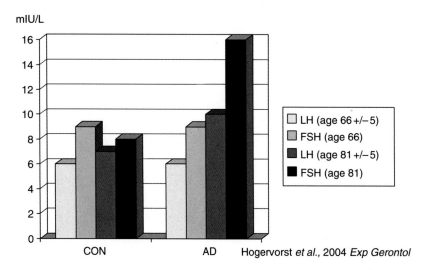

Fig. 18.3 Gonadotropin levels are higher in older cases with AD than controls, suggesting perhaps an age-accelerated hormonal change in AD.

Legend:
- LH (age 66 +/−5)
- FSH (age 66)
- LH (age 81 +/−5)
- FSH (age 81)

CON   AD   Hogervorst *et al.*, 2004 *Exp Gerontol*

known to increase SHBG levels [12, 13], to lower the free androgen index and to increase gonadotropin levels [14]. In OPTIMA, lower TSH with normal thyroxine levels indicative of subclinical hyperthyroidism were found to be more common in AD cases compared to controls [15]. Subclinical hyperthyroidism was in fact shown to more than double the risk for AD. Low TSH levels have been associated with acute and chronic systemic illness, wasting, and with the actions of glucocorticosteroid, dopamine, and other psychoactive medication (e.g., lithium) and are more prevalent with increasing age [16]. However, the association between low TSH and dementia remained when these factors were controlled for. Similar findings have been reported in other cohorts [17–19]. In a sub-study from the Medical Research Council Cognitive Function and Ageing Study (MRC-CFAS), we also found that high normal free thyroxine and non-significantly lowered TSH levels in healthy participants (without dementia, organic mental disease, frailty, psychiatric and overt thyroid disorders) were risk factors for a substantial drop in cognitive function (of 4 points on the MMSE), which is possibly indicative of a dementia process [20].

In OPTIMA, free testosterone levels were independently associated with TSH levels in controls (independent from age, BMI, etc.) [7]. It could thus be hypothesized that subclinical hyperthyroidism (e.g., in response to underlying morbidity associated with increased risk for dementia) initially increases SHBG and subsequently lowers FT. Analyses of

OPTIMA data also showed that increased levels of gonadotropins (luteinizing hormone, or LH, and follicle stimulating hormone, or FSH) were independent risk factors for dementia. This increase in gonadotropin levels seen in AD cases with age may be an appropriate response to lowered testosterone levels and could indicate that the hypothalamic-pituitary-gonadal axis is still intact in dementia. This argues against the hypothesis that low testosterone and low TSH are comorbid features of general brain degenerative processes.

Gonadotropin and total testosterone levels were particularly different in cases and controls over 80 years of age [7] (Fig. 18.3). Follicle Stimulating Hormone and Luteinizing Hormone levels increase with age [21]. A study by Bowen *et al.* [22] also reported higher gonadotropin levels in their institutionalized cases with dementia who were on average 85 years of age. This interaction with age could possibly also explain why Short *et al.* [23] found higher LH and FSH in women with AD not using estrogen replacement therapy (ERT) compared to controls not using ERT, but not between the groups who were using ERT as, in general, women using ERT are younger compared with those who are not. In addition, their results became non-significant when they controlled for age. These data combined could suggest that particularly in the older cases with dementia, levels of gonadotropin are higher than those of controls. These data taken together could tentatively point to an age-accelerated endocrinological change process in AD with an earlier lowering of TSH, an earlier increase in SHBG, an earlier lowering of FT, and an earlier than normal increase in gonadotropin levels, which would be a response to the lowered FT levels.

The age-accelerated hormonal change hypothesis thus contrasts with the central hypothesis that suggests that a lowering of sex steroids follows low levels of gonadotropins induced by pathological processes in the brain related to dementia.

Implications for treatment: gonadotropin lowering or testosterone treatment?

Several groups using animal and cell culture studies found that LH can be neurotoxic and it was postulated that lowering LH levels should be a major target to treat AD (see Chapters 25 and 27). This can be achieved by a drug called leuprolide acetate, which decreases gonadotropin levels, but unfortunately also decreases sex steroids. Perhaps thus unsurprising, several treatment studies showed that memory in those treated with leuprolide acetate decreased. Memory is one of the first functions to show a decline in AD [24, 25]. Some of the negative treatment studies were done in men with prostate cancer [26, 27], although others found that some aspects of memory were improved [28, 29]. For women without dementia, leuprolide has only shown negative effects on memory [30–33]; although in women with AD positive effects of leuprolide acetate have been recorded (see Chapter 26).

In contrast to leuprolide, testosterone treatment decreases both gonadotropin and SHBG levels. This could have indirect positive effects by decreasing the toxicity of high levels of gonadotropins, and also by increasing bioavailable estrogen levels. An important experimental study by Monique Cherrier and her group [34] showed that men need estrogen to show improved verbal memory after testosterone treatment. Men were given a drug to inhibit the conversion of testosterone into estradiol (an aromatase inhibitor, as the enzyme aromatase is responsible for the conversion of testosterone into estradiol in the brain and in Sertoli cells). Those men did not show the verbal memory improvement of other men who were given testosterone treatment without this drug. It has been hypothesized that brain aromatase could be neuroprotective by increasing the local estrogen levels in injured neurons.

Genetic polymorphisms related to sex steroids and AD

Aromatase is encoded by the CYP19 gene (which is located at chromosome 15q21.1). Studies have found CYP19 polymorphisms to be associated with estradiol levels [35] and with risk of AD [36]. A study by Christian Pike's group [37] found that brain levels of testosterone (but not estradiol) were lowered in men during normal aging. Furthermore, they also found that brain levels of testosterone (but again not estradiol) were significantly lower in men with AD, and in those men with mild neuropathological changes who had not yet developed dementia, when compared with controls. If anything, levels of estradiol were somewhat but non-significantly elevated in AD, suggestive of CYP19 polymorphisms playing a role in AD, as mentioned above.

There are several other genetic polymorphisms that have been found to play a role in sex steroid function and which were different between AD cases and controls.

APOE ε4 is a known risk factor for AD. In OPTIMA, men who had not developed AD (yet?) but who carried the APOE ε4 allele, already had lower levels of testosterone than controls who did not carry the allele [38]. Burkhardt et al. [39] found (in a group of n = 45 healthy men, older than 55 years of age without dementia) that those who did not carry the APOE ε4 allele performed better on a visual memory test, if they had high free testosterone levels. Those who carried the allele actually performed worse with higher free testosterone levels. We were able to replicate these results in men without dementia from the MRC Foresight Challenge cohort (unpublished results, Hogervorst 2007, Royal Society of Medicine meeting February, see Fig. 18.4).

A study by Raber et al. [40] found that genetically modified female mice that carried the ε4 allele showed reduced levels of androgen receptors (AR) in the cortex. Testosterone treatment in these mice increased the AR receptors.

However, in OPTIMA and several other cohorts, women with AD were actually found to have higher levels of sex steroids than controls, so it is unclear how these data for females should be interpreted.

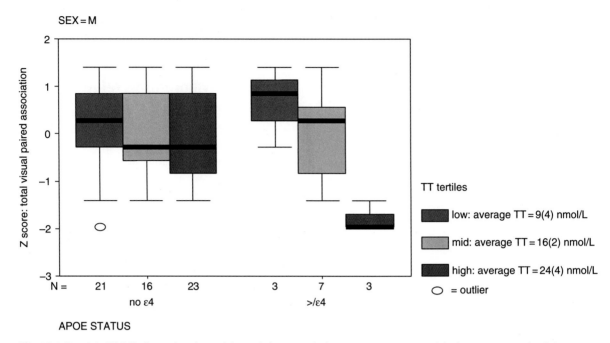

Fig. 18.4 Foresight MRC Challenge data showed that verbal memory had negative associations with higher testosterone levels in men (Hogervorst, 2002). Further analyses showed that in healthy older men (74 (6) years of age), visual memory performance showed an interaction of APOE × TT (beta = 0.96, p < 0.05, which was independent of age, education, SHBG, TT, TT², FAI, APOE, and BMI). Men who carried the ε4 allele had worse visual memory performance when they had higher total testosterone (TT) levels. (See color plate section.)

Lengths of CAG (glutamine) repeat polymorphism of the AR gene can influence androgen activity. It is thought that longer repeat lengths may be associated with decreased androgen sensitivity (linear effect). Yaffe *et al.* [41] reported that 301 community-dwelling elderly white men with greater CAG repeat length were more likely to have lower scores on cognitive tests. However, in OPTIMA men with AD were more likely to carry the short allele (≤20 CAG repeats) version of this polymorphism when compared with controls (adjusted OR = 2.5, 95% CI 1.2–5.0) [42]. The combination of the short allele variant and low testosterone levels was found to increase the risk for AD in men (but not in women) by a factor of 4, compared with men with long alleles and high testosterone levels [43]. It could thus be hypothesized that low testosterone levels in AD might be a natural adaptation to more sensitive AR. However, according to Beilin *et al.* [44] the relation between CAG repeat length and transcriptional activity is cell and tissue specific. It is therefore difficult to judge whether effects in the prostate (on which most research is based) are also true in the brain, on which little research of this polymorphism has been done. Krithivas *et al.*

[45] reported that age-related decline in testosterone is faster in those men with short CAG repeat lengths. This would tie in with our theory of age-related cognitive decline in men with AD.

Concluding remarks

So, in sum, we are left with several questions for future research. First, do lower TT, FT, TSH, and higher SHBG and LH levels at an earlier age in men with AD suggest an accelerated age-related endocrinological change? If this is so, what are the proposed mechanisms? Is subclinical hyperthyroidism, related to underlying morbidity, the driver of this accelerated change in other hormone levels? Could genetic polymorphisms be responsible for this? Do APOE ε4, AR CAG short alleles, and certain CYP19 variants predispose to earlier lowering of FT levels, which, when combined with a decrease of AR in the brain, creates a "double whammy" and therefore increases the risk for AD? Are there any genetic protective mechanisms (APOE ε2)? Is there an optimum FT level depending on age and does this interact with genotype? These factors remain to be investigated and need to be replicated in larger cohorts. Other chapters have discussed the various issues raised in this chapter in more detail.

Acknowledgments

The OPTIMA team, nurses, participants, in particular Professor David Smith, Elizabeth King, and Dr. Marc Combrinck. In addition, we would like to express our gratitude to Professor Pike, Dr. Moffat, and Dr. Almeida for their discussions and input. This work was supported with grants from the Alzheimer's Association, ART, NL Hersenstichting, Bristol-Myers Squibb, the MRC, the Blaschko Fellowship, Somerville College, Richard Bowen (Voyager Pharm), and RIA/Help the Aged.

References

1. Ahlbom E, Prins GS, Ceccatelli S. Testosterone protects cerebellar granule cells from oxidative stress-induced cell death through a receptor mediated mechanism. *Brain Res*. 2001;**892**:255–62.

2. Hammond J, Le Q, Goodyer C, *et al*. Testosterone mediated neuroprotection through the androgen receptor in human primary neurons. *J Neurochem*. 2001;**77**:1319–26.

3. Pike CJ. Testosterone attenuates b-amyloid toxicity in cultured hippocampal neurons. *Brain Res*. 2001;**919**:160–5.

4. Lessov-Schlaggar CN, Reed T, Swan GE, *et al*. Association of sex steroid hormones with brain morphology and cognition in healthy elderly men. *Neurology*. 2005;**65**(10):1591–6.

5. Hogervorst E, Williams J, Budge M, *et al*. Serum total testosterone is lower in men with Alzheimer's disease. *Neuroendocrinology Lett*. 2001;**22**(3):163–8.

6. Roth M, Huppert FA, Tym E, Mountjoy C. *CAMDEX: The Cambridge Examination for Mental Disorders of the Elderly*. Cambridge: Cambridge University Press, 1988.

7. Hogervorst E, Bandelow S, Combrinck M, Smith AD. Low free testosterone is an independent risk factor for Alzheimer's disease. *Exp Gerontol*. 2004;**39**(11/12):1633–9.

8. Moffat SD, Zonderman AB, Metter EJ, *et al*. Free testosterone and risk for Alzheimer disease in older men. *Neurology*. 2004;**62**(2):188–93.

9. Paoletti AM, Congia S, Lello S, *et al*. Low androgenization index in elderly women and elderly men with Alzheimer's disease. *Neurology*. 2004; **62**(2):301–3.

10. Svartberg M, Midtby M, Bonaa KH, *et al*. The associations of age, lifestyle factors and chronic disease with testosterone in men: the Tromso Study. *Eur J Endo*. 2003;**149**(2):145–52.

11. Hoskin EK, Tang MX, Manly JJ, Mayeux R. Elevated sex-hormone binding globulin in elderly women with Alzheimer's disease. *Neurobiol Aging*. 2004; **25**(2):141–7.

12. Brenta G, Schnitman M, Gurfinkiel M, *et al*. Variations of sex hormone-binding globulin in thyroid dysfunction. *Thyroid*. 1999;**9**(3):273–7.

13. Skjoldebrand-Sparre L, Kollind M, Carlstrom K. Ovarian ultrasound and ovarian and adrenal hormones before and after treatment for hyperthyroidism. *Gynecol Obstet Invest*. 2002;**54**(1):50–5.

14. Zahringer S, Tomova A, von Werder K, *et al*. The influence of hyperthyroidism on the hypothalamic-pituitary-gonadal axis. *Exp Clin Endocrinol Diabetes*. 2002;**108**(4):282–9.

15. van Osch LA, Hogervorst E, Combrinck M, Smith AD. Low thyroid-stimulating hormone as an independent risk factor for Alzheimer disease. *Neurology*. 2004; **62**(11):1967–71.

16. Demers LM, Spencer CA. NACB, Biochemistry TNAoC, Laboratory Medicine Practice Guidelines. Laboratory support for the diagnosis and monitoring of thyroid disease. Available at http://www.nacb.org/lmpg/thyroid_LMPG_PDF.stm.

17. Kalmijn S, Mehta KM, Pols HAP, *et al*. Subclinical hyperthyroidism and the risk of dementia. The Rotterdam study. *Clin Endocrinol*. 2000;**53**:733–7.

18. Wahlin A, Wahlin TBR, Small BJ, Backman L. Influences of thyroid stimulating hormone on cognitive functioning in very old age. *J Gerontol Ser B Psychol Sci*. 1998;**53**(4):P234–P239.

19. Wahlin A, Bunce D, Wahlin TB. Longitudinal evidence of the impact of normal thyroid stimulating hormone variations on cognitive functioning in very old age. *Psychoneuroendocrinology*. 2005;**30**(7):625–37.

20. Hogervorst E, Matthews F, Huppert FA, Brayne C. Thyroid function and cognitive decline in the MRC Cognitive Function & Ageing Study. *Psychoneuroendocrinology*. 2008;**33**(7):1013–22.

21. Tsitouras PD, Bulat T. The aging male reproductive system. *Endocrinol Metab Clin North Am*. 1995; **24**:297–315.

22. Bowen RL, Isley JP, Atkinson RL. An association of elevated serum gonadotropin concentrations and Alzheimer disease ? *J Neuroendocrinol*. 2000;**12**(4):351–4.

23. Short RA, Bowen RL, O'Brien PC, Graff Radford NR. Elevated gonadotropin levels in patients with Alzheimer disease. *Mayo Clin Proc*. 2001;**76**(9):906–9.

24. Schrijnemaeckers AMC, De Jager CA, Hogervorst E, Budge MM. Cases with Mild Cognitive Impairment and Alzheimer's disease fail to benefit from repeated exposure to episodic memory tests as compared with controls. *J Clin Exp Neuropsychol*. 2006;**28**(3):438–55.

25. DeJager CA, Hogervorst E, Combrinck M, Budge MM. Sensitivity and specificity of neuropsychological tests for mild cognitive impairment, vascular cognitive impairment and Alzheimer's disease. *Psychol Med*. 2003;**33**(6):1039–50.

26. Almeida OP, Waterreus A, Spry N, Flicker L, Martins RN. One year follow-up study of the association between chemical castration, sex hormones, beta-amyloid, memory and depression in men. *Psychoneuroendocrinology*. 2004;**29**(8):1071–81.

27. Green HJ, Pakenham KI, Headley BC, *et al.* Quality of life compared during pharmacological treatments and clinical monitoring for non-localized prostate cancer: a randomized controlled trial. *BJU Int*. 2004; **93**(7):975–9.

28. Cherrier MM, Rose AL, Higano C. The effects of combined androgen blockade on cognitive function during the first cycle of intermittent androgen suppression in patients with prostate cancer. *J Urol*. 2003;**170**(5):1808–11.

29. Salminen EK, Portin RI, Koskinen A, Helenius H, Nurmi M. Associations between serum testosterone fall and cognitive function in prostate cancer patients. *Clin Cancer Res*. 2004;**10**(22):7575–82.

30. Grigorova M, Sherwin BB, Tulandi T. Effects of treatment with leuprolide acetate depot on working memory and executive functions in young premenopausal women. *Psychoneuroendocrinology*. 2006;**31**(8):935–47.

31. Sherwin BB, Tulandi T. "Add-back" estrogen reverses cognitive deficits induced by a gonadotropin-releasing hormone agonist in women with leiomyomata uteri. *J Clin Endocrinol Metab*. 1996;**81**(7):2545–9.

32. Newton C, Slota D, Yuzpe AA, Tummon IS. Memory complaints associated with the use of gonadotropin-releasing hormone agonists: a preliminary study. *Fertil Steril*. 1996;**65**(6):1253–5.

33. Varney NR, Syrop C, Kubu CS, *et al.* Neuropsychologic dysfunction in women following leuprolide acetate induction of hypoestrogenism. *J Assist Reprod Genet*. 1993;**10**(1):53–7.

34. Cherrier MM, Matsumoto AM, Amory JK, *et al.* The role of aromatization in testosterone

supplementation: effects on cognition in older men. *Neurology*. 2005;**64**(2):290–6.

35. Tworoger SS, Chubak J, Aiello EJ, *et al.* Association of CYP17, CYP19, CYP1B1, and COMT polymorphisms with serum and urinary sex hormone concentrations in postmenopausal women. *Cancer Epidemiol Biomarkers Prev*. 2004;**13**(1):94–101.

36. Iivonen S, Corder E, Lehtovirta M, *et al.* Polymorphisms in the CYP19 gene confer increased risk for Alzheimer disease. *Neurology*. 2004;**62**(7): 1170–6.

37. Rosario ER, Chang L, Stanczyk FZ, Pike CJ. Age-related testosterone depletion and the development of Alzheimer disease. *JAMA*. 2004;**292**(12):1431–2.

38. Hogervorst E, Lehmann DJ, Warden DR, McBroom J, Smith AD. Apolipoprotein E epsilon4 and testosterone interact in the risk of Alzheimer's disease in men. *Int J Geriatr Psychiatry*. 2002;**17**(10):938–40.

39. Burkhardt MS, Foster JK, Clarnette RM, *et al.* Interaction between testosterone and apolipoprotein E epsilon4 status on cognition in healthy older men. *J Clin Endocrinol Metab*. 2006;**91**(3):1168–72.

40. Raber J, Bongers G, LeFevour A, Buttini M, Mucke L. Androgens protect against apolipoprotein E4-induced cognitive deficits. *J Neurosci*. 2002;**22**(12):5204–9.

41. Yaffe K, Edwards ER, Lui LY, *et al.* Androgen receptor CAG repeat polymorphism is associated with cognitive function in older men. *Biol Psychiatry*. 2003;**54**(9):943–6.

42. Lehmann DJ, Butler HT, Warden DR, *et al.* Association of the androgen receptor CAG repeat polymorphism with Alzheimer disease in men. *Neurosci Lett*. 2003;**340**(2):87–90.

43. Lehmann DJ, Hogervorst E, Warden DR, *et al.* The androgen receptor CAG repeat and serum testosterone in the risk of Alzheimer's disease in men. *J Neurol Neurosurg Psychiatry*. 2004;**75**(1):163–4.

44. Beilin J, Ball EM, Favaloro JM, Zajac JD. Effect of the androgen receptor CAG repeat polymorphism on transcriptional activity: specificity in prostate and non-prostate cell lines. *J Mol Endocrinol*. 2000; **25**(1):85–96.

45. Krithivas K, Yurgalevitch SM, Mohr BA, *et al.* Evidence that the CAG repeat in the androgen receptor gene is associated with the age-related decline in serum androgen levels in men. *J Endocrinol*. 1999; **162**(1):137–42.

19 Androgens and cognitive functioning in women

Barbara B. Sherwin

Editors' introduction

The extent to which testosterone and other androgens might affect cognitive skills in women is not yet well understood. In this chapter, Sherwin reviews changes in endogenous androgens over a woman's lifespan and research findings germane to androgens and cognitive skills in women. For younger women, there is evidence that cyclical changes during the menstrual cycle affect cognitive performance, although it is not possible to tease out effects of testosterone from those of estradiol. In older women, the relation between testosterone levels and cognitive test scores is inconsistent. The ratio of estradiol to testosterone may be important in modulating sex-advantaged cognitive functions in women, with a lower ratio leading to relatively impaired performance on cognitive tasks in which women typically excel.

Introduction

Although a considerable amount of knowledge has accumulated concerning the effects of estrogens on neuroanatomy and neurophysiology and its resultant influences on cognitive functioning in women, very little is known of the possible effects of androgens on cognition in women. It is possible that the lesser interest in the functional role of androgens in women is due to the fact that it is not critical for reproductive events such as menstrual cycles and pregnancy. Nonetheless, it is now clear that androgens, particularly testosterone, are important for sexual desire and interest in women even though levels needed to elicit these behaviors are one-tenth to one-fifteenth of those of the normal male testosterone range. This chapter will review the changes in androgen production that occur during the female lifespan, the effects

of androgens on the brain, and the extant clinical literature on androgens and cognition to determine whether testosterone levels within the menstrual cycle range of values play a role in cognitive functioning in women.

Changes in androgens during the female lifespan

The three sources of androgens in women are the adrenal cortex, the ovarian theca/stromal cells, and the peripheral conversion of circulating androgenic prohormones. The adrenal gland produces about 95% of circulating serum dehydroepiandrosterone sulfate, and 50% of dehydroepiandrosterone. Dehydroepiandrosterone sulfate circulates unbound to protein, has limited androgenic action, and primarily acts as a circulating prohormone for the production of dehydroepiandrosterone and the more potent downstream androgens [1]. Androstenedione is produced in almost equal measure by the adrenal cortex and the ovary, and about 40% is produced through peripheral conversion of dehydroepiandrosterone [2]. Testosterone, the most clinically relevant circulating androgen, is produced by the adrenal cortex (25%), by the ovary (25%), and by peripheral conversion of androstenedione (50%) [2]. Dihydrotestosterone, the most potent androgen, is produced almost exclusively in target tissues by 5α-reductase acting on circulating testosterone.

During reproductive life, changing patterns of ovarian cyclicity, particularly the luteinizing hormone surge at midcycle, affect the production of androgens in women. The midcycle luteinizing hormone (LH) surge causes the ovarian thecal/stromal cells to produce testosterone and androstenedione. This results

---

Hormones, Cognition and Dementia: State of the Art and Emergent Therapeutic Strategies, ed. Eef Hogervorst, Victor W. Henderson, Robert B. Gibbs, and Roberta Diaz Brinton. Published by Cambridge University Press.
© Cambridge University Press 2009.

in the midcycle peak in circulating testosterone and androstenedione levels [2].

With increasing age, a decline in the production of all androgens occurs. The decline in the adrenal androgens, dehydroepiandrosterone sulfate and dehydroepiandrosterone, is steepest in the early reproductive years with a flattening out in midlife [3]. Since the great majority of circulating testosterone in women is derived from metabolic transformation of the adrenal androgens, not surprisingly, levels of testosterone decline as well. By the age of 40 years, a woman's serum testosterone level (mean of 0.61 nmol/L) is approximately half of that of a woman of 21 years of age (mean of 1.3 nmol/L) [4]. Because sex hormone binding globulin (SHBG) levels do not change over time, the % of free testosterone (the amount of testosterone not bound to SHBG and therefore available for biological activity) does not vary significantly with age [4].

The ovarian production of androgens also changes with increasing age. With follicular depletion and the onset of the perimenopause, ovarian estradiol production declines precipitously leading to loss of negative feedback at the level of the pituitary and hypothalamus. Consequently, the higher LH and FSH (follicular stimulating hormone) levels that occur during the peri- and postmenopause drive the ovarian thecal/stromal cells to produce increasing amounts of testosterone [5]. Moreover, the finding that the postmenopausal ovary continues to secrete androgens for some time is underlined by the discovery that serum levels of testosterone and androstenedione decrease significantly following bilateral oophorectomy [6] and levels of total and free testosterone are lower in older oophorectomized women compared to age-matched intact women [7]. No changes in androgen production occur in association with the menopausal transition itself [2, 3].

The neurobiology of androgens

Androgen receptors and estrogen receptors are widely distributed throughout the brain. They are present in brain areas involved in endocrine and reproductive functions, but are also found in areas believed to be involved in cognitive function, mood regulation, and aggressive behaviors. In the rat brain, androgen receptors are located in the deep layers of the cerebral cortex, amygdala, hippocampus, lateral septum, and in various nuclei of the hypothalamic region, including the nucleus basalis of Meynert, the diagonal band of Broca, the bed nucleus of the stria terminalis, and the mammillary bodies [8–11]. Several human studies have observed similar patterns of distribution of androgen receptors in the cerebral cortex [12–15], hippocampal formation [12, 15–17], amygdala [12, 18], and the hypothalamus [12, 18, 19]. Although androgen receptors and estrogen receptors tend to be co-localized, the relative distribution of the two receptors is different [11].

Like estrogens, androgens modulate the activity of a variety of neurotransmitter systems. Changes in circulating testosterone levels, via gonadectomy and/or exogenous testosterone administration, caused alterations in the cholinergic [20], the serotonergic [21], and the dopaminergic systems [22], although it is not always clear whether these changes are a result of the actions of testosterone or of its metabolite, estradiol.

Androgens also influence brain morphology by regulating dendritic length and synapse formation [23]. Castration of adult male rats caused a reduction in dendritic spine synapse density in CA1 hippocampal pyramidal cells, and was reversed by either testosterone or dihydrotestosterone administration [24]. Treatment of ovariectomized female rats with either testosterone or dihydrotestosterone significantly increased spine density, whereas priming with an aromatase inhibitor blocked the effect, suggesting that it was estradiol converted from testosterone that was responsible for the effect [24].

A functional magnetic resonance imaging study was undertaken to determine the effect of estradiol and testosterone on brain activation patterns in six surgically menopausal women. They received treatment with transdermal estradiol 0.05 mg/day for 12 weeks and, then, the addition of 1.25 g of a 1% topical testosterone gel daily for an additional 6 weeks [25]. At baseline, the untreated women had significantly decreased areas of brain activation while they viewed both erotic and neutral pictures compared to age-matched premenopausal women as measured by functional imaging. Following six weeks of treatment with estradiol alone, there was an increase in brain activation in response to both the neutral and to the erotic stimuli, especially in the left superior parietal and fusiform gyrus, and in limbic system structures. The addition of testosterone during the last six weeks of treatment was associated with even more brain activation areas; the erotic stimuli elicited increased areas of activation of the bilateral medial frontal and superior temporal gyri but also greater limbic system response, specifically in the parahippocampal gyrus and thalamus compared to treatment with estradiol alone. Since some of the brain areas activated by estradiol plus testosterone therapy are also important for specific cognitive functions, these findings provide reason to believe that testosterone may be important for certain cognitive functions in women.

Organizational and activational effects of the sex hormones

Although there are no qualitative differences in cognitive skills between the sexes, quantitative differences have been consistently found. Whereas women tend to excel on tasks of verbal skills and memory, on perceptual speed and accuracy, and on fine motor skills (female-typical skills), men tend to outperform women on tests of visual memory and on mathematical and spatial ability (male-typical skills) [26]. Although the effect sizes of these sexual dimorphisms in cognitive function are moderate (0.5–1.0 SD), they have been found consistently in studies that have attempted to document them. These sex differences in cognitive functioning are thought to occur as a result of the exposure of the fetal brain to differential levels of the sex hormones during prenatal life. These so-called organizational effects of sex hormones are thought to alter the structure and/or function of specific brain areas during fetal life permanently, perhaps by directing the development of certain neural pathways. It is thought that, postpubertally, the increased production of each of the sex hormones amplifies the neural "hard-wiring" laid down prenatally under its influence, usually referred to as the activational effect of that hormone. Therefore, this psychoendocrine theory proposes that, during prenatal life, the presence of significant quantities of a sex hormone organizes neural substrates for a certain behavior or function that becomes manifest after puberty under the influence of high circulating levels of that same hormone.

An impressive amount of evidence is available to support this psychoendocrine theory of the genesis of sex differences in cognition. Perhaps the most compelling support comes from studies of individuals who have a genetic disorder that resulted in their having been exposed to abnormal levels of sex hormones during prenatal life. For example, girls with

congenital adrenal hyperplasia have a 21-hydroxylase deficiency that prevents them from synthesizing cortisol [27]. This deficiency results in high adrenocorticotropic hormone levels and, consequently, in an overproduction of adrenal androgens so that the brains of affected females are exposed to high levels of androgens prenatally. If the prenatal sex hormone environment contributes to cognitive sex differences as the psychoendocrine theory proposes, it would be predicted that, compared with normal controls, girls with congenital adrenal hyperplasia would have better performance on tests of male-typical cognitive functions such as enhanced spatial ability. Indeed, these girls performed better on tests of spatial ability and worse on tests of verbal ability compared with their unaffected sisters [28]. The superior spatial skills of girls with congenital adrenal hyperplasia were later confirmed using spatial tasks that normally show sex differences [29]. Finally, in two methodologically rigorous investigations, girls with congenital adrenal hyperplasia performed significantly better on three separate tests of spatial ability compared with their unaffected female relatives [30]. When CYP21, the 21-hydroxylase gene whose defect is considered to cause congenital adrenal hyperplasia, was genotyped and used to determine the degree of fetal androgen exposure in girls with this disorder, a dose–response relationship was evident between disease severity and degree of masculinization of behavior of the affected girls [31]. Therefore, the combined evidence of these studies involving congenital adrenal hyperplasia suggests that prenatal exposure of genetic females to excessive amounts of androgens masculinizes their cognitive profile.

Studies that investigate the effect of a sex hormone on an aspect of behavior in individuals with a normal prenatal history are said to examine the activational effects of that hormone; these refer to hormonal effects that result from current, circulating levels of hormones. However, it is beginning to appear as though this traditional view of activational effects of hormones may need to undergo modification in light of evidence that the administration of a hormone for some period of time during adulthood may have enduring beneficial effects many years following its discontinuation [32].

A hypothesis that derives from this literature on the organizational and activational effects of sex hormones on behavior relevant to this review is that, in adulthood, estrogen would have its most profound effect on cognitive tasks, such as verbal skills and memory, perceptual speed and accuracy, and fine motor skills, in which females are known to excel. If this is true, then the administration of estrogen to postmenopausal women should preferentially enhance female-typical cognitive skills.

Human studies

Menstrual cycle studies

Since hormone levels fluctuate widely over the course of the menstrual cycle and testosterone levels peak at midcycle, some have used it as a model to study the activational effects of sex hormones on cognition. Unfortunately, numerous methodological limitations of these studies, the most common of which is the failure to characterize menstrual cycle phases reliably, limit the usefulness of their findings. Nonetheless, there is a moderate degree of consistency among their results. The majority of studies found that women perform better on tasks that measure visuospatial abilities during the menstrual phase of the cycle, when levels of all sex hormones are lowest, than at any other cycle phase [33]. In contrast, performance on female-favoring tasks, such as verbal fluency, appears to be enhanced during the periovulatory and luteal phase of the cycle (when estradiol levels are highest) compared to the menstrual phase, although not all findings are in agreement [34]. It is possible to conclude, however, that menstrual cycle studies show that performance on female-favoring tasks is enhanced during phases in which estradiol levels are high whereas performance on male-favoring tasks is optimal in the presence of very low levels of estradiol.

Correlational studies

The findings of correlational studies that have investigated whether there are positive associations between levels of circulating testosterone in women and their scores on a variety of cognitive tests are inconsistent. Although the cognitive sex differences hypothesis would predict that higher serum levels of testosterone would facilitate performance on tasks in which males typically excel, numerous studies have failed to find a significant positive relationship between testosterone levels and performance on tasks of visuospatial abilities in women [35–38]. In contrast, in untreated 68-year-old women, a positive

association between estradiol and testosterone levels and scores on tests of verbal memory occurred [39], whereas another study found significant positive correlations between free testosterone levels and two tests of verbal memory in 72-year-old estrogen-treated women [40]. On the other hand, several studies have reported negative correlations between verbal memory scores and total testosterone levels in untreated 75-year-old women [41] and in an age-controlled study of women [42]. These findings suggest that relatively higher levels of testosterone may dampen the performance of women on tasks in which they typically excel.

Randomized controlled trials

Randomized controlled trials are thought to provide higher quality evidence than correlational studies because of their ability to control factors other than the independent variable that could influence the outcome measures. In a cross-over study, premenopausal women who needed to undergo a hysterectomy and bilateral oophorectomy for benign disease were tested before surgery, again after three months of treatment with either a combined estradiol-plus-testosterone drug, estradiol-alone, testosterone-alone, or placebo and, for a third time, three months after they had been crossed-over to a different treatment for three months [43]. The scores of the women who had been treated with placebo decreased significantly postoperatively on tests of short- and long-term memory and on a test of logical reasoning coincident with a significant decrease in their serum levels of both estradiol and testosterone. However, the scores of women who had randomly received either estradiol-plus-testosterone, estradiol-alone, or testosterone-alone postoperatively did not differ on any of the tests compared to their preoperative performance when their ovaries had been intact. Although this suggests that testosterone is equally efficacious as estradiol in protecting verbal memory and working memory in surgically menopausal women, it must be considered that testing was performed six days following the administration of this intramuscular drug (given every four weeks) when testosterone levels were maximal and somewhat exceeded the upper limit of the female physiological range. Therefore, it remains a possibility that it was the estradiol aromatized from the high levels of testosterone that actually protected verbal and working memory functions in that study. It needs to be considered, therefore, that testosterone might protect against a decline in verbal and working memory that occurs following a surgical menopause only when administered in supraphysiological doses.

In a second cross-over study, a single dose of 0.5 mg sublingual testosterone or placebo was given to 15 young, healthy women within 10 days after their last menstruation in successive months [44]. In a prior study, this dose of testosterone had been shown to cause a ten-fold increase in total testosterone in plasma within 15 minutes of administration and returned to baseline within 90 minutes. The women were tested 4–5 hours following administration of the drug or placebo. Visuospatial ability (measured by the Mental Rotations Test) improved significantly following testosterone administration compared to placebo. The fact that serum levels of estradiol and testosterone were not assayed in this study moderates the confidence in these findings.

A recent randomized controlled trial was undertaken to determine whether inhibiting the conversion of testosterone to estradiol modifies the effects of testosterone on cognition in women. Sixty-one healthy estradiol-treated postmenopausal women (mean age of 54 years) were administered 400 μL of a 0.5% testosterone gel daily and were randomized to receive either an aromatase inhibitor (letrozole 2.5 mg/day) or a placebo tablet for 16 weeks coincident with testosterone treatment [45]. Significant improvements occurred in immediate and delayed visual and verbal recall in both testosterone-treated groups irrespective of whether the aromatase inhibitor or placebo was co-administered. Although this suggests that estradiol was not involved in the cognitive improvements seen in these postmenopausal women, it is important to remember that they had been receiving exogenous estradiol treatment both before and during administration of testosterone and the aromatase inhibitor or administration of placebo, and this may have been sufficient to maintain scores on visual and verbal memory. In contrast to these findings in postmenopausal women, an improvement in performance on tests of verbal memory following testosterone treatment in hypogonadal men was impaired by the addition of an aromatase inhibitor, implying that estradiol, converted from the exogenous testosterone, was critical in the cognitive improvements in verbal memory that occurred in these hypogonadal men with testosterone treatment alone.

Recently, an attempt was made to further investigate the possible effects of androgens on cognition in women by studying women with polycystic ovary disease. This syndrome affects 4 to 7% of all women [46] and is associated with endocrine abnormalities including chronically elevated free testosterone levels. Women with polycystic ovary syndrome typically experience anovulation or oligomenorrhea, and estrogen levels remain stable within the early follicular range [47]. Twenty-nine women with polycystic ovary syndrome (and elevated free testosterone levels) performed significantly worse on tests of verbal fluency, verbal memory, manual dexterity, and visuospatial memory compared to healthy control women with free testosterone levels within the normal female range [48]. See Figs. 19.1 and 19.2. No differences in performance between the groups were found on tests of mental rotations, spatial visualization, spatial perception, or perceptual speed. These findings therefore suggest that high levels of free testosterone in women are associated with poorer performance on cognitive tasks that tend to show a female advantage. On the other hand, the women with polycystic ovary syndrome and high free testosterone levels did not outperform the healthy control group on male-favoring tasks, as had been expected. Confirmation of these findings came from a recent internet-based study of polycystic ovary syndrome women (self-reported medical confirmation of their diagnosis) and control women who were administered the mental rotation test and the word recognition task via the web [49].

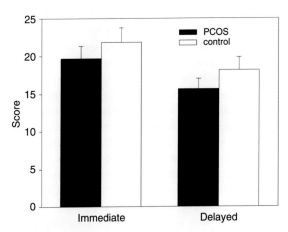

Fig. 19.1 Mean scores +/− SEM on the immediate and delayed trials of the Logical Memory Test. The differences in scores between the PCOS women and the controls for both trials are significant at the 0.05 level [48].

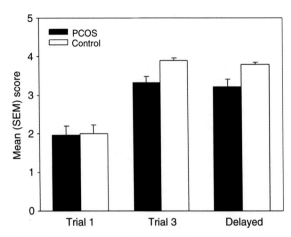

Fig. 19.2 Mean scores +/− SEM across trials for the difficult (unassociated) items of the Paired Associates Test in PCOS women compared to controls. The between-group differences in scores in Trial 3 and on the delayed recall trial were significant at the 0.05 level [48].

Similar to the Schattmann and Sherwin [48] findings, women with polycystic ovary syndrome performed more poorly than the healthy control women on tasks considered to demonstrate a female advantage but their scores did not differ from those of the control women in tasks that show a male advantage.

A randomized trial investigated whether the pharmacological manipulation of the high free testosterone levels in women with polycystic ovary syndrome might affect their performance on cognitive tests. Nineteen women with polycystic ovary syndrome were tested at baseline and, again, following 14 weeks of randomly assigned treatment with either an anti-androgen (cyproterone acetate) plus estrogen or with a placebo [50]. Hormone treatment resulted in a significant reduction in free testosterone levels and in an increase in scores on a test of verbal fluency compared to their own pretreatment performance, but no changes occurred in their scores on tests of visuospatial ability, verbal memory, or manual dexterity. One possible explanation for the findings that treatment with anti-androgen plus estrogen did not reverse the deficits in all cognitive domains that were evident in these women at baseline [48] may relate to the fact that polycystic ovary syndrome is a chronic endocrine disorder that typically starts around menarche so that alterations in the cognitive profile may require a duration of treatment longer than 14 weeks in the face of their chronically elevated testosterone levels.

Summary and conclusions

Although there is relatively little information on the possible influence of testosterone on aspects of cognition in women, it is possible to draw some tentative conclusions from the available studies. First, androgen receptors are present in areas of the brain that are important for cognition, and one small study shows increased brain activation in areas known to subserve certain cognitive functions. Second, testosterone up-regulates neurotransmitter systems that have been implicated in memory. Therefore, the findings from basic neuroscience provide biological plausibility for the possible influence of testosterone on aspects of cognition in women.

Studies on girls with congenital adrenal hyperplasia provide evidence that the exposure of female fetal brains to excessive amounts of androgen prenatally organizes their cognitive profile along masculine lines in that they perform better on tasks in which males typically excel compared to females with a normal prenatal history.

Results of studies that have investigated the activational effects of testosterone on cognition in women are somewhat inconsistent because of the variety and ages of the populations studied, the failure, in some, to control for hormonal status by measuring serum levels of the sex hormones, and because of the use of different drugs and different measuring instruments across studies. Nonetheless, some patterns emerge from these data. Most, but not all, studies have found better performance in women on visuospatial tasks, in which men typically excel, during the menstrual phase of the cycle when levels of both estradiol and testosterone are low and better performance on female-favoring tasks, such as verbal fluency, when estradiol levels are high (ovulatory and mid-luteal phases). This suggests that higher levels of estradiol enhance female-favoring tasks and its relative absence favors better performance on male-favoring tasks. Such a formulation is difficult to prove in menstrual cycle studies because testosterone levels always fluctuate in association with estradiol levels precluding an independent assessment of testosterone on cognitive functions using this model.

Results of correlational studies are also mixed and somewhat more problematic because some investigated untreated women whereas others studied women on estrogen therapy. Second, it is not at all clear that serum levels of sex steroid hormones reflect actual levels available to the brain. Despite these issues, several studies have reported that relatively higher levels of testosterone are associated with worse performance on tasks in which women typically excel.

In summary, the evidence thus far fairly consistently suggests that, in adult life, it is likely the ratio of estradiol/testosterone, and not absolute levels of testosterone alone, that determines the effect of testosterone on sex-specific cognitive functions in women. This conclusion is derived from the consistency in findings using different experimental paradigms that higher levels of testosterone within the physiological range in women do not seem to affect cognitive tasks in which males typically excel. However, there is fairly consistent evidence that a lower estradiol/testosterone ratio impairs performance on cognitive tasks in which women typically excel. However, more well controlled studies are needed in order to draw firm conclusions regarding the role of androgens on aspects of cognitive functioning in women.

References

1. Burger NZ, Johnson JV. Androgen production in women. In Tulandi T, Gelfand MM, eds. *Androgens and Reproductive Aging*. Boca Ratan, FL: Taylor & Francis, 2006, pp. 1–4.

2. Burger HG. Androgen production in women. *Fertil Steril*. 2002;77:S3–S5.

3. Davison SL, Davis SR. Androgens in women. *J Steroid Biochem Mol Biol*. 2003;85:363–6.

4. Zumoff B, Strain GW, Miller LK, *et al.* Twenty-four hour mean plasma testosterone concentration declines with age in normal premenopausal women. *J Clin Endocrinol Metab*. 1995;80:1429–30.

5. Adashi EY. The climacteric ovary as a functional gonadotropin-driven androgen-producing gland. *Fertil Steril*. 1994;62:20–7.

6. Judd H, Lucas WE, Yen SSC. Effect of oophorectomy on circulating testosterone and androstenedione levels in patients with endometrial cancer. *Am J Obstet Gynecol*. 1974;118:793–8.

7. Labrie F, Belanger A, Cusan L, *et al.* Marked decline in serum concentrations of adrenal C-19 sex steroid precursors and conjugated androgen metabolism during aging. *J Clin Endocrinol Metab*. 1997;82:2396–402.

8. Clancy AN, Bonsall RW, Michael RP. Immunohistochemical labeling of androgen receptors in the brain of the rat and monkey. *Life Sci*. 1992;50:409–17.

9. Gibbs RB. Expression of estrogen receptor-like immunoreactivity by different subgroups of basal forebrain cholinergic neurons in gonadectomized male and female rats. *Brain Res*. 1996;720:61–8.

10. Kerr JE, Beck SG, Handa RJ. Androgens selectively modulate c-fos messenger RNA induction in the rat hippocampus following novelty. *Neuroscience*. 1996;70:757–66.

11. Simerly RB, Chang C, Muramatsu MS, *et al.* Distribution of androgen and estrogen receptor mRNA-containing cells in the rat brain: an in-situ hybridization study. *J Comp Neurol*. 1990;294:76–95.

12. Osterlund MK, Hurd YL. Estrogen receptors in the human forebrain and the relation to neuropsychiatric disorders. *Prog Neurobiol*. 2001;64:251–67.

13. Puy L, MacLusky NJ, Becker L, *et al.* Immunocytochemical detection of androgen receptor in human temporal cortex: characterization and application of polyclonal androgen receptor antibodies in frozen and paraffin-embedded tissues. *J Steroid Biochem Mol Biol*. 1995;55:197–209.

14. Sarrieau A, Mitchell JB, Lal S, *et al.* Androgen binding sites in human temporal cortex. *Neuroendocrinology*. 1990;51:713–16.

15. Taylor AH, Al-Azzawi F. Immunolocalisation of estrogen receptor beta in human tissues. *J Clin Endocr Metab*. 2000;24:145–55.

16. Beyenburg S, Watzka M, Clusmann H, *et al.* Androgen receptor mRNA expression in the human hippocampus. *Neurosci Lett*. 2000;294:25–8.

17. Tohgi H, Utsugisawa K, Yamagata M, *et al.* Effects of age on messenger RNA expression of glucocorticoid, thyroid hormone, androgen, and estrogen receptors in postmortem human hippocampus. *Brain Res*. 1995;700:245–53.

18. Donahue JE, Stopa EG, Chorsky RL, *et al.* Cells containing immunoreactive estrogen receptor-a in the human basal forebrain. *Brain Res*. 2000;856:142–51.

19. Fernández-Guasti A, Kruijver FPM, Fodor M, *et al.* Sex differences in the distribution of androgen receptors in the human hypothalamus. *J Comp Neurol*. 2000;425:422–35.

20. Luine VN, Khylchevskaya RI, McEwen BS. Effect of gonadal steroids on activities of monoamine oxidase and choline acetylase in rat brain. *Brain Res*. 1975;86:293–306.

21. Fink G, Sumner B, Rosie R, *et al.* Androgen actions on central serotonin neurotransmitters: relevance for mood, mental state, and memory. *Behav Brain Sci*. 1999;211:311–52.

22. Bitar MS, Ota M, Linnoila M, *et al.* Modification of gonadectomy-induced increases in brain monoamine metabolism by steroid hormones in male and female rats. *Psychoneuroendocrinology*. 1991;16:547–57.

23. DeVoogd TJ, Nottebohm F. Gonadal hormones induce dendritic growth in the adult brain. *Science.* 1981;**214**:202–4.

24. Leranth C, Hajszan T, MacLusky NJ. Androgen increases spine synapse density in the CA1 hippocampal subfield of ovariectomized female rats. *J Neurosci.* 2004;**24**:495–9.

25. Archer JS, Love-Geffen TE, Herbst-Damm KL, *et al.* Effect of estradiol versus estradiol and testosterone on brain-activation patterns in postmenopausal women. *Menopause.* 2006;**13**:528–37.

26. Halpern DF. *Sex Differences in Cognitive Abilities.* Hillsdale: Lawrence Erlbaum Associates, 1992.

27. White PC, Speiser PW. Congenital adrenal hyperplasia due to 21-hydroxylase deficiencies. *Endocr Rev.* 2000;**21**:245–91.

28. Baker SW, Ehrhardt AA. Prenatal androgen, intelligence and cognitive sex differences. In Friedman RC, Richart RM, Wiele RLV, eds. *Sex Differences in Behavior.* New York: Wiley, 1974, pp. 53–76.

29. Perlman SM. Cognitive abilities of children with hormonal abnormalities: screening by psychoeducational tests. *J Learn Disabil.* 1973;**6**:22–9.

30. Resnick SM, Berenbaum SA, Gottesman II, *et al.* Early hormonal influences on cognitive functioning in congenital adrenal hyperplasia. *Dev Psychol.* 1986;**22**:191–8.

31. Nordenstrom A, Servin A, Bhlin G, *et al.* Sex-typed toy play behavior correlates with the degree of prenatal androgen exposure assessed by CYP21 genotype in girls with congenital adrenal hyperphasia. *J Clin Endocrinol Metab.* 2002;**87**:5119–24.

32. Bagger Y, Tanko L, Alexandersen G, *et al.* Early postmenopausal hormone therapy may prevent cognitive impairment later in life. *Menopause.* 2005;**12**:12–17.

33. Hampson E. Variations in sex-related cognitive abilities across the menstrual cycle. *Brain Cognition.* 1990;**14**:26–43.

34. Maki PM, Rich JB, Rosenbaum RS. Implicit memory varies across the menstrual cycle: estrogen effects in young women. *Neuropsychologia.* 2002;**40**:518–29.

35. Gouchie C, Kimura D. The relationship between testosterone levels and cognitive ability patterns. *Psychoneuroendocrinology.* 1991;**16**:323–34.

36. Hassler M, Gupta D, Wollmann H. Testosterone, estradiol, ACTH and musical, spatial and verbal performance. *Int J Neurosci.* 1992;**65**:45–60.

37. Moffat SD, Hampson E. A curvilinear relationship between testosterone and spatial cognition in humans: possible influence of hand preference. *Psychoneuroendocrinology.* 1996;**21**:323–37.

38. Silverman I, Kastuk D, Choi J, *et al.* Testosterone levels and spatial ability in men. *Psychoneuroendocrinology.* 1999;**24**:813–22.

39. Wolf OT, Kirschbaum C. Endogenous estradiol and testosterone levels are associated with cognitive performance in older women and men. *Horm Behav.* 2002;**41**:259–66.

40. Carlson LE, Sherwin BB. Higher levels of plasma estradiol and testosterone in healthy elderly men compared with age-matched women may protect aspects of explicit memory. *Menopause.* 2000;**7**:168–77.

41. Hogervorst E, De Jager C, Budge M, *et al.* Serum levels of estradiol and testosterone and performance in different cognitive domains in healthy elderly men and women. *Psychoneuroendocrinology.* 2004;**29**:405–21.

42. Thilers PP, MacDonald SWS, Herlitz A. The association between endogenous free testosterone and cognitive performance: a population-based study in 35 to 90 year-old men and women. *Psychoneuroendocrinology.* 2006;**31**:565–76.

43. Sherwin BB. Estrogen and/or androgen replacement therapy and cognitive functioning in surgically menopausal women. *Psychoneuroendocrinology.* 1988;**13**:345–57.

44. Aleman A, Bronk E, Kessels RPC, *et al.* A single administration of testosterone improves visuospatial ability in young women. *Psychoneuroendocrinology.* 2004;**29**:612–17.

45. Shah S, Bell RJ, Savage G, *et al.* Testosterone aromatization and cognition in women: a randomized, placebo-controlled trial. *Menopause.* 2006;**13**:600–8.

46. Asuncion M, Calco RM, Millan JL, *et al.* A prospective study of the prevalence of the polycystic ovary syndrome in unselected Caucasian women from Spain. *J Clin Endocrinol Metab.* 2000;**85**:2434–8.

47. Lobo RA, Carmina E. Polycystic ovary syndrome. In Lobo RA, Mishell DR, Paulson RJ, eds. *Infertility, Contraception and Reproductive Endocrinology*, 4th edn. Malden, MA: Blackwell Science, 1997, pp. 363–83.

48. Schattmann L, Sherwin BB. Testosterone levels and cognitive functioning in women with polycystic ovary syndrome and in healthy young women. *Horm Behav.* 2007;**51**:587–96.

49. Barnard L, Balen AH, Ferriday D, *et al.* Cognitive functioning in polycystic ovary syndrome. *Psychoneuroendocrinology.* 2007;**32**:906–14.

50. Schattmann L, Sherwin BB. Effects of the pharmacologic manipulation of testosterone on cognitive functioning in women with polycystic ovary syndrome: a randomized, placebo-controlled treatment study. *Horm Behav.* 2007;**51**:579–86.

Chapter 20

The role of estradiol in testosterone treatment

Monique M. Cherrier

Editors' introduction

Cherrier describes several mechanisms by which testosterone can affect the brain and other target tissues. By binding to classic intracellular androgen receptors, testosterone regulates transcription of target genes. Rapid, non-genomic effects of testosterone may involve membrane receptors. Dihydrotestosterone, a testosterone metabolite, is a more potent ligand for the androgen receptor. Testosterone can also be converted to estradiol, and estradiol in turn can affect the brain by binding to estrogen receptors or by acting through non-genomic mechanisms. In this chapter, Cherrier also reviews clinical research on testosterone and cognition, focusing on studies in men in which these different modes of testosterone action can – in part – be teased apart. Her review emphasizes studies that look specifically at potential mediating effects of estradiol. MMC supported in part by NIA R01AG027156.

Testosterone: mechanisms of action in the central nervous system

Several central nervous system functions are regulated by testosterone and other gonadal steroids. Examples include prenatal sexual differentiation of the brain, adult sexual behavior, gonadotropin secretion, and cognition. The effects of testosterone are mediated through the androgen receptor that is widely, but selectively, distributed throughout the brain [1]. Castration rapidly decreases androgen receptor expression in the brain, and testosterone up-regulates neural androgen receptor in a dose-dependent manner in both male and female mice [2–5]. Testosterone also acts via rapid, non-genomic methods of action through G-protein-coupled,

agonist-sequestrable testosterone membrane receptors that initiate a transcription-independent signaling pathway affecting calcium channels [6–9]. Thus androgen effects on the brain may occur rapidly through non-genomic mechanisms or within the traditional longer time frame of genomic to protein transformation mechanisms.

Another important aspect of testosterone action is its active metabolism in vivo. In the body, testosterone is converted to estradiol by the enzyme cytochrome P450 aromatase, and to dihydrotestosterone by the enzymes 5α-reductase type I and type 2. Estradiol formed from testosterone may then act on target organs via intracellular estrogen receptors alpha and beta. Dihydrotestosterone is not aromatizable and therefore cannot be further metabolized into estradiol. Dihydrotestosterone binds to androgen receptors with greater affinity than testosterone and therefore is sometimes considered a more potent androgen. Both estradiol and dihydrotestosterone are also widely distributed throughout the male brain. Androgen effects on cognition may therefore occur through testosterone directly or via its active metabolites, estradiol and dihydrotestosterone (Fig. 20.1) [3, 10–16].

Androgen receptors and aromatase activity in mice, rats, and monkeys have been shown to be widely distributed throughout the hypothalamus and limbic system in hormone-sensitive brain circuitry structures that serve essential roles in the central regulation of both reproductive function and cognition. For example, castration in male rats produces androgen sensitive increases in dopamine axon density in the prefrontal cortex, and it produces significant decreases in cholinergic neurons in the anterior cingulate, posterior parietal cortex, and medial septum

Hormones, Cognition and Dementia: State of the Art and Emergent Therapeutic Strategies, ed. Eef Hogervorst, Victor W. Henderson, Robert B. Gibbs, and Roberta Diaz Brinton. Published by Cambridge University Press.
© Cambridge University Press 2009.

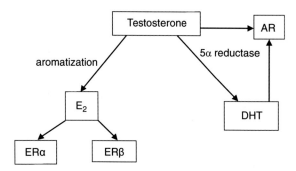

Fig. 20.1 Pathway of androgen metabolism and action in the central nervous system from testosterone through dihydrotestosterone (DHT) via 5α reductase and estradiol (E₂) via aromatase. Androgen receptor (AR), estrogen receptor alpha (ERα), and beta (ERβ).

[17–21]. Testosterone supplementation increases neuronal spine density in the hippocampus in gonadectomized animals [22]. The prefrontal cortices are involved in cognitive, affective, and memory functions, and gonadectomized rats demonstrate impairments in learning a maze, which are restored by testosterone administration [23]. These effects appear to be selective for the memory aspects of maze performance, as gonadectomy did not affect performance on a motor task [23].

Studies of testosterone replacement in mice and rats have generally supported a positive relationship between testosterone manipulation and cognitive task performance. Studies of age-accelerated mice and young rats have found beneficial effects of testosterone on avoidance learning and memory tasks, with other studies failing to find beneficial effects of testosterone on learning and memory. Differences in these studies may be due to the dose level of testosterone, as a recent study found a beneficial effect of testosterone on spatial memory at a modest dose but detrimental effects on spatial memory at higher doses [24, 25]. In addition, the type of memory assessed may also contribute to differences among studies. Development of a working memory water maze task, which separates working memory (a form of scratch pad or temporary memory) from reference memory (a form of declarative, or long-term, memory), found older male rats given testosterone demonstrate a beneficial increase in working memory capacity compared to older sham-operated rats and rats treated with dihydrotestosterone treated [26]. This finding suggests that changes in cognition from androgen supplementation or replacement may be selective to

frontal brain regions that underlie working memory and other executive functions, and this region may be more responsive to estradiol.

However, more recently, there is evidence that both androgens and estrogens may modulate spine synapse density in this region. Greater spine synapse density allows for better communication between neighboring neurons and may represent a mechanism by which new memories are made [27]. Intact and gonadectomized wild type rats were compared with testicular feminization mutant animals replaced with dihydrotestosterone or estradiol [28]. These mutant animals have a defective androgen receptor that reduces the binding capacity of the receptor to approximately 10–18% of wild type animals [29]. As reported previously, wild type animals after castration demonstrate a significant decline in spine synapse density in the medial prefrontal region, and density is restored to normal levels with dihydrotestosterone. However, estradiol administration to testicular feminization mutant rats also significantly increased spine synapse density. These results suggest that for males spine synapse density in the medial prefrontal region may be influenced by both androgens and estrogens. In contrast, previous work has shown that androgens but not estradiol affect spine synapse remodeling in the hippocampus of male rats [30]. Thus, effects of androgens and estrogens on cognition in male animals may be both hormone and task specific.

Cognitive changes from androgen supplementation in healthy younger men, women, and transsexuals

Cognitive changes from exogenously manipulated androgen levels have been examined in healthy young men, women, transsexuals, and hypogonadal males. For example, Gordon and Lee examined cognitive performance in a group of healthy young men in response to administration of testosterone enanthate [31]. They administered a low dose of testosterone enanthate (10 mg) to young men, who were tested with a battery of cognitive tests immediately after injection and four hours later. They reported no appreciable effects from hormone administration; participants demonstrated the same improvement from baseline to the second test session during the placebo condition as in the testosterone condition. However, no hormone values were reported. Therefore the relationship between cognition and hormone levels is unknown.

In contrast, a group of female-to-male transsexuals administered testosterone demonstrated improved spatial abilities but decreased verbal abilities [32]. In a subsequent study by the same research group, beneficial effects of androgen treatment on spatial abilities were again confirmed in female-to-male transsexuals and remained over a period of one-and-a-half years. However, male-to-female transsexuals treated with androgen blockade and estrogen showed opposite effects [33]. As expected, untreated male-to-female transsexuals had higher scores on visuospatial tasks than untreated female-to-male transsexuals; after three months of cross-sex hormone treatment, the group differences disappeared. The study of Slabbekoorn and colleagues indicates that testosterone had an enhancing effect, which was not quickly reversible, on spatial ability performance, but it had no deleterious effect on verbal fluency in female-to-male transsexuals. In contrast, male-to-female transsexuals demonstrated improved verbal memory in response to estrogen treatment, with no differences between the treatment and control groups on tests of attention, mental rotation, or verbal fluency [34].

However, not all studies have found support for cognitive changes from cross-gender hormone treatment [32]. It has been suggested that results from transsexual studies may be affected by co-morbid psychiatric or mood conditions. However, at least one study has reported no appreciable differences between the hormone treated and wait list groups on mood measures [34]. Postma and colleagues found in a population of healthy young women that short-term testosterone administration (0.5 mg testosterone cyclodextrine) resulted in improved spatial memory compared to placebo on some measures but not on others [35]. A recent neuroimaging study of male-to-female and female-to-male transsexuals found a significant increase in task-related brain activation for a language task in both groups; language activation in this study correlated with estradiol levels. An increase in brain activation was not found for a spatial task. However, post-treatment testosterone levels correlated with task-related mental rotation activity [36]. There were no significant changes in a lateralization index.

Overall, the results from exogenous manipulation of androgens and estradiol levels in healthy young men and women suggest that androgens may exert beneficial effects on spatial abilities, whereas estrogens may mediate verbal abilities. However, findings to date remain equivocal, and differences among studies due to study design, study population, and sometimes lack of documented change in hormone levels continue to make cross-study comparisons challenging.

Testosterone supplementation in older, eugonadal men

Serum levels of total testosterone and bioavailable testosterone (testosterone that is not bound to sex hormone binding globulin) decrease with age in men. Although this decrease is gradual, it is associated in some studies with decreased muscle mass, osteoporosis, decreased sexual activity, increased incidence of depression, decreased functional ability, and changes in cognition. Androgen therapy in normal older men has demonstrated benefits on bone mass, muscle strength, sexual functioning, and physical functioning [37]. Although the effects of estradiol on physiology are less well known in men, there are some effects on cardiovascular risk and bone that have become clearer in recent years. Animal and human studies suggest that both androgens and estrogens play a role in maintaining bone health in men. Osteoblasts express androgen and estrogen receptors [38–40]. In adult men, a correlation between estradiol levels and fractures has been reported [41], and men with mutations in the estrogen receptor gene are osteoporotic [42]. Epidemiological studies suggest that androgen levels within the normal range or slightly above normal range are associated with beneficial lipid profiles, whereas low androgen levels are associated with adverse lipid profiles (low high density lipoprotein, high low density lipoprotein). Testosterone treatment generally results in a mixed effect, with lowering of both lipids [43, 44]. Oral estrogens raise serum high density lipoprotein and triglyceride levels and decrease total cholesterol and low density lipoprotein levels in older men [45]. However, lowering estradiol by using an aromatase inhibitor in men does not change lipid profiles [46].

In addition to peripheral physiological effects, age-related declines in testosterone levels may affect cognitive abilities. Studies examining exogenous testosterone administration in older men have produced mixed results. Studies utilizing testosterone undecanoate are not included in this section, as circulating testosterone levels do not appear to be robustly or reliably increased from baseline in these studies. Sih and colleagues, using a double-blind placebo controlled design, gave older hypogonadal men biweekly injections of 200 mg testosterone cypionate for twelve months. Fifteen men were randomly assigned to receive placebo, and 17 men were randomly assigned to receive testosterone [47]. The men were in good general health with a mean age of 68 years. Tests of verbal and visual memory were administered prior to treatment and again after six months. Although grip strength improved, memory measures remained unchanged. Lack of significant findings in this study may be due to a non-significant change in testosterone levels from baseline or to assessment of cognition during nadir periods of testosterone levels. Janowsky and colleagues found improvements in spatial abilities in a double-blind study using daily 15 mg testosterone skin patches [48]. In this study, 56 healthy older men, mean age 67 years, were randomized to placebo or testosterone for three months. Prior to and after three months of treatment, participants were administered a battery of tests measuring semantic knowledge, constructional ability, verbal memory, fine motor coordination, and divided attention. The treatment group demonstrated improvement on a measure of visuoconstructional ability. In a second study, Janowsky and associates found weekly testosterone enanthate 150 mg injections improved spatial working memory in a group of healthy older males [49]. These improvements were evident compared to an age-matched placebo group and exceeded practice effects demonstrated by young men without testosterone treatment.

Working memory refers to the ability to maintain information in mind while simultaneously manipulating or updating information as needed. It is the scratchpad of the mind, and therefore improvements in working memory can affect a number of cognitive and day-to-day tasks. Consistent with these results, we have reported significant improvements in spatial and verbal memory in a group of healthy older men in response to short-term administration of testosterone enanthate [50]. Twenty-five healthy older men, mean age 68 years, were randomized to 100 mg testosterone enanthate or placebo. They received treatment for six weeks followed by six weeks of washout. Participants were administered a comprehensive battery of tests including verbal and spatial memory, spatial abilities, verbal fluency, and selective attention. Testosterone-treated participants demonstrated significant improvements on spatial memory (recall of a walking route), spatial ability (block construction), and verbal memory (recall of a short story). Improvements in spatial memory for a task that utilizes navigation in three-dimensional space, and verbal memory have not been previously reported. Although improvements were not found for all cognitive measures, we did not expect changes on measures of verbal fluency or selective attention.

However, a recent study suggested that testosterone supplementation may have adverse effects on cognition. In eugonadal older men, Maki and colleagues reported a decline in short-delay verbal memory with six months of testosterone treatment, and a decrease in relative task-associated brain activation in the temporal cortex – a brain region associated with memory functions [51]. Other areas of cognitive function remained stable, and there were also areas of increased task-associated activation, such as bilateral prefrontal cortex, which is associated with executive functions.

In all of these previous studies using testosterone administration, due to the natural conversion of testosterone into estradiol, changes in cognition may in fact be mediated in whole or in part by the subsequent rise in estradiol levels. The next sections will address additional studies in castrated and hypogonadal populations, as well as a study that systematically manipulated both testosterone and estradiol levels.

Castration and cognition in men

Several studies have examined relatively healthy men undergoing androgen deprivation treatment, and two studies have examined the addition of estrogen to the castrated state. Salminen and colleagues used a computerized battery and paper tests to examine 26 men prior to the start of combined androgen deprivation treatment (flutamide plus a luteinizing-hormone releasing hormone analog) and again after 6 and 12 months of treatment. They found a significant decline in attention (digit symbol test) and working memory (subtraction task), and improvement on an object recall (location memory) task. These changes were significantly related to declines in testosterone levels [52, 53]. In that sample, a correlation was found between estradiol levels and the decline in visual memory and speeded recognition of numbers and an improvement in verbal fluency [54]. Although the results suggest a relationship between estradiol levels and cognition, the correlation is within the context of the absence of androgens. A similar prospective study involved 40 men evaluated prior to the start of combined treatment and again after weeks 4, 12, 24, and 36 of treatment, at which point treatment was discontinued. Cognitive evaluations administered 42, 48, and 54 weeks after baseline found a significant improvement on the overall score for a computerized battery and a verbal list learning task [55]. This finding suggests that androgen deprivation therapy may have been suppressing practice effects that became evident with cessation of androgen deprivation therapy.

A six-month study of 62 men with more advanced prostate cancer randomly assigned to cyproterone acetate, to a luteinizing-hormone releasing hormone agonist, or to no treatment, along with a sample of healthy community-dwelling men, found significant declines in verbal memory in the luteinizing-hormone releasing hormone group compared to the no-treatment group, and declines in both treatment groups for sustained attention (digit symbol) [56, 57]. Significant differences were evident at nearly all time points between the prostate cancer groups and the healthy, community-dwelling group.

In a similar study, we examined cognitive changes in response to intermittent androgen suppression in 19 participants and 15 healthy age-matched controls. The men undergoing intermittent androgen suppression had no evidence of metastases following primary therapy (radiation, brachytherapy, or prostatectomy) and were treated with nine months of combined therapy (leuprolide and flutamide) followed by an off-treatment period of variable length [58]. Participants in this study were captured prior to and during their first cycle of treatment. Cognitive function tests were administered twice, before baseline and at baseline, to reduce practice effects, after nine months of androgen suppression, and three months after cessation of androgen deprivation. The intermittent androgen suppression group evidenced a significant decrease compared to baseline for performance on the mental rotation test ($p < 0.05$). We also observed a significant increase in the number of words recalled on a word list test during the washout three months after cessation.

Two studies have examined the addition of an estrogen to ongoing castration treatment. A study of 27 community-dwelling men who were either starting or already receiving luteinizing-hormone releasing hormone treatment for prostate cancer were enrolled

into a nine-week randomized trial of 1 mg/day of micronized 17-β estradiol or placebo [59]. Although all subjects showed a practice effect or improvement on delayed recall of a word list task, only those subjects in the estradiol-treated group evidenced an improvement on the Trail Making Test part A and the Stroop test. A study of men who recently stopped androgen deprivation therapy and were given transdermal estradiol (0.6 mg/week patch) for four weeks found improvements in verbal memory as measured by a story recall task as compared to men who continued androgen deprivation therapy [60]. These results are similar to those of Almeida and colleagues in which cognition changed once androgen ablation treatment ceased. These studies suggest that estradiol may in fact modulate cognitive abilities in men, particularly when androgen levels are low. Further, they suggest that estradiol may mediate attention and verbal memory as suggested by some studies in women.

Testosterone supplementation in older hypogonadal men

Several studies have examined androgen supplementation in older hypogondal men. Kenny and colleagues assessed 44 older (65–87 years) hypogonadal men randomized to placebo or testosterone patch for one year [61]. Significant improvement associated with testosterone levels was observed on a measure of divided attention (Trail Making Test Part B) in the treatment group. Both the treatment and placebo group demonstrated improvement on a measure of complex attention. We have also observed improvement in cognition in a group of older hypogonadal men given testosterone or dihydrotestosterone gel [62]. Twelve older (mean age 57 years) hypogonadal men were given testosterone gel and a battery of cognitive tests assessing verbal and spatial memory, language, and attention at baseline and again at days 90 and 180 of treatment. In addition to robustly raised testosterone and estradiol levels, a significant improvement in verbal memory compared to baseline was evident at day 180. A beneficial increase in spatial memory was also evident, which, however, did not reach statistical significance. In a separate study, nine older hypogonadal men (mean age 74) were randomized to receive dihydrotestosterone or placebo gel. Participants were given a comprehensive cognitive battery at baseline and after 30 and 90 days of treatment. Dihydrotestosterone gel significantly increased dihydrotestosterone levels and decreased testosterone levels compared to baseline. Spatial memory improved significantly. Results from these two studies suggest that aromatization of testosterone to estradiol may regulate verbal memory in men, whereas non-aromatizable androgens may regulate spatial memory [62].

A recent study of testosterone supplementation in older (65–80 years) hypogonadal men given testosterone or testosterone combined with finasteride (a 5α-reductase inhibitor) found improved working memory (digits backwards) in the testosterone group compared to the testosterone and finasteride group and the placebo group after 36 months of treatment. Verbal memory was improved in the testosterone and finasteride group [63]. However, the authors concluded that testosterone replacement does not improve cognition, as no improvements were seen on the other cognitive measures. This improvement in verbal memory observed in the testosterone and finasteride group may be secondary to changes in estradiol, as the testosterone plus finasteride group evidenced a significant increase in estradiol levels compared to the placebo group and the testosterone group.

In addition to cognitive changes measured by psychometric tests, two recent studies provide some evidence that androgen supplementation may change or optimize brain metabolism. Cerebral perfusion, assessed by single-photon emission computed tomography, increased in the superior frontal gyrus and midbrain of seven older (aged 58–72) hypogonadal men treated with testosterone for 3 to 5 weeks, with increases in midbrain perfusion after 12 to 14 weeks of treatment [64]. Although objective assessment of cognitive function was not included, responses to a questionnaire indicated that the increases in brain perfusion were coincident with self-reported increases in cognitive function. These findings are consistent with increases in brain metabolism assessed with positron emission tomography in four young hypogonadal men given testosterone therapy [65].

Testosterone treatment in men with Alzheimer's disease or mild cognitive impairment

Although observational studies suggest that lower testosterone levels may increase risk for developing Alzheimer's disease (AD), there are few studies that have examined whether testosterone supplementation may benefit Alzheimer's disease patients. Findings to date are mixed. Tan and Pu treated ten male patients with AD who also met criteria for hypogonadism [66]. Participants were given 200 mg testosterone every two weeks. A comprehensive cognitive test battery was administered at baseline and after three, six, and nine months of treatment. Alzheimer's disease patients demonstrated a significant improvement at months three, six, and nine compared to baseline and compared to the placebo group. A randomized study of testosterone supplementation in 16 eugondal AD patients treated with 75 mg daily of testosterone gel for 24 weeks found no changes in cognition but improvement on a quality-of-life measure [67].

Older adults who experience age-associated decrements in memory but do not meet criteria for AD are now defined with a new diagnostic category termed mild cognitive impairment (MCI). Approximately 50 to 70% of these individuals progress to develop AD, and therefore MCI is often considered a prodromal condition to AD. A study of older hypogonadal men who also met criteria for MCI found no significant changes on mood or cognitive measures in response to testosterone supplementation for 12 weeks [68]. A study of eugondal men with either MCI or AD given 100 mg of testosterone enanthate weekly for six weeks found an improvement in spatial memory compared to baseline, but no changes in other cognitive domains [69]. Thus, it is difficult to determine whether testosterone supplementation benefits cognition in AD or MCI patients. As with the studies of older men and hypogonadal men, the findings in AD and MCI patients are mixed and have generally involved small sample sizes. However, evidence does not yet suggest that testosterone supplementation worsens cognition.

Estradiol versus testosterone

Studies of estradiol supplementation to castrated men provide a good model for examining the role of estradiol in cognition in men. However, one study from our laboratory has attempted to examine the relative role of testosterone versus estradiol by using an aromatase inhibitor to block conversion of testosterone to estradiol. We recruited 60 healthy community-dwelling volunteers, aged 50 to 90 years, who were randomized to receive weekly intramuscular injections of either 100 mg testosterone enanthate plus daily oral placebo pill (testosterone group, N = 20); or 100 mg

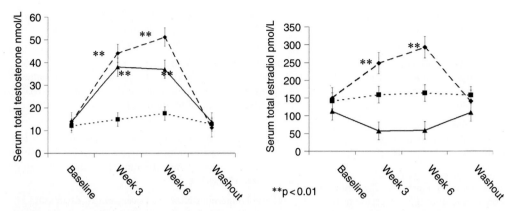

Fig. 20.2 (left) Mean serum total testosterone levels (nmol/L) and (right) serum total estradiol levels (pmol/L) in treatment (testosterone and anastrazol-testosterone) and placebo groups. Solid line with triangles represents the anastrazol-testosterone group; dashed lines with diamonds represents the testosterone group; and the dashed lines with squares represent the placebo group. Error bars represent standard error of measurement. Total testosterone increased at weeks three and six in the testosterone and anastrazol-testosterone groups compared to baseline (p < 0.01) and compared to placebo (p < 0.01). An interaction effect was also evident (p < 0.01). Estradiol levels increased at weeks three and six of treatment in the testosterone group compared to baseline (p < 0.01). Estradiol levels decreased in the anastrazol-testosterone group compared to placebo (p < 0.05) at weeks three and six although change from baseline at weeks three and six did not reach significance (p < 0.06). An interaction effect was also evident (p < 0.01).

testosterone enanthate plus 1 mg daily of oral anastrozole, an aromatase inhibitor, to block the conversion of testosterone to estradiol (testosterone-anastrozole group, N = 19); or saline injection and placebo pill (placebo group, N = 21) for six weeks [70]. Cognitive evaluations using a battery of neuropsychological tests were conducted at baseline, week three, and week six of treatment, and after six weeks of wash-out. Circulating total testosterone was raised from baseline an average of 238% in both the testosterone and testosterone-anastrozole groups. Estradiol increased by an average of 81% in the testosterone group and decreased by 50% in the testosterone-anastrozole group during treatment (Fig. 20.2). Significant improvements in spatial memory were evident in both the treatment groups. However, only the group with elevated estradiol levels (testosterone group) demonstrated significant verbal memory improvement. These results suggest that in healthy older men, improvement in verbal memory induced by testosterone administration depends upon aromatization of testosterone to estradiol, whereas improvement in spatial memory occurs in the absence of increases in estradiol.

Summary and conclusion

Previous studies suggest that testosterone administration may have beneficial effects on spatial and verbal memory, although findings across studies are inconsistent; a recent study indicates a potential adverse effect on cognition. Testosterone is naturally converted

into estradiol in the body. Thus, the role of increased estradiol cannot be ruled out as mediating cognitive changes in studies of testosterone administration in men. In addition, this chapter reviewed both animal and human studies that more clearly indicate a role for estradiol effects on cognition in males independent of androgens. These included studies of men undergoing androgen ablation with estradiol treatment and male-to-female transsexuals. In another study, testosterone was administered along with an aromatase inhibitor, which blocks the conversion of testosterone into estradiol. Potential beneficial effects of androgen supplementation and the associated rise in estradiol on cognition may be particularly important for older males, who may have age-related decreases in endogenous testosterone levels, which are predictive of cognitive loss and increased risk for the development of AD. More studies of testosterone supplementation are needed to better evaluate the balance between benefit and risk. This is further emphasized by a recent Institute of Medicine Report that concluded additional studies of testosterone supplementation in older men are needed, and the report noted that cognition should be included among the study outcomes.

References

1. Roselli CE, Klosterman S, Resko JA. Anatomic relationships between aromatase and androgen receptor mRNA expression in the hypothalamus

and amygdala of adult male cynomolgus monkeys. *J Comp Neurol.* 2001;**439**(2):208–23.

2. Brown TJ, Adler GH, Sharma M, Hochberg RB, MacLusky NJ. Androgen treatment decreases estrogen receptor binding in the ventromedial nucleus of the rat brain: a quantitative in vitro autoradiographic analysis. *Mol Cell Neurosci.* 1994;**5**(6):549–55.

3. Lynch CS, Story AJ. Dihydrotestosterone and estrogen regulation of rat brain androgen-receptor immunoreactivity. *Physiol Behav.* 2000;**69**(4/5): 445–53.

4. Singh R, Pervin S, Shryne J, Gorski R, Chaudhuri G. Castration increases and androgens decrease nitric oxide synthase activity in the brain: physiologic implications. *Proc Natl Acad Sci USA.* 2000;**97**(7): 3672–7.

5. Kerr JE, Allore RJ, Beck SG, Handa RJ. Distribution and hormonal regulation of androgen receptor (AR) and AR messenger ribonucleic acid in the rat hippocampus. *Endocrinology.* 1995;**136**(8):3213–21.

6. Lieberherr M, Grosse B. Androgens increase intracellular calcium concentration and inositol 1,4,5-trisphosphate and diacylglycerol formation via a pertussis toxin-sensitive G-protein. *J Biol Chem.* 1994;**269**(10):7217–23.

7. Benten WP, Lieberherr M, Sekeris CE, Wunderlich F. Testosterone induces Ca^{2+} influx via non-genomic surface receptors in activated T cells. *FEBS Lett.* 1997;**407**(2):211–14.

8. Benten WP, Lieberherr M, Stamm O, et al. Testosterone signaling through internalizable surface receptors in androgen receptor-free macrophages. *Mol Biol Cell.* 1999;**10**(10):3113–23.

9. Benten WP, Lieberherr M, Giese G, et al. Functional testosterone receptors in plasma membranes of T cells. *FASEB J.* 1999;**13**(1):123–33.

10. Cyr M, Calon F, Morissette M, et al. Drugs with estrogen-like potency and brain activity: potential therapeutic application for the CNS. *Curr Pharm Des.* 2000;**6**(12):1287–312.

11. Gundlah C, Kohama SG, Mirkes SJ, et al. Distribution of estrogen receptor beta (ERbeta) mRNA in hypothalamus, midbrain and temporal lobe of spayed macaque: continued expression with hormone replacement. *Brain Res Mol Brain Res.* 2000;**76**(2):191–204.

12. Osterlund MK, Gustafsson JA, Keller E, Hurd YL. Estrogen receptor beta (ERbeta) messenger ribonucleic acid (mRNA) expression within the human forebrain: distinct distribution pattern to ERalpha mRNA. *J Clin Endocrinol Metab.* 2000;**85**(10):3840–6.

13. Michael RP, Rees HD, Bonsall RW. Sites in the male primate brain at which testosterone acts as an androgen. *Brain Res.* 1989;**502**(1):11–20.

14. Osterlund MK, Grandien K, Keller E, Hurd YL. The human brain has distinct regional expression patterns of estrogen receptor alpha mRNA isoforms derived from alternative promoters. *J Neurochem.* 2000; **75**(4):1390–7.

15. Ishunina TA, Fisser B, Swaab DF. Sex differences in androgen receptor immunoreactivity in basal forebrain nuclei of elderly and Alzheimer patients. *Exp Neurol.* 2002;**176**(1):122–32.

16. de Fougerolles Nunn E, Greenstein B, Khamashta M, Hughes GR. Evidence for sexual dimorphism of estrogen receptors in hypothalamus and thymus of neonatal and immature Wistar rats. *Int J Immunopharmacol.* 1999;**21**(12):869–77.

17. Nakamura N, Fujita H, Kawata M. Effects of gonadectomy on immunoreactivity for choline acetyltransferase in the cortex, hippocampus, and basal forebrain of adult male rats. *Neuroscience.* 2002;**109**(3):473–85.

18. Kritzer MF. Long-term gonadectomy affects the density of tyrosine hydroxylase- but not dopamine-beta-hydroxylase-, choline acetyltransferase- or serotonin-immunoreactive axons in the medial prefrontal cortices of adult male rats. *Cereb Cortex.* 2003;**13**(3):282–96.

19. Kritzer MF. Effects of acute and chronic gonadectomy on the catecholamine innervation of the cerebral cortex in adult male rats: insensitivity of axons immunoreactive for dopamine-beta-hydroxylase to gonadal steroids, and differential sensitivity of axons immunoreactive for tyrosine hydroxylase to ovarian and testicular hormones. *J Comp Neurol.* 2000; **427**(4):617–33.

20. Kritzer MF, Adler A, Marotta J, Smirlis T. Regionally selective effects of gonadectomy on cortical catecholamine innervation in adult male rats are most disruptive to afferents in prefrontal cortex. *Cereb Cortex.* 1999;**9**(5):507–18.

21. Kritzer MF. Perinatal gonadectomy exerts regionally selective, lateralized effects on the density of axons immunoreactive for tyrosine hydroxylase in the cerebral cortex of adult male rats. *J Neurosci.* 1998; **18**(24):10735–48.

22. Leranth C, Hajszan T, MacLusky NJ. Androgens increase spine synapse density in the CA1 hippocampal subfield of ovariectomized female rats. *J Neurosci.* 2004;**24**(2):495–9.

23. Kritzer MF, McLaughlin PJ, Smirlis T, Robinson JK. Gonadectomy impairs T-maze acquisition in adult male rats. *Horm Behav.* 2001;**39**(2):167–74.

24. Naghdi N, Oryan S, Etemadi R. The study of spatial memory in adult male rats with injection of testosterone enanthate and flutamide into the basolateral nucleus of the amygdala in Morris water maze. *Brain Res.* 2003;**972**(1/2):1–8.

25. Naghdi N, Nafisy N, Majlessi N. The effects of intrahippocampal testosterone and flutamide on spatial localization in the Morris water maze. *Brain Res.* 2001;**897**(1/2):44–51.

26. Bimonte-Nelson HA, Singleton RS, Nelson ME, *et al.* Testosterone, but not nonaromatizable dihydrotestosterone, improves working memory and alters nerve growth factor levels in aged male rats. *Exp Neurol.* 2003;**181**(2):301–12.

27. Woolley CS. Effects of oestradiol on hippocampal circuitry. *Novartis Found Symp.* 2000;**230**:173–80.

28. Hajszan T, MacLusky NJ, Johansen JA, Jordan CL, Leranth C. Effects of androgens and estradiol on spine synapse formation in the prefrontal cortex of normal and testicular feminization mutant male rats. *Endocrinology.* 2007;**148**(5):1963–7.

29. Yarbrough WG, Quarmby VE, Simental JA, *et al.* A single base mutation in the androgen receptor gene causes androgen insensitivity in the testicular feminized rat. *J Biol Chem.* 1990;**265**(15):8893–900.

30. MacLusky NJ, Hajszan T, Prange-Kiel J, Leranth C. Androgen modulation of hippocampal synaptic plasticity. *Neuroscience.* 2006;**138**(3):957–65.

31. Gordon HW, Lee PA. A relationship between gonadotropins and visuospatial function. *Neuropsychologia.* 1986;**24**:563–76.

32. Van Goozen SHM, Cohen-Kettenis PT, Gooren LJG, Frijda NH, Van De Poll NE. Activating effects of androgens on cognitive performance: causal evidence in a group of female-to-male transsexuals. *Neuropsychologia.* 1994;**32**(10):1153–7.

33. Slabbekoorn D, van Goozen SH, Megens J, Gooren LJ, Cohen-Kettenis PT. Activating effects of cross-sex hormones on cognitive functioning: a study of short-term and long-term hormone effects in transsexuals. *Psychoneuroendocrinology.* 1999;**24**(4): 423–47.

34. Miles C, Green R, Sanders G, Hines M. Estrogen and memory in a transsexual population. *Horm Behav.* 1998;**34**:199–208.

35. Postma A, Meyer G, Tuiten A, *et al.* Effects of testosterone administration on selective aspects of object-location memory in healthy young women. *Psychoneuroendocrinology.* 2000;**25**(6):563–75.

36. Sommer IE, Cohen-Kettenis PT, van Raalten T, *et al.* Effects of cross-sex hormones on cerebral activation during language and mental rotation: an fMRI study in transsexuals. *Eur Neuropsychopharmacol.* 2008;**18** (3):215–21.

37. Matsumoto AM. 'Andropause' – are reduced androgen levels in aging men physiologically important? [editorial; comment]. *West J Med.* 1993;**159**(5):618–20.

38. Oursler MJ, Osdoby P, Pyfferoen J, Riggs BL, Spelsberg TC. Avian osteoclasts as estrogen target cells. *Proc Natl Acad Sci USA.* 1991;**88**(15):6613–17.

39. Eriksen EF, Colvard DS, Berg NJ, *et al.* Evidence of estrogen receptors in normal human osteoblast-like cells. *Science.* 1988;**241**(4861):84–6.

40. Colvard DS, Eriksen EF, Keeting PE, *et al.* Identification of androgen receptors in normal human osteoblast-like cells. *Proc Natl Acad Sci USA.* 1989; **86**(3):854–7.

41. Khosla S, Riggs BL. Androgens, estrogens, and bone turnover in men. *J Clin Endocrinol Metab.* 2003; **88**(5):2352.

42. Korach KS, Couse JF, Curtis SW, *et al.* Estrogen receptor gene disruption: molecular characterization and experimental and clinical phenotypes. *Recent Prog Horm Res.* 1996;**51**:159–86; discussion 86–8.

43. Snyder PJ, Peachey H, Berlin JA, *et al.* Effect of transdermal testosterone treatment on serum lipid and apolipoprotein levels in men more than 65 years of age. *Am J Med.* 2001;**111**(4):255–60.

44. Barrett-Connor EL. Testosterone and risk factors for cardiovascular disease in men. *Diabetes Metab.* 1995;**21**(3):156–61.

45. Moorjani S, Dupont A, Labrie F, *et al.* Changes in plasma lipoproteins during various androgen suppression therapies in men with prostatic carcinoma: effects of orchiectomy, estrogen, and combination treatment with luteinizing-hormone-releasing hormone agonist and flutamide. *J Clin Endocrinol Metab.* 1988;**66**(2):314–22.

46. Leder BZ. Testosterone, estradiol and aromatase inhibitor therapy in elderly men. *J Steroid Biochem Mol Biol.* 2007;**106**(1/5):162–7.

47. Sih R, Morley JE, Kaiser FE, *et al.* Testosterone replacement in older hypogonadal men: a 12 month randomized controlled trial. *J Clin Endocrinol Metab.* 1997;**82**(6):1661–7.

48. Janowsky JS, Oviatt SK, Orwoll ES. Testosterone influences spatial cognition in older men. *Behav Neurosci.* 1994;**108**(2):325–32.

49. Janowsky JS, Chavez B, Orowoll E. Sex steroids modify working memory. *J Cogn Neurosci.* 2000;**12**(3):407–14.

50. Cherrier MM, Asthana S, Baker LD, *et al.* Testosterone supplementation improves spatial and verbal memory in healthy older men. *Neurology.* 2001;**57**:80–8.

51. Maki PM, Ernst M, London ED, *et al.* Intramuscular testosterone treatment in elderly men: evidence of memory decline and altered brain function. *J Clin Endocrinol Metab.* 2007;**92**(11):4107–14.

52. Salminen E, Portin R, Korpela J, *et al.* Androgen deprivation and cognition in prostate cancer. *Br J Cancer.* 2003;**89**(6):971–6.

53. Salminen EK, Portin RI, Koskinen A, Helenius H, Nurmi M. Associations between serum testosterone fall and cognitive function in prostate cancer patients. *Clin Cancer Res.* 2004;**10**(22):7575–82.

54. Salminen EK, Portin RI, Koskinen AI, Helenius HY, Nurmi MJ. Estradiol and cognition during androgen deprivation in men with prostate carcinoma. *Cancer.* 2005;**103**(7):1381–7.

55. Almeida OP, Waterreus A, Spry N, Flicker L, Martins RN. One year follow-up study of the association between chemical castration, sex hormones, beta-amyloid, memory and depression in men. *Psychoneuroendocrinology.* 2004;**29**(8):1071–81.

56. Green HJ, Pakenham KI, Headley BC, *et al.* Altered cognitive function in men treated for prostate cancer with luteinizing-hormone-releasing hormone analogues and cyproterone acetate: a randomized controlled trial. *BJU Int.* 2002;**90**(4):427–32.

57. Green HJ, Pakenham KI, Headley BC, *et al.* Quality of life compared during pharmacological treatments and clinical monitoring for non-localized prostate cancer: a randomized controlled trial. *BJU Int.* 2004; **93**(7):975–9.

58. Cherrier MM, Rose AL, Higano C. The effects of combined androgen blockade on cognitive function during the first cycle of intermittent androgen suppression in patients with prostate cancer. *J Urol.* 2003;**170**(5):1808–11.

59. Taxel P, Stevens MC, Trahiotis M, Zimmerman J, Kaplan RF. The effect of short-term estradiol therapy on cognitive function in older men receiving hormonal suppression therapy for prostate cancer. *J Am Geriatr Soc.* 2004;**52**(2):269–73.

60. Beer TM, Bland LB, Bussiere JR, *et al.* Testosterone loss and estradiol administration modify memory in men. *J Urol.* 2006;**175**(1):130–5.

61. Kenny AM, Bellantonio S, Gruman CA, Acosta RD, Prestwood KM. Effects of transdermal testosterone on cognitive function and health perception in older men with low bioavailable testosterone levels. *J Gerontol A Biol Sci Med Sci.* 2002;**57**(5):M321–5.

62. Cherrier MM, Craft S, Matsumoto AH. Cognitive changes associated with supplementation of testosterone or dihydrotestosterone in mildly hypogonadal men: a preliminary report. *J Androl.* 2003;**24**(4):568–76.

63. Vaughan C, Goldstein FC, Tenover JL. Exogenous testosterone alone or with finasteride does not improve measurements of cognition in healthy older men with low serum testosterone. *J Androl.* 2007;**28**(6):875–82.

64. Azad N, Pitale S, Barnes WE, Friedman N. Testosterone treatment enhances regional brain perfusion in hypogonadal men. *J Clin Endocrinol Metab.* 2003;**88**(7):3064–8.

65. Zitzmann M, Weckesser M, Schober O, Nieschlag E. Changes in cerebral glucose metabolism and visuospatial capability in hypogonadal males under testosterone substitution therapy. *Exp Clin Endocrinol Diabetes.* 2001;**109**(5):302–4.

66. Tan RS, Pu SJ. A pilot study on the effects of testosterone in hypogonadal aging male patients with Alzheimer's disease. *Aging Male.* 2003;**6**(1):13–17.

67. Lu PH, Masterman DA, Mulnard R, *et al.* Effects of testosterone on cognition and mood in male patients with mild Alzheimer disease and healthy elderly men. *Arch Neurol.* 2006;**63**(2):177–85.

68. Kenny AM, Fabregas G, Song C, Biskup B, Bellantonio S. Effects of testosterone on behavior, depression, and cognitive function in older men with mild cognitive loss. *J Gerontol A Biol Sci Med Sci.* 2004;**59**(1):75–8.

69. Cherrier MM, Matsumoto AH, Asthana S, *et al.* Testosterone improves spatial memory in men with Alzheimer disease and mild cognitive impairment. *Neurology.* 2005;**64**:2063–8.

70. Cherrier MM, Matsumoto AM, Amory JK, *et al.* The role of aromatization in testosterone supplementation: effects on cognition in older men. *Neurology.* 2005;**64**:290–6.

Endogenous testosterone levels and cognitive aging in men

Scott D. Moffat

Editors' introduction

In this chapter, Moffat reviews observational research in older men that examines serum testosterone concentrations in relation to cognitive aging or Alzheimer's disease (AD) risk. Prospective cohort studies, such as the Baltimore Longitudinal Study of Aging, provide particularly useful data. Despite methodological limitations and conflicting findings, Moffat tentatively concludes that age-associated reductions in testosterone concentrations are a risk factor for cognitive decline and dementia. Cognitive vulnerability may be limited to specific domains of cognitive performance and may be modified by apolipoprotein E genotype. As he suggests, more definitive answers may require well designed randomized clinical trials that target cognitive effects of testosterone therapy. Any future trial must also consider other health outcomes that may be beneficially or adversely affected by testosterone.

Introduction

There has been much interest in the possibility that age-related changes in several endocrine systems may affect cognitive status, cognitive decline, and brain health in the elderly. To date, the endocrine systems that have received the most attention have been the hypothalamic-pituitary-adrenal axis, which regulates cortisol levels, and the hypothalamic-pituitary-gonadal axis, which regulates sex steroid levels. In the latter case, the possible cognitive effects of endogenous estrogen levels in women as well as the effects of its subsequent replacement through exogenous supplementation have received the most research focus. Although testosterone levels in men have more rarely been the subject of inquiry, this field too is now generating considerable interest. This chapter reviews the extant literature on associations between endogenous testosterone levels, cognitive function, and risk for dementia in older men. The results of numerous associational studies are largely mixed with a preponderance indicating that testosterone loss may be a risk factor for cognitive decline and possibly for dementia. This chapter will also discuss some possible reasons for diverging results between studies and suggest ways to improve methodology.

First, it is important to establish that in addition to its well publicized effects on the body periphery, testosterone has important effects on the central nervous system. Most of what we know about direct effects of testosterone on the nervous system come from well controlled experimental studies in non-human species. Researchers from a variety of disciplines have demonstrated that androgens have effects on myriad behavioral systems. These include sexual and maternal behavior, activity levels, aggression and play, and song production in songbirds [1] Testosterone may act on androgen receptors in the nervous system not only as testosterone but also after conversion to dihydrotestosterone by 5α-reductase. Testosterone may also act on brain estrogen receptors after conversion to estradiol by aromatase. Thus, testosterone may interact not only with androgen receptors but also with estrogen receptors, and hence, testosterone administration may in some circumstances parallel the effects of estrogens throughout the nervous system.

Of particular interest to researchers investigating hormonal contributions to human abilities is the observation that regions of the rat brain thought to subserve aspects of spatial learning and memory, including the hippocampus, have been shown to be affected by gonadal hormones. The hippocampus

---

contains high concentrations of androgen receptors [2]. Testosterone administration to females during critical periods of development enhances spatial learning, while castration in males impairs maze learning [3, 4]. These observations are similarly of interest to researchers interested in cognitive aging because of the prominent role of the hippocampus in human memory function and the focus of the aging literature on human memory loss.

Also of importance to researchers interested in the possible protective effects of testosterone on cognitive and brain aging is that the early organizational effects of testosterone on the development of the hypothalamus [5], the cerebral cortex [6], and the hippocampus [3] is most often neurotrophic. That is, early administration of testosterone tends to promote larger neural structures. This clearly raises the question of whether testosterone may exert neurotrophic or neuroprotective effects into later adult life. Several observations suggest that this indeed may be the case.

For example, testosterone loss in aging mice is associated with spatial learning deficits, which are reversed by testosterone administration [7]. Androgen treatment prevents N-methyl-D-aspartate (NMDA) excitotoxicity in hippocampal neurons [8] and may facilitate recovery after injury by promoting fiber outgrowth and sprouting [9]. Administration of testosterone increases nerve growth factor levels in the hippocampus, and induces an up-regulation of nerve growth factor receptors in the forebrain [10]. Testosterone decreases β-amyloid secretion from rat cortical neurons [11] and reduces β-amyloid induced neurotoxicity in cultured hippocampal neurons [12]. Rosario and colleagues [13] reported that in a transgenic mouse model of AD, gonadectomy in male mice resulted in increased accumulation of β-amyloid and decrease performance on a hippocampal-dependent cognitive measure. These observations of inhibitory effects of testosterone on the expression of β-amyloid are critical, as β-amyloid is one of the principal neuropathological hallmarks of AD. There has now been at least one study in humans that investigated the effects of testosterone on human neural tissue. Hammond and colleagues [14] found that testosterone was protective of human primary neurons in culture, providing the most direct evidence for neuroprotective effects of testosterone on human neural tissue.

Taken together, these findings suggest that testosterone may exert important neurotrophic and possibly neuroprotective effects. Additionally, studies in non-human species compellingly demonstrate that testosterone affects various aspects of behavior, including learning and memory. It is therefore reasonable to investigate whether the decline in testosterone levels as men age may impact their cognitive and neural processing. The corollary of this idea is that if loss of endogenous testosterone impairs brain function, then its supplementation from exogenous sources could prove to be a viable treatment for cognitive decline.

Endogenous testosterone concentrations and cognitive aging in men without dementia

As men age, they experience a considerable drop in the levels of testosterone [15, 16]. Total testosterone levels decline by approximately 50% from ages 30 to 80 [16], and as many as 68% of men over age 70 can be classified as hypogonadal based on their endogenous free testosterone concentrations [15]. This progressive loss of testosterone with age in men, often called the "andropause," may have significant physiological consequences. These include decreased muscle mass, reduced bone density, and sexual dysfunction [17, 18]. Among men with suspected andropause, memory loss was reported by 36% of patients. In fact, memory loss was the third most commonly reported symptom after sexual dysfunction (46%) and general weakness (41%) [19].

Several investigations examining the association between testosterone levels and cognition have been studies in young adult men and women [20, 21, 22]. However, there is now a growing literature that examines the association between testosterone levels and cognition in older men. This literature is quite varied along a number of key dimensions of study design and sample composition, and thus it is not entirely surprising that the results of these studies have been variable. Although there are some studies reporting associations between testosterone levels and cognitive function in women, the present chapter focuses only on those studies that have evaluated testosterone loss in elderly men.

Table 21.1 summarizes the results from existing studies examining the association between endogenous testosterone levels, cognitive performance, and cognitive decline across a number of cognitive domains in older men. In Table 21.1, a positive sign

Table 21.1 Association between endogenous testosterone levels, cognitive performance and cognitive decline across a number of cognitive domains in older men.

Authors	N	Age	Years follow-up	Total T/Free T	Cognitive status	Verbal memory	Visual memory	Working memory	Spatial cognition	Speed	Exec. function
Aleman (2001) [23]	25	69	0	TT		0					
Barrett-Connor (1999) [24]	547	70	0	TT	−	+		+		0	
				FT	−	+		+		0	
Burkhardt (2005)[a] [25]	45	72	0	TT							
				FT	+/0	0		+/−			+/−
Driscoll (2005) [26]	35	52	0	TT					+		
Fonda (2005) [27]	981	63	0	TT		0	0	0	0	0	
				FT				0	0	0	
Geerlings (2006) [28]	2,974	77	6	TT	0						
				FT							
Hogervorst (2004) [29]	145	74	0	TT	0	0	0	0	+	+	
				FT							
Martin (2007) [30]	1,046	54	0	TT			−			+	−
				FT			−			+	−
Moffat (2002) [31]	320	64	10	TT	0	0	0	0	0	0	
				FT	0	+	+	0	+	+	
Morley (1997) [32]	56	20–84	0	TT	0	+	+			0	+
Muller (2005) [33]	395	60	0	TT	0	0				0	+
				FT	0	0				0	0

199

Table 21.1 (cont.)

Authors	N	Age	Years follow-up	Total T Free T	Cognitive status	Verbal memory	Visual memory	Working memory	Spatial cognition	Speed	Exec. function
Perry (2001) [34]	78	66	0	TT							
				FT						0	+
Thilers (2006) [35]	1,107	62	0	TT		+			+		
				FT	0						
Wolf (2002) [36]	30	69	0	TT		0	0		0		0
				FT		0	0				
Yaffe (2002) [37]	310	73	0	TT	0					0	
				FT	+					+	
Yeap (2008) [38]	2,932	70–89	0	TT	0						
				FT	+						

Note:

[a] direction of relationships varied as a function of apolipoprotein E genotype status.

N: number of men on which primary data analyses were performed.

Years follow-up: number of years over which participants were followed in longitudinal study design. Cross-sectional studies are noted by 0 years follow-up.

TT, FT: results in each cognitive domain for total testosterone (TT) and free testosterone (FT).

+ : significant effect in study in which higher levels of testosterone were associated with higher cognitive performance.

− : significant effect in study in which higher levels of testosterone were associated with lower cognitive performance.

0 : effect in study in which there was null finding relating testosterone to cognitive performance.

Blank cells reflect cognitive domains that were not assessed.

(+) indicates a result showing that higher endogenous testosterone was associated with better cognitive performance; a negative sign (−) indicates results showing that higher endogenous testosterone was associated with poorer cognitive performance; and a zero (0) indicates that the findings were not statistically significant. The first observation that can be made in examining the table is that there is great variation along a number of critical study parameters. First, there is little uniformity in selection of cognitive domains to be assessed.[1] Moreover, even when the same construct was assessed in a study (e.g., verbal memory), there is little uniformity in the selection of a specific assessment instrument. Other key sources of variability include sample sizes and average age of the study population. Sample age may be a critical factor as there may exist a "window of opportunity" in the elderly during which steroids may exert positive effects on brain and cognitive function. Once this window closes, steroids may no longer exert effects or may even become detrimental [39, 40] (see Chapter 4).

I would argue that the greatest drawback in the literature relating testosterone levels to cognitive function are those related to the measurement of testosterone. In particular, there are inherent and serious limitations in relating a single testosterone measurement to any behavioral variable. A single measure (usually taken in the morning after an overnight fast) is subject to major sources of error variance. This problem limits our ability to detect significant relationships when they are truly there (type II error) and may create spurious significant findings when they may be truly absent (type I error). Major sources of measurement error are detailed by Carruthers [17] and include circadian and circannual variation, diet, exercise, alcohol consumption, smoking habits, as well as others. Also of considerable importance is that while we are measuring peripheral blood levels of androgens, we are interested in brain levels, and there is some disagreement on the magnitude of the correlation between blood and cerebrospinal fluid levels of steroids [41, 42]. Virtually nothing is known about the relationship between blood levels of steroids and intracellular concentrations. These and other factors conspire to produce considerable error variance, and are likely a major source of the variability in outcomes observed in Table 21.1.

Another observation that needs to be made regarding the literature relating endogenous testosterone concentrations to cognitive function in men is the dearth of longitudinal studies. Longitudinal designs are important, as these allow each individual to serve as his own control. This design also helps to address the serious shortcomings noted above of relying on a single androgen "snapshot" to infer longer term androgen status in any given man. Although this approach still does not completely overcome the unknown relations between peripheral and central nervous system steroid levels, one can be more confident in the classification of a man as having "high testosterone" if he measures with high testosterone levels over multiple assessments over a longer time period. Another advantage of the longitudinal design is that it allows us to assess within-individual *rates of change* in cognitive function, which may be an important factor in determining who may be at greatest risk for later acquisition of AD.

In the Baltimore Longitudinal Study of Aging, we investigated the cognitive and neural consequences of testosterone loss in aging men. In the first study [31], we investigated age-associated decreases in endogenous testosterone concentrations and declines in neuropsychological performance among 407 men aged 50 to 91 years. The men in the study were followed *longitudinally* for an average of ten years, with assessments of multiple cognitive domains and contemporaneous determination of serum total testosterone, sex hormone binding globulin, and a calculated free testosterone index. Also of note is that this study included multiple serial measures of testosterone, which were averaged in order to achieve a more reliable index of individual differences in long-term androgen exposure. In this study, higher free testosterone was associated with higher scores on visual and verbal memory and visuospatial functioning and with a reduced rate of decline in visual memory. No relations were observed between testosterone and measures of verbal knowledge, general mental status, or depressive symptoms. These results suggest a possible beneficial effect of high circulating free testosterone concentrations in older men on specific domains of cognitive performance and cognitive decline.

---

[1] Cognitive domains listed in the table do not necessarily cover all domains assessed in each study. The most common domains assessed across studies were selected for presentation. The Trail Making Test was included in the "Speed" construct.

In another longitudinal design based on the Honolulu-Asia Aging Study, a sample of 2,974 men were followed for an average of 6.1 years [28]. Consistent with the results from Moffat and colleagues [31], free testosterone levels were not associated with rate of change in general cognitive status as assessed by the Cognitive Abilities Screening Instrument. Results from any additional cognitive instruments from this study were not reported.

Much more numerous than the few longitudinal studies in the literature are the cross-sectional studies, which relate testosterone concentrations to cognitive function at a single point in time. Although a formal meta-analysis of these data is beyond the scope of this chapter, a number of observations can be made. First, there are numerous null findings in all cognitive domains, which may reflect either a true absence of a relationship or may reflect limitations of the cross-sectional study design noted above. Among those studies that reported statistically significant results, there are clearly more positive than negative findings. That is, there are more findings suggesting that higher levels of endogenous testosterone are beneficial to cognitive function than there are those suggesting the opposite. This is particularly true for the domains of verbal memory, spatial cognition, and speed (which includes the Trail Making test), for which there are several cross-sectional studies reporting positive effects and none reporting a negative relationship.

Clearly, the results of these studies are not dispositive. Association between testosterone levels and cognitive outcome in men is an area of much ongoing work and the subject of considerable debate. The literature in the field could be advanced with the publication of more longitudinal studies. Of course, even longitudinal studies do not answer the question of causality. It is possible that low testosterone levels or free testosterone levels may serve as a marker for, rather than a causative factor in, age-related cognitive decline. Most importantly, the literature relating testosterone to cognitive outcome in cross-sectional studies could also be improved by incorporating multiple blood draws taken over a longer time span to increase the reliability and validity of testosterone measurement.

Another critical element that may account for variability among studies is individual differences in particular subject characteristics. The most obvious one is age at assessment, as it is conceivable that steroids may have different or even opposite effects within an individual at different ages of their lifespan [39, 40]. Other important variables often go unassessed, and a recent study by Burkhardt attests to the potential importance of apolipoprotein E genotype status as a determinative factor [25]. This study showed that higher levels of free testosterone were associated with better cognitive function in men who were not ε4 carriers. In contrast, carriers of the ε4 allele showed exactly the opposite relationship; higher free testosterone levels were associated with lower scores on tests of executive functioning and working memory. This result suggests that variation in a single gene may reveal opposite findings in sub groups. It would be fascinating to know whether apolipoprotein E genotype status in the other studies reported in Table 21.1 could help resolve discrepancies.

Endogenous testosterone concentrations and risk for Alzheimer's disease and dementia in men

A related question concerning cognitive aging is whether age-related testosterone decline may be a risk factor for the development and diagnosis of AD. Results from studies relating testosterone concentrations to risk for AD are presented in Table 21.2. In general, there have been two approaches to this domain of research. One approach has been to select participants who have already been diagnosed with AD and compare their endogenous androgen levels with case controls who have not been diagnosed with AD or other dementia. Some recent cross-sectional studies have used this approach and reported lower testosterone concentrations in men diagnosed with AD [51, 45, 46, 47]. One study [49] found the opposite result, with AD cases having higher endogenous testosterone levels than controls. As discussed by Hogervorst and Bandelow [54], this study was unique in that it contained a large sample of case controls who were hypogonadal, calling into question the generalizability of the findings.

A problem with studies assessing androgen levels in individuals who have already been diagnosed with AD is that the observed differences in testosterone levels could be a consequence rather than a cause of the disease. For example, degenerative brain changes in AD could potentially alter hypothalamic-pituitary-gonadal axis function and result in altered steroid

Table 21.2 Studies relating testosterone concentrations and risk of Alzheimer's disease in older men.

Authors	N	Age	Years follow-up	Total T Free T	Risk for dementia	Risk for Alzheimer's disease	Risk for mild cognitive impairment
Moffat (2004) [43]	574	66	19.1	TT	0	0	
				FT	0	+	
Bowen (2000) [44]	69	85	0	TT	+		
				FT			
Geerlings (2006) [28]	2,974	77	6	TT			
				FT	0	0	
Hogervorst (2001) [45]	80	75	0	TT		+	
				FT			
Paoletti (2004) [46]	64	75	0	TT		0	
				FT		+	
Watanabe (2004) [47]	134	74	0	TT	+	+	
				FT			
Ravaglia (2007) [48]	376	74	4	TT			
				FT	0	0	
Pennanen (2004) [49]	30	72	0	TT	−	−	
				FT	−	−	
Rosario (2004)[a] [50]	45	72	0	TT		+	
				FT			
Hogervorst (2004) [51]	210	73	0	TT		+	
				FT		0	
Rasumuson (2002) [52]	55	76	0	TT			
				FT		0	
Chu (2008) [53]	203	75	0	TT		0	0
				FT		+	+

Note:
[a] brain levels of T
N: number of men on which primary data analyses were performed.
Years follow-up: number of years over which participants were followed in longitudinal study design. Cross-sectional studies are noted by 0 years follow-up.
TT, FT: results in each cognitive domain for total testosterone (TT) and free testosterone (FT).
+ : effect in study in which higher levels of testosterone were associated with lower risk for disease.
− : effect in study in which higher levels of testosterone were associated with higher risk for disease.
0 : effect in study in which there was null finding relating testosterone to cognitive performance.
Blank cells reflect cognitive domains that were not assessed.

hormone levels. Thus, it is important to evaluate hormone levels *prior* to the diagnosis of AD to be more certain that lower androgen levels do not follow central nervous system changes in AD.

The second approach to studying testosterone levels in association with risk for AD or dementia has been the prospective longitudinal design. In this approach, testosterone levels are assessed at baseline in individuals who do not have dementia. These individuals are then followed and evaluated for "conversion" to AD and the probability of subsequent AD diagnosis is related to earlier testosterone levels. There are, to my knowledge, only three studies that have used this approach. In one study from the Baltimore Longitudinal Study of Aging, testosterone concentrations were quantified in individuals prior to dementia diagnosis [43]. This was done by restricting assays only to those blood samples that were provided two, five, and ten years prior to AD diagnosis. Results revealed lower free testosterone levels in individuals diagnosed with AD compared to controls. More specifically, the results of this study revealed an approximately 26% reduction in the risk for AD for each ten unit increase in free testosterone. These results were robust with respect to restricting testosterone values to two, five, and ten years prior to AD diagnosis. The restriction of testosterone observations to as long as 10 years *prior* to AD diagnosis makes it less likely that the reduced testosterone concentrations observed in AD cases were a result of AD pathology. This study provides evidence that altered testosterone levels in AD may precede rather than follow diagnosis. Indeed it suggests that lower testosterone levels may be evident quite early in those individuals who go on to develop dementia years later. In this study, care was taken to control for health-related factors that may potentially affect testosterone concentrations or cognitive performance.

In two other longitudinal prospective studies, calculated free testosterone levels were not found to be associated with later dementia diagnoses. Geerlings *et al.* [28], followed 2,974 male participants for an average of six years and found no association with baseline testosterone levels. Ravaglia [48] followed 376 men for four years and similarly found no associatation with baseline testosterone levels. These three studies [28, 43, 48] are consistent in that none report that higher levels of testosterone may increase risk for AD. They are in conflict in that one study [43] reported a protective effect while two others reported null results [28, 48]. Similarities between the studies include the relatively large sample sizes and use of prospective design. However, there are also substantial differences between these studies, which may help to explain divergent results. First of all, in the study by Moffat and colleagues [43] the average age of the men (66 years) was younger and the duration of follow-up (19 years) longer than in the studies by Geerlings and

colleagues [28] (mean age = 77 years; six years follow-up) and by Ravaglia and colleagues [48] (mean age = 74 years; four years follow-up). Moreover, Moffat *et al.* used multiple assays of testosterone over time to compute a long-term average testosterone exposure. As in the literature on cognitive function, it is also possible that other unmeasured subject characteristics, such as apolipoprotein E genotype, may play an important mediating role, and future studies incorporating these measures may help to resolve differences between studies.

Another interesting possibility in explaining differences between studies is that relations between testosterone, cognitive function, and dementia could be mediated in part by age-related alterations in levels of gonadotropins. In response to lower testosterone with age in men, the pituitary gland may increase secretion of luteinizing hormone and follicle stimulating hormone to increase androgen levels [16]. One hypothesis argues that high levels of gonadotropins may have direct and deleterious effects on brain function [55]. Levels of gonadotropins were found to be increased in men with AD compared with age-matched controls [56]. These data could be interpreted to suggest that high levels of gonadotropins, rather than low levels of testosterone per se, may be critical. Of course hypotheses regarding the role of testosterone and gonadotropins in human aging need not be mutually exclusive. Low levels of testosterone may prove to be a risk factor for brain health by virtue of depriving the brain of an important neuroprotective agent, and high levels of gonadotropins could represent a concomitant risk factor.

In conclusion, data from extant epidemiologic studies are mixed both in the domain of relating testosterone levels to cognitive function in non-demented men as well as evaluating testosterone as a risk factor for AD. It could be cautiously concluded that the preponderance of the data are more consistent with a positive impact of testosterone levels on cognitive decline and risk for dementia. However, we are far from concluding unequivocally that high endogenous testosterone levels may enhance brain and cognitive function. It is important to note that all of the studies reviewed in this chapter are associational in design. Despite the fact that many of these studies controlled for many potentially confounding variables, controlling for these factors after the fact in advanced statistical models does not substitute for random assignment. This is true in both cross-sectional and longitudinal studies, although longitudinal designs offer considerable advantages.

To overcome the drawbacks that are inherent in associational studies, it is essential to perform randomized intervention studies to more conclusively investigate the possible cognitive effects of testosterone. In particular, what is needed in this field are large, well controlled intervention studies assessing the effects of testosterone intervention on multiple body systems. Currently there is some cause for optimism that testosterone may aid the treatment of cognitive and neural dysfunction in some aging men. However, even if testosterone were unequivocally shown to enhance cognitive and brain function, these results would still have to be balanced with the possible consequences on other body systems.

References

1. Becker JB, Breedlove SM, Crews D. *Behavioral Endocrinology*. Cambridge, MA: MIT Press.

2. Kerr JE, Allore RJ, Beck SG, Handa RJ. Distribution and hormonal regulation of androgen receptor (AR) and AR messenger ribonucleic acid in the rat hippocampus. *Endocrinology*. 1995;**136**(8):3213–21.

3. Roof RL, Havens MD. Testosterone improves maze performance and induces development of a male hippocampus in females. *Brain Res*. 1992;**572**(1/2): 310–13.

4. Williams CL, Meck WH. The organizational effects of gonadal steroids on sexually dimorphic spatial ability. *Psychoneuroendocrinology*. 1991;**16**(1/3):155–76.

5. Jacobson CD, Csernus VJ, Shryne JE, Gorski RA. The influence of gonadectomy, androgen exposure, or a gonadal graft in the neonatal rat on the volume of the sexually dimorphic nucleus of the preoptic area. *J Neurosci*. 1981;**1**(10): 1142–7.

6. Diamond MC. Hormonal effects on the development of cerebral lateralization. *Psychoneuroendocrinology*. 1991;**16**(1–3):121–9.

7. Flood JF, Farr SA, Kaiser FE, La Regina M, Morley JE. Age-related decrease of plasma testosterone in SAMP8 mice: replacement improves age-related impairment of learning and memory. *Physiol Behav*. 1995;**57**(4):669–73.

8. Pouliot WA, Handa RJ, Beck SG. Androgen modulates N-methyl-D-aspartate-mediated depolarization in CA1 hippocampal pyramidal cells. *Synapse*. 1996;**23**(1):10–19.

9. Morse JK, DeKosky ST, Scheff SW. Neurotrophic effects of steroids on lesion-induced growth in the hippocampus. II. Hormone replacement. *Exp Neurol*. 1992;**118**(1):47–52.

10. Tirassa P, Thiblin I, Agren G, *et al*. High-dose anabolic androgenic steroids modulate concentrations of nerve growth factor and expression of its low affinity receptor (p75-NGFr) in male rat brain. *J Neurosci Res*. 1997;**47**(2):198–207.

11. Gouras GK, Xu H, Gross RS, *et al*. Testosterone reduces neuronal secretion of Alzheimer's beta-amyloid peptides. *Proc Natl Acad Sci USA*. 2000;**97**(3):1202–5.

12. Pike CJ. Testosterone attenuates beta-amyloid toxicity in cultured hippocampal neurons. *Brain Res*. 2001; **919**(1):160–5.

13. Rosario ER, Carroll JC, Oddo S, LaFerla FM, Pike CJ. Androgens regulate the development of neuropathology in a triple transgenic mouse model of Alzheimer's disease. *J Neurosci*. 2006;**26**(51): 13384–9.

14. Hammond J, Le Q, Goodyer C, *et al*. Testosterone-mediated neuroprotection through the androgen receptor in human primary neurons. *J Neurochem*. 2001;**77**(5):1319–26.

15. Harman SM, Metter EJ, Tobin JD, Pearson J, Blackman MR. Longitudinal effects of aging on serum total and free testosterone levels in healthy men. Baltimore Longitudinal Study of Aging. *J Clin Endocrinol Metab*. 2001;**86**(2):724–31.

16. Lamberts SW, van den Beld AW, van der Lely AJ. The endocrinology of aging. *Science*. 1997;**278**(5337): 419–24.

17. Carruthers M. *Androgen Deficiency in the Adult Male*. London, UK: Taylor & Francis.

18. Gruenewald DA, Matsumoto AM. Testosterone supplementation therapy for older men: potential benefits and risks. *J Am Geriatr Soc*. 2003;**51**(1): 101–15; discussion 115.

19. Tan RS. Memory loss as a reported symptom of andropause. *Arch Androl*. 2001;**47**(3): 185–9.

20. Christiansen K, Knussmann R.. Sex hormones and cognitive functioning in men. *Neuropsychobiology*. 1987;**18**(1):27–36.

21. Gouchie C, Kimura D. The relationship between testosterone levels and cognitive ability patterns. *Psychoneuroendocrinology*. 1991;**16**(4):323–34.

22. Moffat SD, Hampson E. A curvilinear relationship between testosterone and spatial cognition in humans: possible influence of hand preference. *Psychoneuroendocrinology*. 1996;**21**(3):323–37.

23. Aleman A, de Vries WR, Koppeschaar HP, *et al*. Relationship between circulating levels of sex hormones and insulin-like growth factor-1 and fluid intelligence in older men. *Exp Aging Res*. 2001; **27**(3): 283–91.

24. Barrett-Connor E, Goodman-Gruen D, Patay B. Endogenous sex hormones and cognitive function

in older men. *J Clin Endocrinol Metab*. 1999;**84**(10): 3681–5.

25. Burkhardt MS, Foster JK, Clarnette RM, *et al.* Interaction between testosterone and apolipoprotein E epsilon4 status on cognition in healthy older men. *J Clin Endocrinol Metab*. 2006;**91**(3):1168–72.

26. Driscoll I, Hamilton DA, Yeo RA, Brooks WM, Sutherland RJ. Virtual navigation in humans: the impact of age, sex, and hormones on place learning. *Horm Behav*. 2005;**47**(3):326–35.

27. Fonda SJ, Bertrand R, O'Donnell A, Longcope C, McKinlay JB. Age, hormones, and cognitive functioning among middle-aged and elderly men: cross-sectional evidence from the Massachusetts Male Aging Study. *J Gerontol A Biol Sci Med Sci*. 2005; **60**(3):385–90.

28. Geerlings MI, Strozyk D, Masaki K, *et al.* Endogenous sex hormones, cognitive decline, and future dementia in old men. *Ann Neurol*. 2006;**60**(3):346–55.

29. Hogervorst E, De Jager C, Budge M, Smith AD. Serum levels of estradiol and testosterone and performance in different cognitive domains in healthy elderly men and women. *Psychoneuroendocrinology*. 2004;**29**(3):405–21.

30. Martin DM, Wittert G, Burns NR, Haren MT, Sugarman R. Testosterone and cognitive function in ageing men: data from the Florey Adelaide Male Ageing Study (FAMAS). *Maturitas*. 2007;**57**(2):182–94.

31. Moffat SD, Zonderman AB, Metter EJ, *et al.* Longitudinal assessment of serum free testosterone concentration predicts memory performance and cognitive status in elderly men. *J Clin Endocrinol Metab*. 2002;**87**(11):5001–7.

32. Morley JE, Kaiser F, Raum WJ, *et al.* Potentially predictive and manipulable blood serum correlates of aging in the healthy human male: progressive decreases in bioavailable testosterone, dehydroepiandrosterone sulfate, and the ratio of insulin-like growth factor 1 to growth hormone. *Proc Natl Acad Sci USA*. 1997; **94**(14):7537–42.

33. Muller M, Aleman A, Grobbee DE, de Haan EH, van der Schouw YT. Endogenous sex hormone levels and cognitive function in aging men: is there an optimal level? *Neurology*. 2005;**64**(5):866–71.

34. Perry PJ, Lund BC, Arndt S, *et al.* Bioavailable testosterone as a correlate of cognition, psychological status, quality of life, and sexual function in aging males: implications for testosterone replacement therapy. *Ann Clin Psychiatry*. 2001;**13**(2):75–80.

35. Thilers PP, Macdonald SW, Herlitz A. The association between endogenous free testosterone and cognitive performance: a population-based study in 35 to 90 year-old men and women. *Psychoneuroendocrinology*. 2006;**31**(5):565–76.

36. Wolf OT, Kirschbaum C. Endogenous estradiol and testosterone levels are associated with cognitive performance in older women and men. *Horm Behav*. 2002;**41**(3):259–66.

37. Yaffe K, Lui LY, Zmuda J, Cauley J. Sex hormones and cognitive function in older men. *J Am Geriatr Soc*. 2002;**50**(4):707–12.

38. Yeap BB, Almeida OP, Hyde Z, *et al.* Higher serum free testosterone is associated with better cognitive function in older men, while total testosterone is not. The Health in Men Study. *Clin Endocrinol (Oxf)*. 2008;**68**(3):404–12.

39. Brinton RD. Investigative models for determining hormone therapy-induced outcomes in brain: evidence in support of a healthy cell bias of estrogen action. *Ann N Y Acad Sci*. 2005;**1052**:57–74.

40. Sherwin BB. Estrogen and memory in women: how can we reconcile the findings? *Horm Behav*. 2005; **47**(3):371–5.

41. Guazzo EP, Kirkpatrick PJ, Goodyer IM, Shiers HM, Herbert J. Cortisol, dehydroepiandrosterone (DHEA), and DHEA sulfate in the cerebrospinal fluid of man: relation to blood levels and the effects of age. *J Clin Endocrinol Metab*. 1996;**81**(11):3951–60.

42. Mulchahey JJ, Ekhator NN, Zhang H, *et al.* Cerebrospinal fluid and plasma testosterone levels in post-traumatic stress disorder and tobacco dependence. *Psychoneuroendocrinology*. 2001;**26**(3):273–85.

43. Moffat SD, Zonderman AB, Metter EJ, *et al.* Free testosterone and risk for Alzheimer disease in older men. *Neurology*. 2004;**62**(2):188–93.

44. Bowen RL, Isley JP, Atkinson RL. An association of elevated serum gonadotropin concentrations and Alzheimer disease. *J Neuroendocrinol*. 2000;**12**(4): 351–354.

45. Hogervorst E, Williams J, Budge M, *et al.* Serum total testosterone is lower in men with Alzheimer's disease. *Neuroendocrinol Lett*. 2001;**22**(3):163–8.

46. Paoletti AM, Congia S, Lello S, *et al.* Low androgenization index in elderly women and elderly men with Alzheimer's disease. *Neurology*. 2004;**62**(2):301–3.

47. Watanabe T, Koba S, Kawamura M, *et al.* Small dense low-density lipoprotein and carotid atherosclerosis in relation to vascular dementia. *Metabolism*. 2004; **53**(4):476–82.

48. Ravaglia G, Forti P, Maioli F, *et al.* Endogenous sex hormones as risk factors for dementia in elderly men and women. *J Gerontol A Biol Sci Med Sci*. 2007; **62**(9):1035–41.

49. Pennanen C, Laakso MP, Kivipelto M, Ramberg J, Soininen H. Serum testosterone levels in males with Alzheimer's disease. *J Neuroendocrinol*. 2004;**16**(2):95–8.

50. Rosario ER, Chang L, Stanczyk FZ, Pike CJ. Age-related testosterone depletion and the development of Alzheimer disease. *JAMA*. 2004;**292**(12):1431–2.

51. Hogervorst E, Bandelow S, Combrinck M, Smith AD. Low free testosterone is an independent risk factor for Alzheimer's disease. *Exp Gerontol*. 2004;**39**(11/12): 1633–9.

52. Rasmuson S, Nasman B, Carlstrom K, Olsson T. Increased levels of adrenocortical and gonadal hormones in mild to moderate Alzheimer's disease. *Dement Geriatr Cogn Disord*. 2002;**13**(2):74–9.

53. Chu LW, Tam S, Lee PW, *et al.* Bioavailable testosterone is associated with a reduced risk of amnestic mild cognitive impairment in older men. *Clin Endocrinol (Oxf)*. 2008;**68**(4):589–98.

54. Hogervorst E, Bandelow S. The controversy over levels of sex steroids in cases with Alzheimer's disease. *J Neuroendocrinol*. 2004;**16**(2):93–4.

55. Meethal SV, Smith MA, Bowen RL, Atwood CS. The gonadotropin connection in Alzheimer's disease. *Endocrine*. 2005;**26**(3):317–26.

56. Bowen RL, Smith MA, Harris PL, *et al.* Elevated luteinizing hormone expression colocalizes with neurons vulnerable to Alzheimer's disease pathology. *J Neurosci Res*. 2002;**70**(3):514–18.

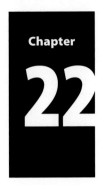
Clinical trials and neuroimaging studies of testosterone in men: insights into effects on verbal memory

Pauline M. Maki

Editors' introduction

Maki reviews randomized clinical trials of testosterone in older men, in which outcomes are based on standard neuropsychological measures or functional brain imaging with positron emission tomography. Her focus is on verbal memory, where deficits may predict the development of Alzheimer's disease (AD). Findings from these clinical studies are contradictory and sometimes confusing. Available evidence, however, suggests improvement of verbal memory, as long as testosterone therapy leads to moderate (but not large) increases in concentrations of estradiol or total testosterone. Maki believes estradiol may be a key determinant. For elderly men from the Baltimore Longitudinal Study of Aging, results of positron emission tomography link higher levels of testosterone to increased activity in brain areas involved in higher-order cognitive function. Of note, supraphysiological exogenous testosterone in one study was associated with decreased hippocampal activity and decreased verbal memory. Further research may help to understand more fully the impact of testosterone on brain function and the mechanisms by which testosterone can lead to beneficial and detrimental cognitive effects.

Background

There is great interest in testosterone as a potential modulator of brain aging in elderly men. This interest stems from preclinical studies that have identified mechanisms through which testosterone can influence the neuropathological cascade of events underlying the development of AD, as well as from clinical studies that find beneficial effects of testosterone on memory. However, a recent report of a negative impact of testosterone on memory and the brain regions subserving memory raises questions about the safety and efficacy of certain testosterone regimens in certain populations of men [1]. This recent report, coupled with recent findings that certain formulations of hormone therapy lead to declines in verbal memory [2] and increase a woman's risk of dementia [3], suggests a need for a better understanding of the potential beneficial and detrimental effects of testosterone on memory and brain function.

This chapter integrates findings from randomized clinical trials of testosterone and memory with findings from a randomized trial that used both neuroimaging and neuropsychological assessments to simultaneously identify the neural targets of testosterone supplementation in healthy elderly men and characterize its effects on memory performance. The general aim of the chapter is to demonstrate the utility of studies combining standardized cognitive assessments and functional neuroimaging in understanding the effects of testosterone on brain function in men. More specifically, the aims are: (1) to investigate the effects of testosterone supplementation on cognitive test performance, particularly verbal memory; (2) to investigate the effect of testosterone supplementation on patterns of brain activation during performance of a verbal memory task; and (3) to relate the observed changes in brain function to observed changes in verbal memory and hormone levels.

Biological plausibility

Longitudinal studies indicate that men experience a gradual loss of testosterone as they age [4–6]. Neuropathological evidence suggests that testosterone levels in the brain also decrease with age [7]. Several reports

---

associate low levels of endogenous testosterone with the development of AD. Serum levels of testosterone are reported to be lower in men with AD compared to controls [8], and low levels of free testosterone in aging men increase dementia risk and memory decline later in life [9, 10]. Men with a neuropathological diagnosis of AD and men with mild neuropathological markers of AD have lower brain levels of testosterone compared with neuropathologically normal men [7].

Basic science and human studies suggest that androgens may alter dementia risk by preventing brain deposition of β-amyloid protein, the neuropathological hallmark of AD. For example, androgen depletion via gonadectomy in rodents increases brain levels of β-amyloid, and supplementation with 5α-dihydrotestosterone, an active metabolite of testosterone, reverses that effect [11]. Testosterone supplementation reduces neuronal secretion of β-amyloid peptides and increases secretion of non-amyloidogenic soluble amyloid precursor protein peptides, possibly through conversion to estradiol [12, 13]. In humans, suppression of endogenous testosterone with androgen blockade therapy (i.e., flutamide and leuprolide) increased plasma β-amyloid levels [14, 15]. Plasma β-amyloid levels were negatively associated with verbal memory, but verbal memory improved upon discontinuation of the blockade [15]. Together, these studies suggest that testosterone may decrease risk for AD and verbal memory decline by increasing the activity of the α-secretase pathway and thereby decreasing the amount of β-amyloid deposition.

Effects of testosterone supplementation on verbal memory and other cognitive tests

The effects of testosterone on cognitive function in elderly men have been examined in eight randomized, placebo-controlled clinical trials [16–24]. Of these trials, five have investigated the effects of testosterone on verbal memory [17, 18, 21, 23, 24]. Two of these trials found no significant effect of testosterone on verbal memory [17, 18]. The first of these "neutral" studies was a study of 56 men (mean age 67 years; range 60–75 years) with normal baseline testosterone values randomized to receive either scrotal testosterone (15 mg/day) or placebo for three months [16].

Although a significant benefit was observed on a test of visuospatial function (i.e., the Block Design Test), no effect was observed on a standardized measure of verbal memory, the California Verbal Learning Test. The longest trial to date found no effect of 12 months of treatment with a larger dose of testosterone cypionate (200 mg intramuscularly every 14–17 days) on verbal memory (i.e., the Rey Auditory Verbal Learning Test), non-verbal memory, or verbal fluency test in 22 healthy men (mean age 65) with low baseline testosterone levels [18].

Three studies from the same laboratory have demonstrated reliable improvements in verbal memory, as well as visuospatial skills, with weekly injections of testosterone enanthate [21, 23, 24]. The first study involved 25 men with normal baseline testosterone values (mean age 67 years, range 50–80) and reported an improvement in verbal memory (i.e., story recall) over time in the group randomized to receive 100 mg intramuscular testosterone enanthate weekly for six weeks, but not in the placebo group [21]. Treatment-related improvements were also evident on measures of visuospatial memory (i.e., Walking Route) and visuospatial function (i.e., Block Design). A second study aimed to determine if the beneficial effects of testosterone enanthate on verbal memory were due to the conversion of testosterone to estradiol. That study paralleled the previous study in design but included a third treatment arm, 100 mg intramuscular testosterone enanthate weekly plus 1 mg oral anastrozole (an aromatase inhibitor) [23]. Sixty healthy elderly men participated (mean age 65 years; range 50–85). Verbal memory (i.e., story recall) was improved following testosterone enanthate treatment only without an aromatase inhibitor, suggesting that the conversion of testosterone enanthate to estradiol modulated the beneficial effects on verbal memory. Both the testosterone enanthate alone intervention and the testosterone enanthate with anastrazole intervention led to improved visuospatial performance, but this effect was significant only after 12 weeks in the testosterone-alone intervention. No significant effects were evident on tests of verbal fluency, selective attention (i.e., Stroop) or working memory (i.e., Self-Ordered Pointing Test). The third study examined the relationship between the magnitude of increase in testosterone and the magnitude of cognitive change [24]. Fifty-seven healthy, eugonadal men (mean age 67 years, range 50–85) were randomized to receive weekly injections of 50, 100, or 300 mg testosterone enanthate or placebo (saline) injection for six weeks. Neuropsychological assessments were completed at baseline, treatment week 3, treatment week 6, and post-treatment (i.e., after six weeks of wash-out). Because the 50 mg dose did not significantly increase testosterone levels, the cognitive results were analyzed not as a function of treatment arm but rather as a function of "change groups." There were three change groups, one showing no increase in testosterone (i.e., 0–10 nmol/L), one showing a moderate increase in testosterone (11–50 nmol/L), and another showing a large increase in testosterone (>50 nmol/L). Men with moderate increases in testosterone showed improvement on a test of spatial/navigational memory (i.e., Route Test) and a test of verbal memory (i.e., Word List). Importantly, however, men with large increases in testosterone showed no improvement in performance. Change in estradiol predicted change in performance on the word list test. Thus, these studies suggest that testosterone produces reliable improvements in verbal memory, and that this improvement is related to increases in estradiol with treatment.

The only study to demonstrate a negative impact of testosterone supplementation on verbal memory function was a randomized, double-blind, placebo-controlled crossover trial involving 15 cognitively normal men (mean age 73.9 years, range 66–86) [1]. Participants were randomized to receive testosterone enanthate (200 mg injections every other week for 90 days) crossed-over with placebo (intramuscular sesame oil vehicle) with a 90-day wash-out between treatments. The primary outcome was a standardized verbal memory test, the California Verbal Learning Test, though measures of working memory and attention, psychomotor speed, and figural memory were also obtained. Results revealed a significant worsening of short-delay verbal recall during treatment compared to placebo, $p < 0.05$, with a medium effect size, Cohen's $d = 0.59$. Treatment did not significantly affect performance on any other cognitive test. (Neuroimaging data are discussed below.) There was no significant relationship between the change in magnitude in estradiol, total testosterone, or free testosterone and change in cognitive test performance. However, free testosterone was assayed by an analog method that underestimates true free testosterone levels.

The reason for the variable effects across clinical trials of testosterone supplementation is difficult to determine. Trials vary with respect to treatment type and duration, individual cognitive tests, timing of cognitive testing in relation to intramuscular (IM) injections, and subject characteristics, particularly age, differed across studies. One trial demonstrated that the relationship between testosterone treatment and verbal memory depended on the magnitude of increase in testosterone and the magnitude of cognitive change [24].

To determine whether there is a systematic relationship between changes in total testosterone and estradiol, and changes in verbal memory across trials, we identified total testosterone values at baseline and post-treatment in each of the trials described above. The findings are shown in Figs. 22.1 and 22.2. Each study except the negative crossover study in older men [1] generally supports the view that there is no change in verbal memory with minimal or large increases in total testosterone. (The Janowsky, 1994, study [17] presented only free testosterone values.) In light of impressive evidence that changes in verbal memory following testosterone supplementation are due to changes in estradiol [23], it is helpful to explore the magnitude of increase in estradiol across those clinical trials. The two studies that found no increase in verbal memory with testosterone found no significant change in estradiol [17, 18]. All of the trials reporting improvements in verbal memory with testosterone showed an increase in estradiol [21, 23, 24]. However, an increase in estradiol of a similar magnitude was also evident in the crossover study that showed a negative impact of testosterone on verbal memory [1]. Thus, with one notable exception [1], the data support the view that testosterone treatments that produce moderate increases in total testosterone and estradiol are associated with enhanced verbal memory. Such an analysis might be taken with caution, however, since peripheral hormone levels have been shown to be an imprecise marker of brain hormone levels [25].

Another possibility is that the older age of the men in the crossover trial may account in part for the negative impact of exogenous testosterone on verbal memory. The mean age in that trial was 74 years (range 66–86), whereas in previous trials the mean age was generally around 65 years, with lower limits of 50 years. There is evidence from other physiological systems that testosterone may be less effective in older men. For example, older men do not always show an increase in bone mineral density in response to testosterone supplementation [26] [27], whereas

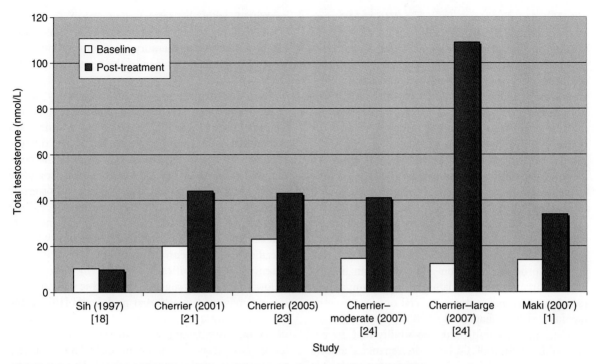

Fig. 22.1 Total testosterone at baseline and post treatment: results from randomized clinical trials.

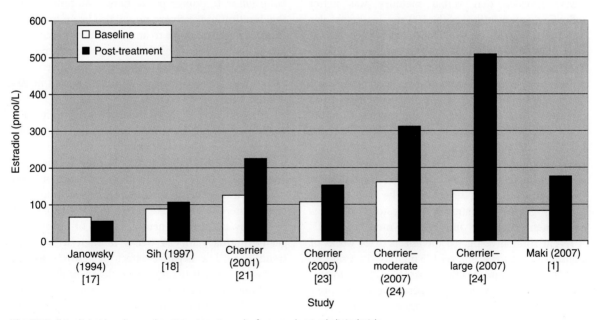

Fig. 22.2 Estradiol at baseline and post-treatment: results from randomized clinical trials.

younger men generally show benefits [28]. A recent review of randomized clinical trials of testosterone therapy found that younger, but not older, men show an increase in mood and sexual function with supplementation [29]. However, testosterone supplementation in older men is effective in improving body composition, and older men respond similarly to younger men to graded doses of testosterone

[30, 31]. Age differences in response to testosterone treatment may in part reflect the poorer clearance of testosterone in older men and may relate to increases in adverse events in this population [31, 32]. Moreover, the effect of total testosterone on health in older men may be reduced by age-related increases in sex hormone binding globulin, which would decrease the amount of free testosterone available to cross the blood–brain barrier [33].

A corollary to the view that testosterone effects on memory depend on age is the view that testosterone effects depend on the health of the cell. Such a view has been proposed for estrogen effects on the hippocampus, the structure that mediates performance on verbal memory. This view is called the healthy cell bias and asserts, at a simplistic descriptive level, that estrogen promotes function and survival in healthy hippocampal cells but in damaged hippocampal cells estrogen over time is not beneficial or is even detrimental [34] (see Chapter 6).

One study contradicts the possibility that the age or health of the cell explains discrepancies among studies. A clinical trial involving men with AD or mild cognitive impairment (MCI) (mean age = 76 years) revealed that verbal memory was better following intervention with 100 mg intramuscular testosterone enanthate weekly for six weeks compared with placebo [35]. There was no significant change over time in the testosterone group alone, so it is unclear whether the group differences reflected a decline in the placebo group, an improvement from treatment, or a combination of the two. One important limitation to that study, however, was the short trial duration of six weeks. An initial benefit of estrogen on cognitive function is observed in women with AD, even though no benefit or a trend toward harm is observed following several months of treatment [36]. Longer term treatment with testosterone does not benefit cognitive function in men with AD. A recent study investigated the effects of 24 weeks of transdermal testosterone gel (75 mg/day) in a sample of AD patients and healthy controls [37]. Testosterone supplementation had no effect on verbal memory in men with AD (mean age = 69.8 years). Moreover, among the healthy men, who were younger than the AD patients, both placebo-treated (n = 14; mean age = 61.2) and testosterone-treated men (n = 15; mean age = 63.6) showed an improvement in verbal memory over time, but the magnitude of improvement was twice as great in the placebo group

compared with the testosterone group (p = 0.10). Those data suggest potential negative effects of testosterone gel on verbal memory in eugonadal men who were younger than the men in the negative crossover trial.

Two final explanations for the discrepancy among trials are notable. One is the possibility that the timing of cognitive testing in relation to IM injections is a critical determinant of performance. The other is that the duration of treatment is critical. In the positive studies using IM injections [21, 23, 24], cognitive testing was undertaken during peak testosterone levels (23–48 hours following injection of 100 mg testosterone enanthate). The timing of memory assessments in relation to the IM injection was not specified in the neutral 12-month study, but the absence of a significant increase in testosterone following treatment suggests that testing was not done immediately post-injection at peak levels [18]. In the study showing a negative impact of testosterone on verbal memory, testing was undertaken during nadir levels (7–10 days after injection of 200 mg testosterone enanthate) following the peak [1]. Thus, it may be the dramatic decrease in sex hormone levels that contributed to poorer performance. As noted above, the duration of treatment might also be an important factor. The duration of treatment in the negative trial [1] was twice as long as the duration of treatment in the positive trials [21, 23, 24], twelve weeks versus six weeks. The longest trial (12 months) showed neutral effects [18].

In summary, there is a reliable improvement in verbal memory across three studies involving weekly injections of testosterone enanthate (100 mg) for six weeks in healthy men [21, 23, 24] and in men with AD or MCI [35]. Those findings contrast with evidence of a detrimental effect of biweekly intramuscular testosterone enanthate (200 mg) for 12 weeks [1] in healthy older men, neutral effects of testosterone gel (75 mg/day) for 24 weeks in men with AD, a trend toward a negative effect of testosterone gel (75 mg/day; p = 0.10) for 24 weeks in healthy eugonadal men, and neutral effects of scrotal testosterone (15 mg/day) for three months, or testosterone cypionate (200 mg IM every 14–17 days) for 12 months. It is unclear whether the findings differ because of the specific type of supplementations, the duration of supplementation, the age or health of the participants, or the timing of testing in relation to treatment. Testosterone supplementation may confer benefits to verbal memory in older men provided that the treatment is given in low dosages over short intervals. Yet to be fully determined is the impact of prolonged treatment on verbal memory.

Effects of testosterone on brain function in elderly men: implications for memory

Neuroimaging techniques, including functional magnetic resonance (MRI) imaging and positron emission tomography (PET), provide insights into the effects of hormonal supplementation on brain function. Our understanding of the effects of testosterone on the neural circuitry underlying verbal memory performance is currently limited to two PET studies, each involving elderly men. One of these studies used PET and bolus-injected [15-O] water to measure regional cerebral blood flow during a resting condition in relation to endogenous testosterone levels [38]. The other study used PET and [18-F] fluorodeoxyglucose (FDG) to investigate changes in neural circuitry during performance of a verbal memory test [1]. Each of these studies will be reviewed in turn.

The effect of changes in endogenous testosterone with age on brain function, cognition, and AD risk has been investigated in three studies from the Baltimore Longitudinal Study of Aging [9, 10, 38]. In each of these studies, testosterone levels were estimated from 24-hour urine specimens collected over several years, and free testosterone was estimated based on total testosterone levels and sex hormone binding globulin. The first study focused on risk of AD and involved a sample of 574 men with hormone samples collected over an average of 19 years [10]. Longitudinal increases in free testosterone – which crosses the blood–brain barrier – predicted a decreased risk of AD. The second study examined changes in endogenous testosterone over an average ten-year interval in relation to cognitive test performance in a sample of 407 men [9]. Higher free testosterone was associated with better performance on a variety of cognitive functions, including verbal memory, figural memory, mental rotations (i.e., a visuospatial ability that favors men), and psychomotor speed. The third study examined brain function using PET and involved a sample of 40 elderly men with samples over an average of 14 years [38]. Free testosterone levels predicted regional cerebral blood flow during a resting condition in several brain areas subserving memory and other cognitive functions. A higher free testosterone index was associated with increased blood flow in the bilateral hippocampus, anterior cingulate gyrus, and right inferior frontal cortex. Total testosterone predicted increased blood flow in the left putamen, bilateral thalamus, and left inferior frontal cortex and decreased blood flow in bilateral amygdala. Together, these three studies suggest that higher levels of endogenous testosterone exert neuroprotective effects on brain areas involved in higher-order cognitive function, including the prefrontal cortex and the hippocampus, and these effects may contribute to improved cognition and lowered risk of AD.

Another PET study investigated the effects of testosterone supplementation on regional glucose metabolism during performance of a verbal recognition test [1]. These effects were evaluated in a randomized double-blind, placebo-controlled cross-over trial involving 15 elderly men, who also participated in neuropsychological evaluations described above. The testosterone intervention involved biweekly injections of testosterone enanthate (200 mg). The verbal recognition task involved an encoding task wherein men studied a series of abstract words to be remembered later, followed by a 30-minute delay, and the activation task, which was a continuous verbal recognition task. The recognition task presented a series of studied and unstudied abstract words and required both recognition of previously studied words (i.e., "yes" or "no" responses on a hand-held button box) and encoding of newly presented words (i.e., initial "no" responses) that reappeared later (and were therefore "yes" responses). Men performed this task over a 30-minute period during FDG uptake and then completed PET scans to examine patterns of regional uptake of FDG during task performance. Two PET sessions were undertaken, one after a three-month placebo phase, and the other after a three-month active treatment phase. The inter-scan interval was six months, including a three-month wash-out phase. The primary hypotheses were that testosterone supplementation would increase regional metabolism in the medial temporal lobe (i.e., hippocampal formation) and in the prefrontal cortex. Note that this hypothesis was based on the expectation that testosterone would enhance verbal memory. As discussed above, testosterone unexpectedly decreased verbal memory performance, as measured by the

California Verbal Learning Test. Thus, it is reasonable to assume that the changes in brain function observed in these men reflected a detrimental effect of testosterone on neural circuitry underlying verbal memory performance.

Figures 22.3 and 22.4 show the changes in regional glucose metabolism associated with testosterone treatment. Results are presented as difference images that show the difference in regional brain function during testosterone treatment compared to placebo in three views – sagittal, axial, and coronal. The brightness in the image reflects the magnitude of the treatment effect; the brighter the regional difference, the larger the effect of treatment. As shown in Fig. 22.3, testosterone supplementation led to a decrease in relative activity (representing regional glucose metabolism) in a medial temporal region that encompassed the right dorsal entorhinal cortex and the amygdala. There was also a trend ($p < 0.05$) toward an increase in relative activity in the left entorhinal cortex, right posterior hippocampus, and right parahippocampal gyrus. As shown in Fig. 22.4, compared to placebo, testosterone treatment led to widespread increases in relative activity in multiple prefrontal regions, including the left medial (Brodmann area 25), superior (Brodmann area 10), and inferior (Brodmann area 45, 46) frontal regions, and right middle (Brodmann area 46) and orbital (Brodmann area 47) regions.

Next a correlational analysis was undertaken to better understand the significance of the changes in brain activity observed with testosterone supplementation. Correlations were conducted to determine whether the magnitude of change in brain function was related to the magnitude of change in hormone levels or the magnitude of change in memory score. For each change score, the placebo value was subtracted from the testosterone value. As shown in Table 22.1, the magnitude of decline in activation in the right amygdala/entorhinal cortex related to the magnitude of decline on the California Verbal Learning Test ($r = 0.45$, $p = 0.10$). This finding suggested that testosterone-induced decreases in the hippocampal formation and amygdala may contribute to decreased verbal memory performance. Changes in activity in the left entorhinal cortex, and left Brodmann area 45, 46, and 47 were each significantly and positively related to changes in free testosterone. Change in activity in the right Brodmann area 47 was positively related to the change in both free testosterone and performance on the activation task. Thus, the only prefrontal area to predict a change in behavior was the Brodmann area 47, orbital frontal cortex.

It is notable that each of the two PET studies – one examining endogenous testosterone and the other examining exogenous testosterone – found changes in hippocampal activity with testosterone, but the studies found effects in opposite directions. High endogenous testosterone was associated with increased hippocampal activity and verbal memory, whereas supraphysiological exogenous testosterone was associated with decreased hippocampal activity and decreased memory. Androgen receptor containing cells are abundant in the hippocampus [39], on the same order of magnitude as the prostate [40], suggesting that the hippocampus may mediate effects of androgens on memory performance. Physiological levels of testosterone help to maintain normal density of dendritic spines in the CA1 region of the hippocampus in non-human primate [41] and rat models [42]. It may be that supraphysiological levels of testosterone in older men negatively influence the function of the hippocampus, thereby negatively impacting verbal memory. In contrast, high endogenous levels of testosterone in older men may positively impact the function of the hippocampus, thereby positively impacting verbal memory.

Both endogenous and exogenous testosterone also impacted function of prefrontal cortex in elderly men. The dorsolateral and orbitofrontal prefrontal cortex subserve memory performance, and these brain regions contain intracellular androgen receptor proteins in neurons and glia [43]. A review of neuroimaging studies found associations between various prefrontal areas and specific aspects of memory performance, specifically between the left Brodmann area 45 and verbal episodic encoding tasks, the right Brodmann area 46 and verbal retrieval, and the left Brodmann area 40 and working memory [44]. Testosterone supplementation primarily led to increases in left hemisphere areas during verbal recognition. This left hemisphere finding is interesting in light of the finding that cortico–cortico projections of androgen-receptor containing neurons are strong within the same hemisphere [45]. It is likely that the verbal recognition task differentially increased activity in the left hemisphere because the test was a verbal test and verbal tests differentially invoke left hemisphere structures.

In the exogenous testosterone supplementation study, the largest area of increase was the left inferior

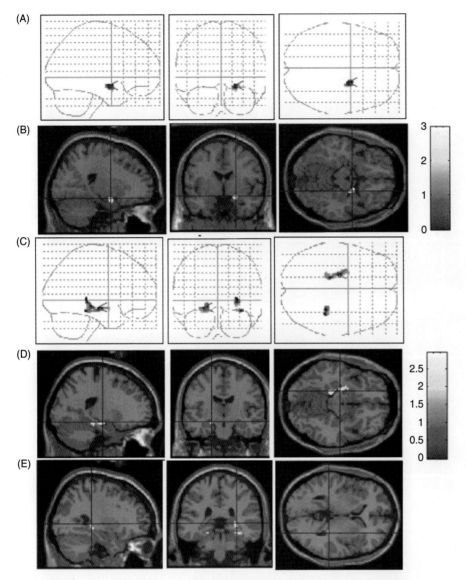

Fig. 22.3 Effects of testosterone on glucose metabolism in the hippocampus and amygdala during performance of a verbal memory task. This figure shows within-subject changes in relative brain activity with testosterone supplementation compared with placebo. Brain areas showing significant changes are labeled with the anatomical location by Brodmann area and Talairach coordinates (x, y, z). Panel A shows glass-brain sagittal, coronal, and axial projections of all medial temporal regions showing significant (p < 0.01) decreases in glucose metabolism with testosterone supplementation compared with placebo. Panel B highlights treatment-related decrease in right entorhinal cortex/amygdala (22, −2, −10). Panel C shows glass-brain projections of all medial temporal regions demonstrating trends (p < 0.05) of increased glucose metabolism with testosterone supplementation compared with placebo. Panel D highlights treatment-related increase in the left entorhinal cortex, Brodmann area 28 (−20, −14, −9) in the crosshairs. Panel E highlights treatment-related increase in the right posterior hippocampus (30, −33, 3) in crosshairs, and the coronal view also shows increase in the right parahippocampal gyrus, Brodmann area 36 (36, −36, −12). Maki, P. M. *et al. Journal of Clinical Endocrinology and Metabolism*. 2007 Nov;92(11):4107–14. © 2007, The Endocrine Society. (See color plate section.)

parietal lobe (Brodmann area 40) – an area that was not shown to be affected by endogenous testosterone. Notably, a similar testosterone-related increase in activation in this area was reported during viewing of visually sexual stimuli in a comparison of hypogonadal men receiving treatment with testosterone compared with controls [46]. Testosterone effects on brain function during the viewing of sexual stimuli were

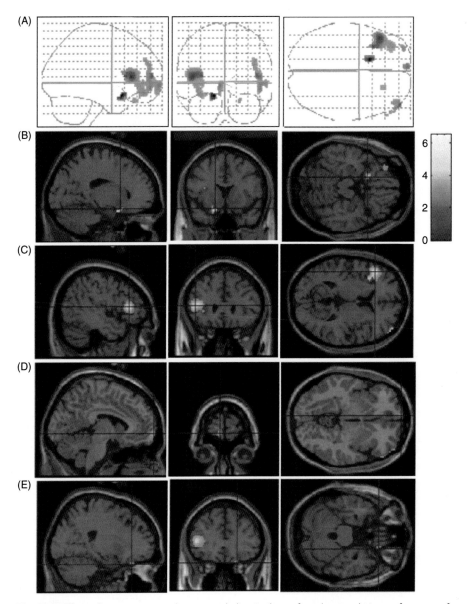

Fig. 22.4 Effects of testosterone on glucose metabolism in the prefrontal cortex during performance of a verbal memory task. This figure shows within-subject increases in relative brain activity with testosterone supplementation compared with placebo. Brain areas showing significant increases are labeled with the anatomical location by Brodmann Area and Talairach coordinates (x, y, z). Panel A shows glass-brain sagittal, coronal, and axial projections of all prefrontal areas showing significant increases in glucose metabolism with testosterone supplementation compared with placebo. Panel B highlights the left medial frontal gyrus, subgenual, Brodmann area 25 (−16, 13, −16), in the crosshairs, and the axial view also shows left superior frontal gyrus, Brodmann area 10 (−32, 60, −3). Panel C highlights the left inferior frontal cortex, Brodmann area 45 and 46 (−46, 28, 8), in the crosshairs, and the axial view also shows increase in the right middle frontal gyrus Brodmann area 46 (48, 55, 5). Panel D highlights the left superior frontal gyrus, Brodmann area 10 (−6, 66, −7). Panel E highlights the right orbitofrontal cortex, Brodmann area 47 (22, 30, −23). Maki, P. M. *et al. Journal of Clinical Endocrinology and Metabolism.* 2007 Nov;92 (11):4107–14. © 2007, The Endocrine Society. (See color plate section.)

similar to those observed in the verbal memory study, but were in the opposite hemisphere, including effects in the insula, orbitofrontal cortex (Brodmann area 47), and the middle temporal gyrus. Testosterone treatment increased activation in those areas in the right hemisphere during processing of sexual pictures and in the left hemisphere areas during processing of written words.

Table 22.1 Relationship between the change in brain activation following testosterone supplementation and the change in hormone levels and memory performance.

Brain region	Direction of treatment effect	HORMONE VALUES			MEMORY PERFORMANCE	
		Estradiol	Total testosterone	Free testosterone	Activation task	California Verbal Learning Test Composite
Right amygdala/ entorhinal	Decrease	0.10	0.27	−0.13	−0.03	0.45
Left entorhinal	Increase[a]	0.00	0.16	0.57*	−0.03	−0.28
Left BA 25	Increase	−0.31	−0.34	−0.05	0.06	−0.04
Left BA 45/46	Increase	0.40	0.56*	0.77**	0.22	0.08
Right BA 46	Increase	0.12	0.34	0.02	0.23	0.22
Left BA 10	Increase	0.20	0.18	−0.02	0.20	0.22
Left BA 10	Increase	0.47	0.26	0.53[a]	0.03	−0.08
Right BA 47	Increase	0.16	0.45	0.57*	0.55*	0.22

Note: *p < 0.05, **p < 0.01. BA = Brodmann area. The first column lists only a priori regions of interest that showed a significant change in metabolism during testosterone treatment compared to placebo. The second column is a reminder of the direction of the change in this region during testosterone treatment compared to placebo. The remaining columns show the magnitude of correlation (Pearson's r) between change scores for each outcome variable, where change scores were calculated by subtracting the placebo score from the testosterone score. For example, the increase in glucose metabolism in the left Brodmann area 45/46 following testosterone treatment (shown in Fig. 22.3C) was positively associated with the increase in serum free testosterone following testosterone treatment (r = 0.56 *p < 0.05) and the increase in total testosterone following treatment (r = 0.77 **p < 0.01).
[a] Trend p < 0.10. Note that correlations are not shown for the right posterior hippocampus and right parahippocampal gyrus – regions showing a trend toward an increase with treatment (p < 0.05) – because not all participants had suprathreshold values for these regions.

In summary, the sparse neuroimaging literature on testosterone and brain function in relation to verbal memory suggests that testosterone impacts the function of the hippocampus, prefrontal cortex, and parietal cortex. The direction of brain changes frequently parallels the direction of behavioral changes, such that testosterone-related decreases in verbal memory are associated with decreases in hippocampal activity and testosterone-related increases in verbal memory are associated with increases in hippocampal activity. Additional studies are needed to elucidate the impact of testosterone on brain function and to better understand the mechanisms by which testosterone can exert positive or negative cognitive effects.

effects of testosterone on verbal memory is important, because decreases in verbal memory are significant early predictors of AD and can predict AD up to ten years before diagnosis [47]. In light of the increased use of testosterone among the elderly male population, there is a pressing need for larger, longer duration clinical trials. The possibility that at least some testosterone regimens can have harmful cognitive effects further underscores the need for additional studies. There is a need for careful consideration of the route of administration, dose, timing of testing in relation to treatment, duration of treatment, and population under study. At the present time, testosterone supplementation is not indicated for the treatment of memory problems or for the prevention of memory loss with age.

General summary

Randomized clinical trials of testosterone supplementation provide contradictory findings regarding effects on verbal memory. An understanding of the

References

1. Maki PM, Ernst M, London ED, *et al.* Intramuscular testosterone treatment in elderly men: evidence of

memory decline and altered brain function. *J Clin Endocrinol Metab*. 2007;**92**(11):4107–14.

2. Resnick SM, Maki PM, Rapp SR, *et al*. Effects of combination estrogen plus progestin hormone treatment on cognition and affect. *J Clin Endocrinol Metab*. 2006;**91**(5):1802–10.

3. Shumaker S, Legault C, Rapp S, *et al*. Estrogen plus progestin and the incidence of dementia and mild cognitive impairment in postmenopausal women: the Women's Health Initiative Memory Study: a randomized controlled trial. *JAMA*. 2003;**289**:2651–62.

4. Morley JE, Kaiser FE, Perry HM, 3rd, *et al*. Longitudinal changes in testosterone, luteinizing hormone, and follicle-stimulating hormone in healthy older men. *Metabolism*. 1997;**46**(4):410–13.

5. Harman SM, Metter EJ, Tobin JD, Pearson J, Blackman MR. Longitudinal effects of aging on serum total and free testosterone levels in healthy men. Baltimore Longitudinal Study of Aging. *J Clin Endocrinol Metab*. 2001 Feb;**86**(2):724–31.

6. Feldman HA, Longcope C, Derby CA, *et al*. Age trends in the level of serum testosterone and other hormones in middle-aged men: longitudinal results from the Massachusetts male aging study. *J Clin Endocrinol Metab*. 2002;**87**(2):589–98.

7. Rosario ER, Chang L, Stanczyk FZ, Pike CJ. Age-related testosterone depletion and the development of Alzheimer disease. *JAMA*. 2004;**292**(12):1431–2.

8. Hogervorst E, Williams J, Budge M, *et al*. Serum total testosterone is lower in men with Alzheimer's disease. *Neuro Endocrinol Lett*. 2001;**22**(3):163–8.

9. Moffat SD, Zonderman AB, Metter EJ, *et al*. Free testosterone and risk for Alzheimer disease in older men. *Neurology*. 2004;**62**(2):188–93.

10. Moffat SD, Zonderman AB, Metter EJ, *et al*. Longitudinal assessment of serum free testosterone concentration predicts memory performance and cognitive status in elderly men. *J Clin Endocrinol Metab*. 2002;**87**(11):5001–7.

11. Ramsden M, Nyborg AC, Murphy MP, *et al*. Androgens modulate beta-amyloid levels in male rat brain. *J Neurochem*. 2003;**87**(4):1052–5.

12. Gouras GK, Xu H, Gross RS, *et al*. Testosterone reduces neuronal secretion of Alzheimer's beta-amyloid peptides. *Proc Natl Acad Sci USA*. 2000;**97**(3):1202–5.

13. Goodenough S, Engert S, Behl C. Testosterone stimulates rapid secretory amyloid precursor protein release from rat hypothalamic cells via the activation of the mitogen-activated protein kinase pathway. *Neurosci Lett*. 2000;**296**(1):49–52.

14. Gandy S, Almeida OP, Fonte J, *et al*. Chemical andropause and amyloid-beta peptide. *JAMA*. 2001;**285**(17):2195–6.

15. Almeida OP, Waterreus A, Spry N, Flicker L, Martins RN. One year follow-up study of the association between chemical castration, sex hormones, beta-amyloid, memory and depression in men. *Psychoneuroendocrinology*. 2004;**29**(8):1071–81.

16. Janowsky JS, Chavez B, Orwoll E. Sex steroids modify working memory. *J Cogn Neurosci*. 2000;**12**(3):407–14.

17. Janowsky JS, Oviatt SK, Orwoll ES. Testosterone influences spatial cognition in older men. *Behav Neurosci*. 1994;**108**(2):325–32.

18. Sih R, Morley JE, Kaiser FE, *et al*. Testosterone replacement in older hypogonadal men: a 12-month randomized controlled trial. *J Clin Endocrinol Metab*. 1997;**82**(6):1661–7.

19. Kenny AM, Bellantonio S, Gruman CA, Acosta RD, Prestwood KM. Effects of transdermal testosterone on cognitive function and health perception in older men with low bioavailable testosterone levels. *J Gerontol A Biol Sci Med Sci*. 2002;**57**(5):M321–5.

20. Kenny AM, Fabregas G, Song C, Biskup B, Bellantonio S. Effects of testosterone on behavior, depression, and cognitive function in older men with mild cognitive loss. *J Gerontol A Biol Sci Med Sci*. 2004;**59**(1):75–8.

21. Cherrier MM, Asthana S, Plymate S, *et al*. Testosterone supplementation improves spatial and verbal memory in healthy older men. *Neurology*. 2001;**57**(1):80–8.

22. Haren MT, Wittert GA, Chapman IM, Coates P, Morley JE. Effect of oral testosterone undecanoate on visuospatial cognition, mood and quality of life in elderly men with low-normal gonadal status. *Maturitas*. 2005;**50**(2):124–33.

23. Cherrier MM, Matsumoto AM, Amory JK, *et al*. The role of aromatization in testosterone supplementation: effects on cognition in older men. *Neurology*. 2005;**64**(2):290–6.

24. Cherrier MM, Matsumoto AM, Amory JK, *et al*. Characterization of verbal and spatial memory changes from moderate to supraphysiological increases in serum testosterone in healthy older men. *Psychoneuroendocrinology*. 2007;**32**(1):72–9.

25. Yue X, Lu M, Lancaster T, *et al*. Brain estrogen deficiency accelerates A-beta plaque formation in an Alzheimer's disease animal model. *Proc Natl Acad Sci USA*. 2005;**102**(52):19198–203.

26. Snyder PJ, Peachey H, Hannoush P, *et al*. Effect of testosterone treatment on bone mineral density in men over 65 years of age. *J Clin Endocrinol Metab*. 1999;**84**(6):1966–72.

27. Liverman CT, Blazer DG. *Testosterone and aging: clinical research directions*. Institute of Medicine Committee on Assessing the Need for Clinical Trials of Testosterone Replacement Therapy. Washington DC: National Academies Press, 2003.

28. Swerdloff RS, Wang C. Androgens and the ageing male. *Best Pract Res Clin Endocrinol Metab.* 2004;**18**(3):349–62.

29. Krause W, Mueller U, Mazur A. Testosterone supplementation in the aging male: which questions have been answered? *Aging Male.* 2005;**8**(1):31–8.

30. Snyder PJ, Peachey H, Hannoush P, *et al.* Effect of testosterone treatment on body composition and muscle strength in men over 65 years of age. *J Clin Endocrinol Metab.* 1999;**84**(8):2647–53.

31. Bhasin S, Woodhouse L, Casaburi R, *et al.* Older men are as responsive as young men to the anabolic effects of graded doses of testosterone on the skeletal muscle. *J Clin Endocrinol Metab.* 2005;**90**(2):678–88.

32. Wang C, Catlin DH, Starcevic B, *et al.* Testosterone metabolic clearance and production rates determined by stable isotope dilution/tandem mass spectrometry in normal men: influence of ethnicity and age. *J Clin Endocrinol Metab.* 2004 ;**89**(6):2936–41.

33. Snyder PJ. Effects of age on testicular function and consequences of testosterone treatment. *J Clin Endocrinol Metab.* 2001;**86**(6):2369–72.

34. Brinton RD. Investigative models for determining hormone therapy-induced outcomes in brain: evidence in support of a healthy cell bias of estrogen action. *Ann N Y Acad Sci.* 2005;**1052**:57–74.

35. Cherrier MM, Matsumoto AM, Amory JK, *et al.* Testosterone improves spatial memory in men with Alzheimer disease and mild cognitive impairment. *Neurology.* 2005;**64**(12):2063–8.

36. Mulnard RA, Cotman CW, Kawas C, *et al.* Estrogen replacement therapy for treatment of mild to moderate Alzheimer disease: a randomized controlled trial. *JAMA.* 2000;**283**:1007–15.

37. Lu PH, Masterman DA, Mulnard R, *et al.* Effects of testosterone on cognition and mood in male patients with mild Alzheimer disease and healthy elderly men. *Arch Neurol.* 2006;**63**(2):177–85.

38. Moffat SD, Resnick SM. Long-term measures of free testosterone predict regional cerebral blood flow patterns in elderly men. *Neurobiol Aging.* 2007;**28**(6):914–20.

39. Simerly RB, Chang C, Muramatsu M, Swanson LW. Distribution of androgen and estrogen receptor mRNA-containing cells in the rat brain: an in situ hybridization study. *J Comp Neurol.* 1990;**294**(1):76–95.

40. Beyenburg S, Watzka M, Clusmann H, *et al.* Androgen receptor mRNA expression in the human hippocampus. *Neurosci Lett.* 2000;**294**(1):25–8.

41. Leranth C, Prange-Kiel J, Frick KM, Horvath TL. Low CA1 spine synapse density is further reduced by castration in male non-human primates. *Cereb Cortex.* 2004;**14**(5):503–10.

42. Leranth C, Petnehazy O, MacLusky NJ. Gonadal hormones affect spine synaptic density in the CA1 hippocampal subfield of male rats. *J Neurosci.* 2003;**23**(5):1588–92.

43. Finley SK, Kritzer MF. Immunoreactivity for intracellular androgen receptors in identified subpopulations of neurons, astrocytes and oligodendrocytes in primate prefrontal cortex. *J Neurobiol.* 1999;**40**(4):446–57.

44. Cabeza R, Nyberg L. Imaging cognition II: an empirical review of 275 PET and fMRI studies. *J Cogn Neurosci.* 2000;**12**(1):1–47.

45. Kritzer M. The distribution of immunoreactivity for intracellular androgen receptors in the cerebral cortex of hormonally intact adult male and female rats: localization in pyramidal neurons making corticocortical connections. *Cereb Cortex.* 2004;**14**(3):268–80.

46. Redoute J, Stoleru S, Gregoire MC, *et al.* Brain processing of visual sexual stimuli in human males. *Hum Brain Mapp.* 2000;**11**(3):162–77.

47. Tierney MC, Yao C, Kiss A, McDowell I. Neuropsychological tests accurately predict incident Alzheimer disease after 5 and 10 years. *Neurology.* 2005;**64**(11):1853–9.

Chapter 23

Testosterone therapy and Alzheimer's disease: potential for treatment and prevention in women

Whitney Wharton, Sanjay Asthana, and Carey E. Gleason

Editors' introduction

Testosterone, an androgen, is viewed as a male hormone and for this reason is less studied in women than in men. In postmenopausal women, testosterone concentrations are affected by a number of factors, including age and whether a woman has undergone oophorectomy. Past hormonal exposures may also be relevant. In this chapter, Wharton, Asthana, and Gleason review research indicating that testosterone affects function of the hippocampus and other brain regions, and that testosterone has actions that might be expected to reduce Alzheimer's disease (AD) risk in women as well as men. Some studies in women suggest a relation between testosterone therapy or testosterone concentrations and performance on cognitive tasks involving visuospatial abilities. Unfortunately, few data are available on testosterone administration in women at risk for AD or with symptoms of this disorder. The authors conclude that further research is warranted on the cognitive effects of testosterone administration in older women, perhaps concurrently with estradiol and perhaps particularly in women who have experienced surgical menopause.

Background

Approximately 1.5 to 3 times more women are diagnosed with AD than men [1]. This may be due to an inherent increased risk for AD in women, possibly brought on by the decline in circulating sex hormone levels at menopause. It is widely hypothesized that the natural decline of sex hormones across the lifespan and the drastic drop during menopause is largely responsible for the acceleration of aging effects on cognition. This decline has received much attention and has led to the investigation of multiple hormone therapy (HT) techniques. It is believed that HT, particularly low-dose formulations of transdermal estradiol, exerts neuroprotective properties and may be protective against the development of AD.

Estrogens are unquestionably the most widely studied sex hormones in women. Much less is known about the physiological and cognitive properties of other sex hormones such as luteinizing hormone, follicle stimulating hormone, and androgens such as dehydroepiandrosterone and testosterone. Although testosterone is one of the most abundant sex hormones in the female body, it is arguably the least studied. Most likely, this is because testosterone is typically thought of as a "male" hormone and there is much controversy surrounding testosterone therapy in women. Testosterone is most often prescribed off-label to women in conjunction with HT in order to treat menopausal symptoms such as hot flashes, decreased energy, and sexual dysfunction. The relationship between testosterone and AD in men is quite different than the relation observed in women. Additionally, there has been significantly more research devoted to examining the relation in men, and these studies are discussed elsewhere in this volume. This chapter will serve to inform the reader about testosterone administration in postmenopausal women. We will focus on the neurophysiological and cognitive implications, as well as the potential neuroprotective properties of testosterone and how these factors relate to possible AD prevention in women.

Testosterone across the lifespan

In women, approximately one-third of circulating testosterone is produced in the ovaries, while the remaining two-thirds comes from peripheral

---

Hormones, Cognition and Dementia: State of the Art and Emergent Therapeutic Strategies, ed. Eef Hogervorst, Victor W. Henderson, Robert B. Gibbs, and Roberta Diaz Brinton. Published by Cambridge University Press.
© Cambridge University Press 2009.

conversion of precursors derived from the adrenal glands and ovaries via aromatization of estradiol [2]. Testosterone levels begin to decline at approximately 25 years of age and continue until age 40. Unlike estradiol and other estrogens, testosterone levels do not markedly drop at the menopausal transition [3, 4]. In fact, some investigators have reported an increase in androgen levels at menopause [3, 4]. Although there does seem to be evidence of a brief elevation in androgen levels, androgen levels subside relatively quickly and testosterone levels fall to levels averaging half of those in younger women. Conversely, women who are surgically menopausal experience a drastic 50% decrease in circulating levels of testosterone [5]. In a recent study conducted by Davison, total testosterone, calculated free testosterone, dehydroepiandrosterone sulfate, and androstenedione levels declined steeply with age, with the decline being greater in the earlier than the later decades of life [6]. Furthermore, no marked decline of testosterone was noted at the menopausal transition in intact women, and testosterone was continually produced postmenopausally. On the other hand, women who reported bilateral oophorectomy had significantly lower total testosterone and free testosterone levels than their age-matched, naturally postmenopausal counterparts. Based on these results, age and surgical status likely influence endogenous testosterone levels and should be taken into account when testosterone levels are evaluated in women.

Neurobiology of testosterone
Hormone therapy and the hippocampus

The modulatory effects of exogenous sex hormones on the brain have been well documented. The medial temporal lobes and hippocampus are particularly inundated with estrogen and testosterone receptors. For instance, our laboratory recently explored the effect of long-term hormone therapy on cerebral activation during a functional magnetic resonance imaging verbal encoding task in a group of non-hysterectomized, postmenopausal women [7]. Our comparison of women either naive or exposed to HT revealed a difference in signal change bilaterally in the medial temporal lobes, including the right hippocampus, such that HT-treated women exhibited greater hippocampal activation. More recently, we presented the results of a study in which we examined hippocampal activation in a postmenopausal cohort

at risk for developing AD based on familial history [8]. Our results showed that exposure to HT regimens were associated with an increase in neuronal activation specific to the hippocampus. Additionally, there was a linear relationship between HT treatment duration and hippocampal activation, where women who began HT at the menopausal transition had significantly more hippocampal activation than women who began HT later in life. Our results are supported by previous work in which short-term HT enhanced activation of the neural network underlying working memory [9].

Testosterone and the hippocampus

An abundance of research has examined the relation between individual sex hormones and the neuromodulatory benefits of HT regimens. Like estrogens, there is convincing evidence from basic research that testosterone exerts significant neuromodulatory and neurotrophic effects on the brain. For instance, in men, low levels of testosterone have been linked to an increased risk of developing AD [10]. Additionally, Cherrier et al. have shown that testosterone supplementation not only improves spatial ability in healthy older men, but they reported that testosterone also improves spatial memory in men with AD and mild cognitive impairment [11, 12] (see Chapter 20). As discussed in the preceding paragraph, the hippocampus is one of the brain regions most affected by sex hormones as evidenced by its abundant number of androgen receptors. Importantly, the hippocampus is a region involved in cognitive functioning, particularly memory.

Additionally, it is well established that the hippocampus is particularly affected in AD patients. Testosterone reportedly increases excitatory postsynaptic potential amplitudes and CA1 hippocampal population spike amplitudes [13]. One study found that testosterone therapy prevents N-methyl-D-aspartate (NMDA) excitotoxicity in hippocampal neurons [14] and may facilitate injury recovery by promoting fiber outgrowth and sprouting [15]. Also, administration of testosterone increases nerve growth factor levels in the hippocampus and induces an up-regulation of nerve growth factor receptors in the forebrain [16]. In a small recent study, brain-activation patterns of surgically postmenopausal women were similar to premenopausal women during treatment with estradiol and testosterone but not during treatment with estradiol alone [17]. The authors concluded that agonadal serum hormone levels result in globally decreased brain-activation patterns in postmenopausal women.

In an important study conducted by Leranth involving ovariectomized rats, short-term testosterone administration reversed the loss of CA1 area pyramidal spine synapses [18]. The authors also point out that the neuroprotective effects are not due solely to the aromatization of testosterone to estrogen, as an aromatase-independent testosterone formulation produced the same beneficial outcome. Based on these results, Leranth suggests that testosterone therapy may be as effective as estrogen therapy in reversing the decline in the CA1 region of the hippocampus that occurs in hysterectomized women, and ultimately protecting against the development of AD. Taken together, these results suggest that testosterone is heavily implicated in neuronal protection and facilitation, especially in the hippocampus, via multiple mechanisms. The fact that testosterone has the ability to impart neuromodulatory and neurotrophic effects on the hippocampus, an area principally affected in AD, likely led to the development of research surrounding testosterone's potential influence on AD.

Testosterone and Alzheimer's disease

The hallmarks of AD are senile plaques and neurofibrillary tangles. Senile plaques are composed of aggregated β-amyloid peptide, and neurofibrillary tangles are composed of abnormal filaments consisting primarily of hyperphosphorylated tau protein. Testosterone has been associated with reduced plasma concentrations of β-amyloid [19] and reduced tau phosphorylation [20], suggesting that testosterone may protect against the development of AD. Gouras et al. [21] reported that treatment with testosterone increased secretion of the non-amyloidogenic amyloid precursor protein, thus decreasing the secretion of β-amyloid peptides from rat cerebrocortical neurons. The authors go on to suggest that the results raise the possibility that testosterone supplementation in elderly men may be protective in the treatment of AD.

Other studies have used animal models to investigate the effect of testosterone on AD in women. In a series of comprehensive investigations, Papasozemenos explored the morphology, evolution, and distribution of tau immunoreactivity in animal models of AD. The studies used ovariectomized rats in order to investigate the effect of testosterone on the hyperphosphorylation of tau. In an early study, Papasozemenos showed that androgens, but not estrogens, prevented hyperphosphorylation of tau induced by heat shock, suggesting that testosterone production or secretion may represent a defensive response to various stressful stimuli [20]. In a more recent study, Papasozemenos showed that testosterone, but not 17β-estradiol, prevented hyperphosphorylation of tau by inhibiting the overactivation of glycogen synthase kinase-3β [22]. In this study, testosterone used alone and in conjunction with estradiol, but not estradiol alone, prevented tau hyperphosphorylation. The authors report that testosterone therapy, given in conjunction with an estrogen, might prove beneficial in preventing or treating AD in postmenopausal women.

Taken together, the abovementioned results suggest that testosterone has a direct effect on tau and β-amyloid. Additionally, some basic science research suggests that testosterone may be more beneficial than even 17β-estradiol, the most potent and bioactive of the estrogens. Such research lends support to scientists and clinicians who advocate using testosterone in addition to estrogenic formulations in HT. Although more clinical studies are needed, currently available basic science research suggests that testosterone treatment would likely generate a cognitive benefit in postmenopausal women. Additionally, postmenopausal women diagnosed or "at risk" for developing AD might benefit from a testosterone regimen. Evidence suggests that testosterone may prove to be a successful AD deterrent and possibly even have the capacity to reverse or slow the accumulation and hyperphosphorylation of tau and β-amyloid in women at risk for the disease.

Testosterone in clinical research
Testosterone and methodological issues

Compared to basic scientific research examining the effects of testosterone in animals, clinical neuropsychological studies fall far behind in number and in clarification. Clinical studies are complicated due to a number of methodological issues. The two factors listed as a limitation in virtually every comprehensive literature review examining testosterone in women are (1) the extremely low levels of naturally circulating testosterone in women and (2) the inability to quantify accurately these very small concentrations of testosterone. These two variables affect all age groups and differ considerably across studies. Free testosterone comprises roughly 1% to 2% of total circulating testosterone, while 66% of testosterone is bound to sex hormone binding globulin (SHBG). Due to the latter statistic, any factor influencing SHBG levels will consequently affect testosterone levels, such that increasing SHBG decreases the amount of free testosterone [23]. Importantly, oral estrogens increase SHBG levels, thus lowering the amount of free testosterone. In fact, one investigator suggested that estrogenic therapy alone may produce a significant hypoandrogenic state by inhibiting production or accelerating clearance of adrenal androgens [24].

In addition to small concentrations of endogenous testosterone, the second central difficulty in clinical studies seeking to measure testosterone levels in women is quantifying the very small amounts of testosterone in the presence of steroids with closely related structures. Most often, testosterone is measured by an analog assay or by a free androgen index, which is the ratio of total testosterone to SHBG. The problem with separating and assaying free testosterone is that this method does not allow for approximation of bioavailable testosterone, which is the fraction of testosterone in plasma that can enter cells. The free testosterone index method depends on the amount of testosterone and SHBG. The complication with this method is that free testosterone depends not only on the ratio, but also on the absolute concentration of both testosterone and SHBG [25]. Before investigators are able to assess cognitive and neuroprotective influences of testosterone in women more accurately, we must first reach a consensus regarding an effective and standardized method to measure very low amounts of androgens.

It is also important to note that most research surrounding cognition and exogenous and endogenous testosterone levels in women has been conducted in healthy participants. Exceptions to this trend are studies that have investigated the effect of testosterone administration in women with very low plasma concentrations of androgens, including testosterone. There are some data on androgen deficiency and testosterone treatments in women with anorexia nervosa, hypopituitarism, adrenal insufficiency, human immunodeficiency virus infection, and complete androgen insensitivity syndrome. Although testosterone administration has been explored in these cohorts, no available data exists on exogenous testosterone administration in women diagnosed with, or considered "at risk" for developing AD. As evidenced by basic science and animal research in AD, testosterone treatments could provide the AD population with additional options for slowing or perhaps opposing the neurological effects of AD. Based on the available data, involving AD patient populations in future research pertaining to testosterone administration would greatly benefit our understanding of sex hormones and the brain in a sample that could potentially benefit the most from such treatments.

Testosterone therapy and cognition in young women

In research involving sex hormone levels in younger women, most studies suggest that androgens facilitate visuospatial performance, while acting against tasks involving verbal ability [26]. A few studies examining endogenous testosterone levels in premenopausal women have reported beneficial androgenic effects on cognition. Most relevant to the current chapter, one study reported that spatial performance was superior in women tested during the morning hours when endogenous testosterone levels are high, compared to women tested later in the day when testosterone levels decline [27].

Exogenous androgen administration also seems to facilitate visuospatial performance in young women. For instance, a three-week randomized placebo-controlled study demonstrated that women with anorexia nervosa improved on tasks of spatial ability when treated with transdermal testosterone [28]. Also, Aleman *et al.* reported that Mental Rotation task performance, a test of visuospatial ability, significantly improved after only one administration of testosterone in young women [29]. Recently, our research team demonstrated that the androgenic component in oral contraceptives influences visuospatial task performance in young women. The most androgenic progestins are derived from testosterone, while the less androgenic, more "natural" progestins are derived from soy and wild yam plants. Our results showed that the more androgenic the oral contraceptive, the better the participants performed on visuospatial tasks. Furthermore, the young women taking oral contraceptives with an "anti-androgenic" component performed worse on the Mental Rotation task than women taking more androgenic oral contraceptives, as well as women who were naturally cycling

223

[26]. There seems to be a clear relationship between endogenous and exogenous testosterone levels and cognitive functioning in young women, such that testosterone facilitates performance on tasks measuring visuospatial ability. It is unclear exactly which factors contribute to the disparate results seen in older participants, though age, menopause and prior oral contraceptive use are likely involved.

Testosterone therapy and cognition in postmenopausal women

Research investigating the relationship between cognitive performance and testosterone therapy in postmenopausal women is limited and arguably more complicated than studies involving younger women. In addition to the two methodological issues relating to low testosterone levels and precision in testosterone measurement discussed above, additional and potentially problematic variables affect older, postmenopausal women specifically. One such factor is surgical status. Bilateral oophorectomy results in the loss of ovarian androgen and androgen precursor production in both postmenopausal and premenopausal women [25]. Plasma androgen concentrations are lower in postmenopausal oophorectomized women than in postmenopausal women who have not undergone oophorectomy.

As suggested by the Endocrine Society Clinical Practice Guidelines on androgen therapy in women, investigators should consider age, surgical status, and years since oophorectomy when conducting testosterone therapy research in postmenopausal women. We would also like to suggest that duration and generation of past hormonal contraceptive treatment be considered. As discussed above, our laboratory recently reported significant effects of the androgenic components in oral contraceptives on Mental Rotation task performance [26]. Because these effects were observed in young women taking oral contraceptives for a relatively short duration, there is a high probability that oral contraceptives taken over many years may have an even more influential effect. More specifically, the androgens in oral contraceptives may have the capacity to alter a woman's hormonal profile and impact endogenous hormone levels, or potentially mediate the way in which a woman responds to exogenous hormone administration later in life. Partially based on aforementioned factors, only a handful of studies have examined the effect of

endogenous testosterone levels in postmenopausal women, and none have employed an AD cohort. Many times, measurement of endogenous androgen levels in older women is conducted in order to serve as a control for studies examining exogenous HT administration. As endogenous measurements are not the primary outcome variable, between-group comparisons are rarely conducted, and even less often discussed at length. In light of this trend, one exploratory study examined the relation between endogenous sex hormone levels and cognitive performance in elderly women [30]. The authors reported that testosterone levels were positively correlated with verbal fluency. A more recent but very similar study confirmed these results, reporting that endogenous testosterone levels are highly correlated with estradiol levels and are associated with better verbal memory [31].

These results are in contrast to aforementioned studies examining the relation between endogenous and exogenous testosterone levels and cognition in younger women. As discussed earlier, testosterone levels are associated with improved visuospatial performance and hindered verbal performance in younger women, which is a very different picture than the one just described in postmenopausal women. While a cross-sectional, large-scale study examining testosterone across a wide age range would likely shed light on this issue, we suspect that the resulting pattern is the result of multiple factors such as surgical status, conversion of testosterone to estradiol, and between-study methodological differences. Other possible explanations that might explain the differences just described include cyclical hormone variation and/or that the ratio of estrogen to testosterone may be important. Although such postulations are beyond the scope of this chapter, there are many potential moderating variables concerning the way in which sex hormones relate to each other that have yet to be explored.

Of the few clinical studies examining exogenous testosterone therapy in postmenopausal women, all employed different cognitive tasks, small samples, and only healthy participants. Wisniewski *et al.* (2002) examined the impact of a four-month testosterone or placebo treatment in conjunction with high-dose esterified estrogens [32]. Results revealed a difference between treatment groups on a Building Memory task, where women taking testosterone in conjunction with esterified estrogens outperformed users of esterified estrogens alone. It is important to note that testosterone administration did not improve task performance. Rather, testosterone seemed to protect against the decline in performance observed when participants received esterified estrogens alone. The same study, however, did not find between-group differences on other visuospatial tasks such as Cube Comparisons, a task that is similar to the Mental Rotation task. In this task, both the estrogens group and the estrogens plus testosterone group improved after treatment, but neither improved to the point of significance. Importantly, the analyses did not discriminate between surgical versus naturally postmenopausal participants. As described earlier in the chapter, characterization of testosterone is greatly different between these two groups and should be taken into account in future studies. Overall, the author concluded that the addition of testosterone to high-dose HT exerts a protective effect on memory.

In a double-blind cross-over study, Regenstein *et al.* reported a significant benefit of testosterone treatment on an attention shift task, a test that assesses complex information processing [33]. No effect of testosterone was observed for tasks believed to be female dominant (Finger-Tapping test and verbal fluency); visual discrimination, as measured in the side or direction conditions; or measures of sleep, mood, or exercise. The authors propose that the effect of testosterone on attention shift alone suggests that testosterone may specifically influence working memory, purposive direction of attention, rejection of irrelevant information, spatial sense, or response inhibition. The authors also noted that hysterectomy status did not affect any of the outcome measures.

Some research, however, does not support a relation between cognitive performance and testosterone therapy. Sherwin reported a positive effect of testosterone on verbal ability but not on overall cognitive function, in a well designed cross-over study utilizing intramuscular testosterone injections [34] (see Chapter 19). Inconsistent experimental results (e.g., [34]) surrounding testosterone therapy and cognitive task performance in postmenopausal women could be due to a number of different mechanisms. One factor is the overall aging effect [35], which is a common confounding variable in studies examining postmenopausal participants, and it is not clear when these effects begin [36]. Older populations are more likely to be afflicted with heart disease, hypertension, and other disorders that influence cognition.

It is important to note that studies investigating the protective role of testosterone in women have not been conducted longitudinally. Therefore, this chapter is only able to discuss the short-term effects of testosterone therapy. Due to the limited amount of available data on endogenous testosterone levels in women, it is not surprising that studies involving exogenous testosterone administration are not clearly defined. A recent article published by the Endocrine Society addressed testosterone administration and characterization in women [25]. The article advised against making a diagnosis of androgen deficiency in women due to the lack of clinical and normative data on total and free testosterone levels that are used to define such a disorder.

Future directions of testosterone therapy in women

The progression of testosterone research has followed a similar pattern to estrogen research, but advancements are slow and the issue is controversial. In healthy women, the most common reasons testosterone is prescribed include relief from menopausal symptoms and sexual dysfunction. Unfortunately, very little research has been dedicated to examining the potential salutary cognitive effects of testosterone treatment in women, and the clinical research that has been conducted has utilized only healthy postmenopausal samples. Although the number of postmenopausal women prescribed testosterone is higher than it has ever been, the Food and Drug Administration has yet to approve any form of testosterone treatment for women. This is potentially problematic, as investigators are less likely to spend time and money examining a drug that is used off-label and may not be seen as clinically applicable to the population of interest. Fortunately, clinical studies examining the effects of testosterone on menopausal symptoms are currently underway, which will hopefully bring about more funding and research opportunities relating to the cognitive effects of testosterone in women.

Overall, results of basic scientific and clinical research suggest that there may be a beneficial effect of exogenous testosterone administration in postmenopausal women with AD or at risk for developing AD. Although the specific cognitive domains that could be favorably affected in this population remain unclear, future methodological commonalities and more research overall will likely shed light on this issue. The potential benefits could be similar to the benefits observed in estradiol research within the same population. More specifically, evidence suggests that testosterone administration might be a beneficial addition to an estradiol HT regimen in certain populations, such as surgically menopausal women. Future research should aim to systematically evaluate testosterone therapy in order to more fully understand the effect of androgens in women with and without AD. Longitudinal research in a large, age-matched, surgically menopausal sample, utilizing standardized testosterone measurements, would be optimal. Further research investigating the cognitive and neuroprotective properties of testosterone in women is warranted.

References

1. Twist SJ, Taylor GA, Weddell A, *et al.* Brain oestradiol and testosterone levels in Alzheimer's disease. *Neurosci Lett.* 2000;**286**(1):1–4.

2. NAMS continuing medical education activity. *Menopause.* 2005;**12**(5):496.

3. Burger HG, Dudley EC, Cui J, *et al.* A prospective longitudinal study of serum testosterone, dehydroepiandrosterone sulfate, and sex hormone-binding globulin levels through the menopause transition. *J Clin Endocrinol Metab.* 2000;**85**:2832–8.

4. Overlie I, Moen MH, Morkrid L, *et al.* The endocrine transition around menopause – a five year prospective study with profiles of gonadotropins, estrogens and SHBG among healthy women. *Acta Obstetr Gynecol Scand.* 1999;**78**:642–7.

5. Zumoff B, Strain GW, Miller KL, *et al.* Twenty-four-hour mean plasma testosterone concentration declines with age in normal premenopausal women. *J Clin Endocrinol Metab.* 1995;**80**(4):1429–30.

6. Davison SL, Bell R, Donath S, *et al.* Androgen levels in adult females: changes with age, menopause, and oophorectomy. *J Clin Endocrinol Metab.* 2005;**90**:3847–53.

7. Gleason CE, Schmitz TW, Koscik RL, *et al.* Hormone effects on fMRI and cognitive measures of encoding: importance of hormone preparation. *Neurology.* 2006;**67**:2039–41.

8. Wharton W, Fitzgerald A, Carlsson C, *et al.* Effects of hormone therapy duration on functional MRI activation. *Graylyn Conference in Women's Cognitive Health*, 2007, Abstract.

9. Shaywitz SE, Shaywitz BA, Pugh KR, *et al.* Effect of estrogen on brain activation patterns in postmenopausal women during working memory tasks. *JAMA.* 1999;**281**:1197–202.

10. Hogervorst E, Bandelow S, Combrinck M, *et al.* Low free testosterone is an independent risk factor for Alzheimer's disease. *Exp Gerontol.* 2004;**39**(11/12):1633–9.

11. Cherrier MM, Asthana S, Plymate S. Testosterone supplementation improves spatial and verbal memory in healthy older men. *Neurology.* 2001;**57**:80–8.

12. Cherrier MM, Matsumoto AM, Amory JK, *et al.* Testosterone improves spatial memory in men with Alzheimer disease and mild cognitive impairment. *Neurology.* 2005;**64**:2063–8.

13. Smith MD, Jones LS, Wilson MA. Sex differences in hippocampal slice excitability: role of testosterone. *Neuroscience.* 2002;**109**:517–30.

14. Pouliot WA, Handa RJ, Beck SG. *Synapse.* 1996;**23**:10–19.

15. Morse JK, DeKosky ST, Schett SW. *Exp Neurol.* 1992;**118**:47–52.

16. Tirassa P, Thiblin I, Agren G, *et al. Neurosci Res.* 1997;**47**:198–207.

17. Archer JS, Love-Geffen TE, Herbst-Damm KL, *et al.* NAMS Fellowship findings: effect of estradiol versus estradiol and testosterone on brain-activation patterns in postmenopausal women. *Menopause.* 2006;**13**(3):528–37.

18. Leranth C, Hajszan T, MacLusky NJ. Androgens increase spine synapse density in the CA1 hippocampal subfield of ovariectomized female rats. *J Neurosci.* 2004;**24**(2):495–9.

19. Gandy S, Almeida OP, Fonte J, *et al.* Chemical andropause and amyloid-beta peptide. *JAMA.* 2001;**285**:2195–6.

20. Papasozomenos SC. The heat-shock induced hyperphosphorylation of tau is estrogen-independent and prevented by androgens: implications for Alzheimer's disease. *Proc Natl Acad Sci USA.* 1997;**94**:6612–17.

21. Gouras GK, Xu H, Gross RS, *et al.* Testosterone reduces neuronal secretion of Alzheimer's beta-amyloid peptides. *Proc Natl Acad Sci USA.* 2000;**97**(3):1202–5.

22. Papasozomenos SC, Shanavas A. Testosterone prevents the heat shock-induced overactivation of glycogen synthase kinase-3β but not of cyclin-dependent kinase 5 and c-Jun NH2-terminal kinase and concomitantly abolishes hyperphosphorylation of τ: Implications for Alzheimer's disease. *Proc Natl Acad Sci.* 2002;**99**(3):1140–5.

23. Davison SL, Davis SR. Androgens in women. *J Steroid Biochem Mol Biol.* 2003;**85**:363–6.

24. Simon JA. Safety of estrogen/androgen regimens. *J Reprod Med.* 2001;**46**(3 Suppl.):281–90.

25. Wierman ME, Basson R, Davis SR, *et al.* Androgen therapy in women: an Endocrine Society Clinical Practice guideline. *J Clin Endocrinol Metab.* 2006; **91**(10):3697–710.

26. Wharton W, Hirshman E, Merritt P, *et al.* Oral contraceptives and androgenicity: influences on visuospatial task performance in younger individuals. *Exp Clin Psychopharm.* 2008;**16**(2):156–64.

27. Moffat SD, Hampson E. A curvilinear relationship between testosterone and spatial cognition in humans: possible influence of hand preference. *Psychoneuroendocrinology.* 1996;**21**:323–37.

28. Miller KK, Grieco KA, Klibanski A. Testosterone administration in women with anorexia nervosa. *J Clin Endocrinol Metab.* 2005;**90**:1428–33.

29. Aleman A, Bronk E, Kessels R, *et al.* A single administration of testosterone improves visuospatial ability in young women. *Psychoneuroendocrinology.* 2004;**29**:612–17.

30. Drake EB, Henderson VW, Stanczyk FZ, *et al.* Associations between circulating sex steroid hormones and cognition in normal elderly women. *Neurology.* 2000;**54**:599–603.

31. Wolf OT, Kirschbaum C. Endogenous estradiol and testosterone levels are associated with cognitive performance in older women and men. *Horm Behav.* 2002;**41**:259–66.

32. Wisniewski AB, Nguyen TT, Dobs AS. Evaluation of high-dose estrogen and high-dose estrogen plus methyltestosterone treatment on cognitive task performance in postmenopausal women. *Horm Res.* 2002;**58**:150–5.

33. Regestein QR, Friebely J, Shifren J, *et al.* Neuropsychological effects of methyltestosterone in women using menopausal hormone replacement. *J Womens Health Gend Based Med.* 2001;**10**(7):671–6.

34. Sherwin BB. Estrogen and/or androgen replacement therapy and cognitive functioning in surgically menopausal women. *Psychoneuroendocrinology.* 1988;**13**:345–57.

35. Rosenberg L, Park S. Verbal and spatial functions across the menstrual cycle in healthy young women. *Psychoneuroendocrinology.* 2002;**27**(7):835–41.

36. Sherwin BB. Mild cognitive impairment: potential pharmacological treatment options. *J Am Geriatr Soc.* 2000;**48**(4):431–41.

Endogenous estradiol and dementia in elderly men: the roles of vascular risk, sex hormone binding globulin, and aromatase activity

Majon Muller and Mirjam I. Geerlings

Editors' introduction

In elderly men as in elderly women, endogenous est-radiol may play an important role in age-related cognitive impairment. To explore the relation between estradiol, cognition, dementia, and cerebral atrophy, Muller and Geerlings performed a systematic literature review. In their review, the authors found that most studies in elderly men do not report significant associations between estradiol levels and cognitive performance, cognitive decline, dementia, or brain atrophy. Some studies, however, do imply that higher estradiol levels are potentially detrimental, although to the extent that a relation may exist, the magnitude of risk is likely small. Given the long preclinical phase of Alzheimer's disease (AD), it is difficult to infer caus-ality, even in longitudinal studies with long follow-up. Muller and Geerling indicated that the relation between estradiol and vascular risk merits further study with respect to AD. In addition, they provide evidence that sex hormone binding globulin (SHBG) levels and aromatase activity are relevant to questions of AD pathogenesis.

Introduction

The impact of dementia on society and health care is a growing concern, given the increase of the elderly population. It is expected that with the increase of the elderly population, the prevalence of AD, the most common cause of dementia, will triple to 13 million people in the United States by 2050 [1].

Sex hormones have been identified as factors that modify the risk for dementia. Over the last few decades the number of published studies on the association of exogenous and endogenous levels of estrogens with dementia strongly increased. Earlier observational studies in postmenopausal women found reduced risk for cognitive decline and dementia with higher levels of estrogen [2, 3], findings that are biologically plausible and supported by findings in experimental studies. These in vivo and in vitro experimental studies report that estrogens maintain the production of neurotrophins and the regulation of their receptors responsible for cognition, improve blood flow, modify the processing of amyloid precur-sor protein, increase choline acetyltransferase levels that subsequently increase acetylcholine, and stimu-late neuronal regeneration [4].

More recently, however, higher endogenous levels of estrogens in postmenopausal women have been associated with an increased risk for dementia, poorer memory performance, and smaller hippocampal volumes [5–7]. These findings were confirmed by findings from the Women's Health Initiative Memory Study (WHIMS) where older women who were receiving estrogen therapy had an increased risk for dementia compared with women receiving placebo [8] (see Chapter 1). These unexpected results in women raised interest in the effects of estrogens on cognition and the risk for dementia in older men.

Recent studies showed that endogenous estradiol in elderly men plays an important role in age-related diseases [9, 10]. Endogenous estradiol, the most

Hormones, Cognition and Dementia: State of the Art and Emergent Therapeutic Strategies, ed. Eef Hogervorst, Victor W. Henderson, Robert B. Gibbs, and Roberta Diaz Brinton. Published by Cambridge University Press.
© Cambridge University Press 2009.

Table 24.1 Search terms used in PubMed for estrogens, cognition, dementia, and brain atrophy.

	Search terms
Estrogens	"Estradiol"[Mesh] OR "Estrogens"[Mesh] OR "Estradiol Congeners"[Mesh] OR "estradiol"[Title/Abstract] OR "oestradiol"[Title/Abstract] OR "estrogens"[Title/Abstract] OR "estrogen"[Title/Abstract] OR "oestrogens"[Title/Abstract] OR "oestrogen"[Title/Abstract] OR "female sex hormone"[Title/Abstract] OR "female sex hormones"[Title/Abstract]
Cognition, Dementia	"Delirium, Dementia, Amnestic, Cognitive Disorders"[Mesh] OR "dementia"[Title/Abstract] OR "alzheimer"[Title/Abstract] OR "alzheimers"[Title/Abstract] OR "Alzheimer's disease"[Title/Abstract] OR "cognitive"[Title/Abstract] OR "cognition"[Title/Abstract] OR "memory"[Title/Abstract] OR "amyloid"[Title/Abstract]
Brain atrophy	((ventricle[tiab] OR ventricles[tiab] ventricular[tiab] OR sulcus[tiab] OR sulci[tiab] OR sulcal[tiab]) AND (enlargement[tiab] OR size[tiab] OR dilatation[tiab] OR expansion[tiab])) OR (("atrophy"[MeSH] OR atrophy[tiab]) AND ("brain"[MeSH] OR brain[tiab] OR cerebral[tiab] OR hippocampus[tiab] OR hippocampal[tiab] OR cortical[tiab] OR subcortical[tiab] OR entorhinal cortex[tiab] OR medial temporal lobe[tiab])).

potent estrogen produced in the body, is largely bound to sex hormone binding globulin (SHBG) and albumin, but only the fraction not bound to SHBG is considered to be bioactive. Mean serum estradiol concentrations in elderly men are much higher than in postmenopausal women, and are comparable to estradiol levels of premenopausal women in the early follicular phase of the menstrual cycle. Of the factors influencing plasma estradiol levels in men, plasma testosterone is a major determinant [11]. The relatively strong age-associated decrease in testosterone levels is not observed for plasma estradiol levels, because of increasing aromatase activity with age and the age-associated increase in fat mass [11].

In this chapter we discuss the existing literature on the association of endogenous estradiol with cognition, brain atrophy, and dementia in elderly men. Furthermore, we will discuss the role of vascular factors, SHBG, aromatase activity, and estrogen receptors in this relation.

Estradiol and cognition and dementia in men: review of the literature

Search strategy

We searched PubMed for studies published in English before February 2008 using search terms for estrogens, cognition, dementia, and brain atrophy (Table 24.1). We combined these search terms as follows: estrogens AND (cognition or dementia or brain atrophy) and limited the articles to English language, humans, and male. This search resulted in

440 articles. We screened titles and abstracts and retrieved the full text of 17 articles that examined the relation between endogenous estradiol and cognitive functioning, brain atrophy measures, cognitive decline, or dementia in men. We also included a recently published paper from one of the authors of this chapter. The articles that were excluded were not relevant to the topic, were review articles, were experimental studies, or did not examine endogenous levels of estradiol in a male population. We grouped the articles according to design (cross-sectional or longitudinal) and outcome measure (cognition, dementia, brain atrophy). We recorded the size and mean age of the study population; the mean follow-up duration and proportion lost to follow-up for the longitudinal studies; the covariates that were adjusted for in the analyses; the mean estradiol level of the study population; the assay detection limit; the inter- and intra-assay coefficient of variation; the outcome measures; the number of incident dementia cases if relevant; and the effect estimate and statistical significance. Two studies [5, 12] examined brain atrophy as well as cognition, and these studies are presented twice.

Cross-sectional studies investigating estradiol and cognition or dementia

Table 24.2 presents the characteristics of the seven cross-sectional studies and two case-control studies that investigated the association between estradiol levels and cognition or dementia in men. Of the seven cross-sectional studies, five were population-based,

Table 24.2 Cross-sectional and case-control studies presenting the relation between endogenous estradiol and cognition and dementia.

Study	N	Age, years	Adjustment	E_2, pmol/L mean ± SD/ median (range)	Assay detection limit, pmol/L	Inter/intra assay CV, %	Outcome	Direction of effect	P-value
Aleman et al., 2001 [13] Ambulatory subjects	25	69	2	Total E_2: 97 (60–145)	Total E_2: 40	19/?	Memory Cryst. Intelligence Fluid Intelligence (z-scores)	Total E_2	NS NS NS
Yaffe et al., 2002 [17] Study of Osteoporotic Risk	310	73 ± 7	1, 2, 8	Total E_2: 84 ± 29 Bio E_2: 51 ± 18	Total E_2: 18 Bio E_2: 2	8/5	Mini-Mental State Digit Symbol Substitution Test Trail Making Test Part B	Total/BioE_2 Total E_2↑, Digit Symbol ↓ Bio E_2 Total E_2↑, Trails B ↓ Bio E_2	NS p < 0.001 NS p = 0.002 NS
Wolf & Kirschbaum, 2002 [16] Healthy volunteers	30	69 ± 1	1, 2	Total E_2: 106 ± 9	Total E_2: 29	<10/<10	5 cognitive tests	Total E_2	5 × NS
Den Heijer et al., 2003 [5] Rotterdam Study	202	69 ± 8	1, 2, 3, 4, 5, 6, 7	Total E_2: 45 (0–157) Bio E_2: 34 (0–120) Free E_2: 1.2 (0–4.2)	Total E_2: 5 Bio E_2: calculated Free E_2: calculated	14/18	Delayed recall	Total E_2	β (95%CI) −0.3 (−0.7;0.1)
Hogervorst et al., 2004 [18] Foresight-Challenge Cohort	79	74 ± 6	1	Total E_2: 84 ± 28	Total E_2: 3	13/4	9 cognitive tests	Total E_2 Total E_2↑, visuospatial ↑	8 × NS p = 0.06

Study	N	Age	Confounders	E2 values	CV/assay	Measured	Outcome	Total/Bio E2	Significance
Muller et al., 2005 [15] HAMLET Study	395	60 ± 11	1, 2, 3, 4, 5, 6, 9, 10, 11	Total E_2: 91 ± 23 Bio E_2: 42 ± 12	Total E_2: 20 Bio E_2: calculated	10/?	Mini-Mental State Memory (z-score) Processing/speed (z-score) Executive function (z-score)	Total/Bio E_2	NS NS NS NS
Martin et al., 2007 [14] Florey Adelaide Male Ageing St	1,046	54 ± 11	1, 2, 3, 4, 5, 6, 9, 10, 11	Total E_2: 75 ± 40	unknown	14/?	7 cognitive tests	Total E_2	7 × NS
Senanarong et al., 2002 [19]	20 cases 25 controls	70 ± 8 66 ± 4	1	Total E_2 cases 57 ± 36 Total E_2 controls 81 ± 47	unknown	?/?	Alzheimer's disease	Total E_2↓, Alzheimer's disease ↑	p < 0.05
Paoletti et al., 2004 [20]	32 cases 32 controls	77 ± 2 74 ± 1	–	Total E_2 cases 76 ± 8 Total E_2 controls 54 ± 5	Total E_2: 20	?/?	Alzheimer's disease	Total E_2↑, Alzheimer's disease ↑	p < 0.02

Confounders 1: age; 2: education; 3: smoking; 4: alcohol; 5: body mass index; 6: depression; 7: apolipoprotein E genotype; 8: sex hormone binding globulin; 9: diabetes; 10: hypertension; 11: hyperlipidemia.
Bio = bioavailable; CV = coefficient of variation; E_2 = estradiol; N = number available subjects for analyses; NS = not statistically significant.

one included healthy volunteers, and one included ambulatory male subjects. The case-control studies included patients with AD and healthy controls. The size of the study population varied considerably from 25 to 1,046 subjects. The mean age of the study populations varied from 54 to 77 years, with the majority having study populations of about 70 years of age. Assay detection limits varied significantly between studies and ranged from 3 pmol/L to 40 pmol/L. Also, mean total estradiol levels of the study populations varied between 45 pmol/L and 106 pmol/L. In addition, inter-assay coefficients of variation were relatively high, i.e., between 10% and 20%, in most studies. Intra-assay coefficients of variation were between 4% and 18% but were not reported in five of the nine studies. Some studies directly measured bioactive estradiol (not bound to SHBG) and free estradiol (bound neither to albumin nor SHBG), whereas others calculated bioactive and free estradiol based on total estradiol, SHBG, and albumin levels. Cognitive outcome measures were diverse, and except for one study [5], all analyzed multiple cognitive tests. Most studies adjusted in the analyses for age and education, and three studies also adjusted for vascular risk factors.

The majority of studies did not find a significant association between estradiol levels and cognitive tests [13–16]. One study observed associations with total estradiol but not with bioactive estradiol, with higher total estradiol level being associated with poorer performance on the Digit Symbol Substitution test and poorer performance on the Trail Making Test, Part B [17]. Another study found a borderline significant effect on one out of nine tests, with higher total estradiol being associated with better visuospatial performance [18]. The Rotterdam Scan Study found a borderline significant association between higher total estradiol levels and poorer delayed recall on the 15-word learning test [5]. The two case-control studies found contradictory results. One case-control study found that men with AD had lower levels of estradiol compared to controls [19], while the other case-control study found that men with AD had higher levels of estradiol [20]. The first study only adjusted for age and the second study did not adjust for age or other confounders.

In summary, the majority of the existing cross-sectional and case-control studies do not find an association between levels of endogenous estradiol and cognitive performance in elderly men. The minority of studies that did find significant associations were contradictory in the direction of effect that higher estradiol levels may have on brain function.

Studies investigating estradiol and brain atrophy measures

We retrieved four studies that investigated the relation between estradiol and brain atrophy measures in men. Table 24.3 presents the characteristics of these studies. The Rotterdam Scan Study examined the cross-sectional relation between total, bioactive, and free estradiol levels and hippocampal volumes on magnetic resonance imaging (MRI) in 202 elderly men with a mean age of 69 years [5]. This study did not find an association between any of the estradiol measures and hippocampal volume. Another study in World War II veteran twins found that higher total estradiol levels were associated with smaller right occipital lobe volumes on MRI, but not with any of the other 12 brain volume outcomes measured [12]. It should be noted that the measurement of estradiol was based on blood measurements obtained 10–16 years prior to MRI. The other two studies report findings in very old men from the Honolulu-Asia Aging Study. In one study blood sampling for hormone measurement was performed three years prior to MRI and several outcomes were studied, including atrophy and vascular pathology [21]. After adjustment for several potential confounders, higher bioactive estradiol was associated with cerebral but not hippocampal atrophy on MRI. Also, higher estradiol levels were associated with increased risk for lacunes, but not with large infarcts or white matter lesions. The second study that reported findings from the Honolulu-Asia Aging Study used outcomes evaluated at autopsy on average five years after blood sampling. In this study, men with free estradiol levels in the highest tertile had significantly fewer neurofibrillary tangles, but not fewer diffuse plaques or neuritic plaques than men in the lowest tertile of estradiol [22]. No associations between estradiol level and vascular pathology outcomes were observed.

In summary, so far few studies have investigated the relation between endogenous estradiol levels and brain atrophy measures in elderly men. The majority of studies did not find an association, and those that did find a significant association suggest that higher estradiol levels increase risk for brain atrophy.

Table 24.3 Population-based studies presenting the relation between endogenous estradiol, and imaging and neuropathological markers of dementia.

Study	N	Age, years	Follow-up, years	Adjustment	E_2, pmol/L mean ± SD / median (range)	Assay detection limit, pmol/L	Inter/intra assay CV, %	Outcome	Effect estimate β or RR (95% CI)
Den Heijer et al., 2003 [5] Rotterdam Study	202	69 ± 8	–	1, 2, 3, 4, 5, 6, 7, 8	Total E_2: 45 (0–157) Bio E_2: 34 (0–120) Free E_2: 1.2 (0–4.2)	Total E_2: 5 Bio E_2: calculated Free E_2: calculated	14/18	Hippocampal volumes	Total/Bio/ Free E_2 NS
Lessov-Schlaggar et al., 2005 [12] World War II veteran twins	280	63 ± 3	10–16[†]	1, 2, 6, 8	Total E_2: 141 ± 86	Total E_2: 2	14/11	Volume right occipital lobe 12 other MRI outcome measurements	Total E_2 β –0.14, p < 0.05 12 × NS
Irie et al., 2006 [21] Honolulu-Asia Aging Study	452	82 ± 5	3[†]	1, 2, 7, 8, 9	Total E_2: 98 ± 53 Bio E_2: 64 ± 36	Total E_2: 73** Bio E_2: calculated	5/4	Cerebral atrophy Hippocampal atrophy White matter lesions Lacunes Large infarcts	Bio E_2 2.5 (1.1; 5.6)[††] NS NS 2.0 (1.2; 3.1)[††] NS
Strozyk et al., 2006 [22] Honolulu-Asia Aging Study	232	85 ± 5	5[†]	1, 2, 5, 7, 9, 10, 11, 12, 13, 14	Total E_2: 100 ± 55 Free E_2: 2.4 ± 1	Total E_2: 73** Free E_2: calculated	5/4	Diffuse plaques Neuritic plaques Neurofibrillary tangles Microinfarct Lacunar lesion Ischemic lesion Cerebral amyloid angiopathy	Free E_2 NS NS 0.4 (0.3; 0.7)[††] NS NS NS NS

Note:
[†] Blood sampling number of years prior to outcome measurement.
** Levels of estradiol less than the detection limit of 73 pmol/L were estimated using a curve-fitting program. Although these levels are less precisely measured, the individuals should be correctly ranked relative to the others.
[††] High versus low estradiol tertile.

Confounders 1: age; 2: education; 3: smoking; 4: alcohol; 5: BMI; 6: depression; 7: APOE genotype; 8: intracranial volume; 9: dementia status; 10: diabetes; 11: hyperlipidemia; 12: hypertension; 13: hormone batch; 14: time from blood draw until death.

Bio = bioavailable; CI = confidence interval; CV = coefficient of variation; E_2 = estradiol; MRI = magnetic resonance imaging; N = number available subjects for analyses; NS = not statistically significant; RR = relative risk.

233

Prospective studies investigating estradiol and risk of cognitive decline or dementia

We retrieved seven studies that investigated the longitudinal relation between estradiol levels in men and cognitive decline or risk for developing dementia. Table 24.4 presents the characteristics of these studies. In six studies, the size of the study population varied between 242 and 547 men [6, 12, 23–26], and one study included 2,300 men [27]. The mean age of the majority of populations was 70 years or higher. Follow-up duration in studies varied from 2–6 years, and one study had follow-up of 10–16 years but cognitive testing was performed at follow-up and blood sampling was performed at baseline 10–16 years prior to cognitive testing [12]. As expected loss to follow-up was relatively high in this study (39%). Two other studies also had a relatively high rate of loss to follow-up, but these studies included very old men [24, 27]. The mean level of total estradiol varied from 46 pmol/L to 141 pmol/L across study populations, as did the detection limit of total estradiol, which varied from 2 pmol/L to 73 pmol/L. Interassay coefficients of variation varied between studies from 5% to 17% and intra-assay coefficients of variation varied from 4% to 18%.

Four of the seven studies examined decline in cognition as an outcome measure, of which three examined multiple cognitive outcomes. The first of these four studies used data from the Rancho Bernardo Study and found that higher levels of total and bioactive estradiol on average five years prior to cognitive testing were associated with lower scores on the Mini-Mental State examination, whereas estradiol levels were not significantly associated with scores on 11 other cognitive tests [23]. The second study in World War II veteran twins used 13 cognitive tests as outcome and found that levels of total estradiol 10–16 years prior to cognitive testing were not significantly associated with any of the 13 tests [12]. The third study examining data from the Health ABC Study found that after follow-up that averaged two years, higher levels of bioactive estradiol were associated with a borderline significant reduced risk of memory decline, whereas no significant association was found with decline on the Modified Mini-Mental State examination and decline on a test assessing executive functioning [26]. Finally, unpublished data from the Frail Old Men Study show that higher levels of total and free estradiol were associated with increased risk

of decline on the Mini-Mental State examination after on average four years of follow-up [24].

Three of the seven studies used incident AD and vascular dementia as outcome measures, one of which also examined decline in global cognitive functioning during follow-up. Within the Rotterdam Study no significant association was found between total and bioactive estradiol and risk of AD, but higher levels of total and bioactive estradiol were associated with increased risk of vascular dementia [6]. Within the Honolulu-Asia Aging Study, higher levels of bioactive estradiol were associated with increased risk of AD as well as vascular dementia [27]. Also, higher levels of bioactive estradiol increased the risk for cognitive decline in this study. The third study using data from the Conselice Study did not find associations between levels of total estradiol and risk of AD or vascular dementia [25].

In summary, the results from the prospective studies are conflicting, with some studies finding no association between estradiol levels and risk of cognitive decline and dementia, and other studies finding an increased risk for cognitive decline and dementia in elderly men with higher levels of estradiol.

Validity and reliability of studies

The majority of cross-sectional studies did not find a relation between levels of estradiol and brain outcomes. The results from the prospective studies show either no relation or an increased risk for cognitive decline, brain atrophy, and dementia associated with higher levels of endogenous estradiol. The studies that found evidence suggestive of protective effects of higher levels of estradiol examined multiple outcomes with one outcome being statistically significant [22] or borderline significant [18, 26], and one case-control study found lower levels of estradiol in patients with AD disease compared with controls, but the study sample was small and adjustments were made only for age [19].

It is difficult to detect a pattern that could explain the relative contradictory findings of studies. Although it is generally accepted that estradiol that is not bound to SHBG is biologically active, not all studies examined bioactive estradiol levels. Those that did, did not consistently find significant associations. Furthermore, the outcomes studied are relatively heterogeneous. Most studies looked at cognitive functioning in multiple domains, but it is unclear to

Table 24.4 Population-based longitudinal studies presenting the relation between endogenous estradiol and cognition, cognitive decline, and incident dementia.

Study	N	Age, years	Follow-up, years	Lost to follow-up	Adjustment	E$_2$ (pmol/L) mean (SD)	Assay detection limit, pmol/L	Inter/intra assay CV, %	Outcome	N	Effect estimate β or RR (95% CI)
Barret-Connor, 1999 [23] Rancho Bernardo Study	547	70±8	5†	19%	1, 2, 3, 4, 5, 6	Total E$_2$: 75±25 Bio E$_2$: 49±16	Total E$_2$: 22 Bio E$_2$: 22	7/6 5/4	Mini-Mental State (global) 11 other cognitive tests		Total E$_2$ β −0.62, p < 0.05 Bio E$_2$ β −0.53, p < 0.05 Total/BioE$_2$ 11 × NS
Geerlings et al., 2003 [6] Rotterdam Study	438	69±8	6	0%	1, 2, 3, 4, 5	Total E$_2$: 46±23 Bio E$_2$: 35±18	Total E$_2$: 5 Bio E$_2$: calculated	14/18	Alzheimer's disease	33 10	Total E$_2$ NS Bio E$_2$ NS
									Vascular dementia	10	Total E$_2$ 1.6 (1.1; 2.5) Bio E$_2$ 1.6 (0.9; 2.8)
Lessov et al., 2005 [12] World War II veteran twins	348	63±3	10–16†	39%	1, 2, 3, 4, 6, 7, 18	Total E$_2$: 141±86	Total E$_2$: 2	14/11	13 cognitive tests		Total E$_2$ 13 × NS
Geerlings et al., 2006 [27] Honolulu-Asia Aging Study	2,300	77±4	6	23%	1, 2, 3, 4, 5, 6, 7, 9, 10	Total E$_2$: 95±55 Bio E$_2$: 63±36	Total E$_2$: 73** Bio E$_2$: calculated	5/4	Alzheimer's disease Vascular dementia Decline CASI (global)	134 44	Bio E$_2$ 1.2 (1.0; 1.4) 1.2 (1.0; 1.6) β −0.28, p = 0.002
Yaffe et al., 2007 [26] Health ABC Study	439	75±3	2	7%	1, 2, 8	Bio E$_2$: 31±14	Bio E$_2$: 3	17/8	Decline 3MS (global) Decline SRT (memory) Decline CLOX (executive)	19 17 30	Bio E$_2$ NS 0.5 (0.3; 1.1)†† NS

Table 24.4 (cont.)

Study	N	Age, years	Follow-up, years	Lost to follow-up	Adjustment	E$_2$ (pmol/L) mean (SD)	Assay detection limit, pmol/L	Inter/ intra assay CV, %	Outcome	N	Effect estimate β or RR (95% CI)	
Ravaglia et al., 2007 [25] Conselice Study	376	73 ± 7	4	10%	1, 2, 3, 5, 11, 12, 13, 14, 15	Total E$_2$: 84	Total E$_2$: 37	7/7	Alzheimer's disease Vascular dementia	23 12	Total E$_2$	NS NS
Muller et al., 2009 [24] Frail Old Men Study	242	77 ± 3	4	39%	1, 5, 7, 13, 16, 17, 18	Total E$_2$: 96 ± 48 Free E$_2$: 2.5 ± 1	Total E$_2$: 8 Free E$_2$: calculated	8/5	Decline MMSE (global)	44	Total E$_2$ Free E$_2$	1.6 (1.1; 2.5) 1.5 (1.1; 2.3)

Note:

† Blood sampling number of years prior to outcome measurement.

** Levels of estradiol less than the detection limit of 73 pmol/L were estimated using a curve-fitting program. Although these levels are less precisely measured, the individuals should be correctly ranked relative to the others.

†† High versus low estradiol tertile. In the paper the relative risk of low vs. high tertile is presented: RR 1.9 (0.9; 3.9).

Confounders 1: age; 2: education; 3: smoking; 4: alcohol; 5: BMI; 6: depression; 7: APOE genotype; 8: ethnicity; 9: physical activity; 10: metabolic syndrome; 11: stroke; 12: cardiovascular disease; 13: diabetes; 14: hyperhomocysteinemia; 15: serum creatinine; 16: hyperlipidemia; 17: intima media thickness carotid artery; 18: hypertension.

Bio = bioavailable; CASI = Cognitive Abilities Screening Instrument; CI = confidence interval; CLOX = clock drawing test; CV = coefficient of variation; E$_2$ = estradiol; 3MS = modified Mini-Mental State exam; N = number available subjects for analyses; NS = not statistically significant; RR = relative risk; SD = standard deviation; SRT = simple reaction time.

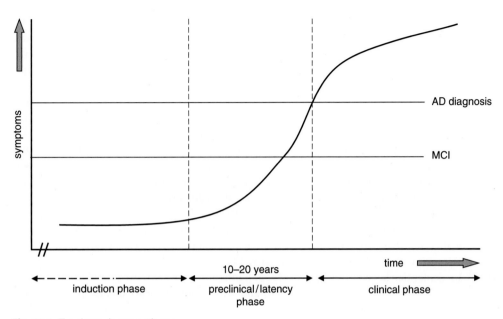

Fig. 24.1 The classic disease pathway.

what extent cognitive impairment or decline in cognitive functioning represents subclinical dementia. Also, the studies that examined brain volumes on MRI did not find an association with hippocampal atrophy, which is considered to be a more specific marker of AD, while higher estradiol was associated with more global cerebral atrophy in one study [21].

To date, three studies have examined incident dementia and its subtypes as outcome. The largest study included 2,300 elderly men from the Honolulu-Asia Aging Study and found a significantly but small increased risk for developing dementia. Per standard deviation increase in estradiol level, the risk for AD and vascular dementia increased by 20%. The findings from this study suggest that if a relation exists between higher estradiol levels and risk of dementia, this risk is small. The other studies had study samples about five times smaller in size, and it is thus possible that lack of statistical power resulted in finding no associations. Also, some studies did not examine the outcome at time of blood sampling, but several years later. This will also have resulted in reduced power to find associations. Another factor that may have resulted in reduced statistical power is the relatively large intra- and interassay coefficient of variation of estradiol measurements. It is worth mentioning that the intra- and interassay variation in the Honolulu-Asia Aging Study were low, i.e., 4% and 5% respectively.

In summary, it is difficult to find a pattern in lack of validity of studies that may explain the relative inconsistency of findings. If a relation exists between estradiol in men and risk of dementia, this risk is small, and it is thus more likely that reduced statistical power due to small sample size and large intra- and interassay variation explain findings of no association.

Time window

Another explanation for finding no associations may be that studies differ in their follow-up period, and estradiol levels are thus measured at varying number of years before clinical onset of dementia. The classic disease pathway offers a way to conceptualize the possible causal role of estradiol in the etiology of dementia (Fig. 24.1). The disease pathway can be separated into the induction phase, which is the period between exposure to the cause and the beginning of pathological changes in the brain, and the latency phase or preclinical phase, which is the period between disease induction and its detection. For AD, both phases might be long, which is confirmed by evidence suggesting that the preclinical phase of AD precedes the diagnosis by ten or more years [28]. Risk factors that most probably act during the induction phase of AD are more likely to be causal factors and

237

usually have strong effects on disease risk, for example, the apolipoprotein E ε4 allele. Risk factors that act during the latency period or preclinical phase are more likely to be factors that have an indirect effect on the true cause and are more likely to be associated with the shift of an asymptomatic state to a diagnosable disease. The follow-up periods of the prospective studies presented in Table 24.4 using dementia diagnosis as outcome variable were four to six years, which means that the estradiol measurements were performed during the latency phase. In other words, endogenous estradiol is probably a factor with an indirect effect on dementia risk and it might modify the relation between the true cause and dementia. An example of this modification could be the interaction of sex hormones with apolipoprotein E genotype in relation to dementia. Several studies have shown that the association between sex hormones and dementia is stronger or different in subjects with the apolipoprotein E ε4 allele compared with those without the ε4 allele [5, 27, 29, 30].

In summary, the inconsistency in the reports of associations between dementia and endogenous estradiol may be related, at least in part, to the fact that they were investigated during the preclinical phase or latency phase of dementia. It is therefore important to be cautious in the interpretation of prospective studies relating baseline risk factors to incident dementia.

The roles of vascular risk, sex hormone binding globulin, aromatase activity, and estrogen receptors

The results of the prospective studies presented in Table 24.4 suggest potential detrimental effects of high estradiol levels on dementia risk. However, because of the relatively short follow-up period of these studies, it could be hypothesized that high estradiol levels are a consequence of preclinical neurodegeneration or a marker for other unmeasured factors that contribute to dementia. A possible "unmeasured factor" is vascular risk.

Vascular risk

It could be hypothesized that endogenous estradiol levels are related to cardiovascular risk and disease, which in their part could lead to increased risk of cerebral small vessel disease, cognitive decline, and dementia [31, 32].

So-called experiments of nature have revealed the importance of estrogens to male cardiovascular function. Estrogen insensitivity, caused by a mutation in the gene encoding aromatase (CYP19) and by a mutation in the estrogen-receptor gene, appears to be associated with glucose intolerance, lipid abnormalities, and atherosclerosis [9]. These findings are confirmed by observational studies showing that *low* estradiol levels in men have been associated with high concentrations of fibrinogen and homocysteine, with unfavorable lipid profiles [9, 33], and with a higher incidence of cardiovascular disease [34].

Most studies, however, describe unfavorable effects of *high* endogenous estradiol levels on vascular risk. High estradiol levels have been associated with obesity, hypertension, diabetes, metabolic syndrome [35–37], inflammation [38], peripheral arterial disease [39], and with coronary heart disease [40]. Recently, prospective studies in elderly men showed that high endogenous estradiol levels were related to increase of the intima media thickness of the common carotid artery [41, 42] and to a higher risk of stroke [43]. This increase in vascular risk and disease in men with high estradiol levels could explain the increased risk of lacunar infarcts on MRI [21], AD [27], and vascular dementia [6] (Tables 24.3 and 24.4).

Sex hormone binding globulin

The relation between high estradiol and dementia risk could also be explained by changes in the balance between estradiol and testosterone. Sex hormone binding globulin, a hepatically secreted protein best known for its role as a binding protein of sex hormones in human plasma, is a major controlling factor in the balance between biologically active testosterone and estradiol [44]. Sex hormone binding globulin prevents hormone binding to the intracellular androgen or estrogen receptors [44, 45]. Although little consensus exists as to what constitutes a normal balance between testosterone and estradiol for an aging man, differences in levels of SHBG resulting in changes in this balance might modify dementia risk. A supporting factor for the possible modifying effect of SHBG on dementia risk is that SHBG increases with age [35], which could indicate that SHBG is a marker for accelerated aging. Furthermore, recent biochemical and molecular analyses of this protein have led to the realization that SHBG functions in much more varied ways [46]. For example, the presence of SHBG and its receptor in human brain tissue suggests its involvement in human neurophysiology, neuroendocrinology, and possibly neuropathology [46, 47]. These findings are supported by findings from cross-sectional and prospective observational studies showing that patients with AD have higher SHBG levels [20, 48, 49], and that subjects with higher SHBG levels had poorer cognitive test scores [17], and an increased risk for incident AD [50]. The finding of increased dementia risk with higher SHBG levels is of interest. However, the exact role of SHBG in the association of endogenous sex hormones with dementia remains to be elucidated.

Aromatase and estrogen receptors

An alternative hypothesis to explain the relation between high estradiol and risk for dementia is that high estradiol levels are a direct result of the neurodegenerative process. Experimental studies in animals demonstrated that after brain injury, aromatase expression in brain astrocytes increased, which in turn increased local estradiol levels to play a role in brain repair [4, 51]. In other words, preclinical neurodegeneration could lead to increased aromatase expression and consequently increase in estradiol production in the brain. However, these changes in brain estradiol levels will probably reflect only small changes in peripheral estradiol levels because the brain is a minor site of aromatization compared to other sites in the body [52]. Nevertheless, if this hypothesis is correct the findings of relatively high levels of estradiol in men who experienced development of dementia were a consequence or an early marker of an incipient dementia process [27].

Another possible explanation for the hypothesis that change in estradiol levels is a consequence of dementia might be that estrogen receptors in the brain tissue of patients with preclinical or clinical AD are less sensitive than receptors in normal brain tissue [53]. This could result in a feedback deficiency, which might increase luteinizing hormone and follicle-stimulating hormone levels and, in turn, increase the conversion from estrone to estradiol.

Recommendations for future research

At present, it is unclear to what extent endogenous estradiol levels modify dementia risk in men. If a relation exists between estradiol and risk of dementia in men, this risk is small, and it is likely that reduced statistical power due to small sample size and large intra- and interassay variation explain findings of no association. Further studies are needed to examine whether there are mechanisms by which estradiol may increase risk for cognitive decline and dementia. An interesting avenue is the possible modifying role of vascular risk in the association of estradiol with dementia. Furthermore, future studies should focus on the role of SHBG, the interrelation between testosterone and estrogen biosynthesis, and the role of aromatase in dementia risk. Future studies examining endogenous estradiol levels in relation to preclinical and clinical markers of dementia should have enough power to make reliable conclusions. Due to the long latency or preclinical phase of AD, longitudinal studies with very long follow-up and with subclinical measures of dementia as outcome variables are necessary to study the possible causal role of estradiol in dementia.

References

1. Cummings JL, Cole G. Alzheimer disease. *JAMA.* 2002;**287**:2335–8.

2. Yaffe K, Lui LY, Grady D, *et al.* Cognitive decline in women in relation to non-protein-bound oestradiol concentrations. *Lancet.* 2000;**356**:708–12.

3. Tang MX, Jacobs D, Stern Y, *et al.* Effect of oestrogen during menopause on risk and age at onset of Alzheimer's disease. *Lancet.* 1996;**348**:429–32.

4. Veiga S, Melcangi RC, Doncarlos LL, Garcia-Segura LM, Azcoitia I. Sex hormones and brain aging. *Exp Gerontol.* 2004;**39**:1623–31.

5. Den Heijer T, Geerlings MI, Hofman A, *et al.* Higher estrogen levels are not associated with larger hippocampi and better memory performance. *Arch Neurol.* 2003;**60**:213–20.

6. Geerlings MI, Launer LJ, de Jong FH, *et al.* Endogenous estradiol and risk of dementia in women and men: the Rotterdam Study. *Ann Neurol.* 2003;**53**:607–15.

7. Geerlings MI, Ruitenberg A, Witteman JC, *et al.* Reproductive period and risk of dementia in postmenopausal women. *JAMA.* 2001;**285**:1475–81.

8. Shumaker SA, Legault C, Kuller L, *et al.* Conjugated equine estrogens and incidence of probable dementia and mild cognitive impairment in postmenopausal women: the Women's Health Initiative Memory Study. *JAMA.* 2004;**291**:2947–58.

9. Muller M, van der Schouw YT, Thijssen JH, Grobbee DE. Endogenous sex hormones and cardiovascular

disease in men. *J Clin Endocrinol Metab.* 2003; **88**:5076–86.

10. Muller M, Grobbee DE, Thijssen JH, van den Beld AW, van der Schouw YT. Sex hormones and male health: effects on components of the frailty syndrome. *Trends Endocrinol Metab.* 2003;**14**:289–96.

11. de Ronde W, Pols HA, van Leeuwen JP, de Jong FH. The importance of oestrogens in males. *Clin Endocrinol (Oxf).* 2003;**58**:529–42.

12. Lessov-Schlaggar CN, Reed T, Swan GE, *et al.* Association of sex steroid hormones with brain morphology and cognition in healthy elderly men. *Neurology.* 2005;**65**:1591–6.

13. Aleman A, de Vries WR, Koppeschaar HP, *et al.* Relationship between circulating levels of sex hormones and insulin-like growth factor-1 and fluid intelligence in older men. *Exp Aging Res.* 2001; **27**:283–91.

14. Martin DM, Wittert G, Burns NR, Haren MT, Sugarman R. Testosterone and cognitive function in ageing men: data from the Florey Adelaide Male Ageing Study (FAMAS). *Maturitas.* 2007;**57**:182–94.

15. Muller M, Aleman A, Grobbee DE, de Haan EH, van der Schouw YT. Endogenous sex hormone levels and cognitive function in aging men. Is there an optimal level? *Neurology.* 2005;**64**(5):866–71.

16. Wolf OT, Kirschenbaum C. Endogenous estradiol and testosterone levels are associated with cognitive performance in older women and men. *Horm Behav.* 2002;**41**:259–66.

17. Yaffe K, Lui LY, Zmuda J, Cauley J. Sex hormones and cognitive function in older men. *J Am Geriatr Soc.* 2002;**50**:707–12.

18. Hogervorst E, De Jager C, Budge M, Smith AD. Serum levels of estradiol and testosterone and performance in different cognitive domains in healthy elderly men and women. *Psychoneuroendocrinology.* 2004;**29**:405–21.

19. Senanarong V, Vannasaeng S, Poungvarin N, *et al.* Endogenous estradiol in elderly individuals: cognitive and noncognitive associations. *Arch Neurol.* 2002;**59**:385–9.

20. Paoletti AM, Congia S, Lello S, *et al.* Low androgenization index in elderly women and elderly men with Alzheimer's disease. *Neurology.* 2004;**62**:301–3.

21. Irie F, Strozyk D, Peila R, *et al.* Brain lesions on MRI and endogenous sex hormones in elderly men. *Neurobiol Aging.* 2006;**27**:1137–44.

22. Strozyk D, White LR, Petrovitch H, *et al.* Sex hormones and neuropathology in elderly men: the HAAS. *Neurobiol Aging.* 2007;**28**(1): 62–8.

23. Barrett-Connor E, Goodman-Gruen D, Patay B. Endogenous sex hormones and cognitive function in older men. *J Clin Endocrinol Metab.* 1999;**84**:3681–5.

24. Muller M, van den Beld AW, Grobbee DE, de Jong FH, Lamberts SW. Sex hormones and cognitive decline in elderly men. *Psychoneuroendocrinology.* 2009; **34**(1):27–31.

25. Ravaglia G, Forti P, Maioli F, *et al.* Endogenous sex hormones as risk factors for dementia in elderly men and women. *J Gerontol A Biol Sci Med Sci.* 2007; **62**:1035–41.

26. Yaffe K, Barnes D, Lindquist K, *et al.* Endogenous sex hormone levels and risk of cognitive decline in an older biracial cohort. *Neurobiol Aging.* 2007; **28**:171–8.

27. Geerlings MI, Strozyk D, Masaki K, *et al.* Endogenous sex hormones, cognitive decline, and future dementia in old men. *Ann Neurol.* 2006;**60**:346–55.

28. Elias MF, Beiser A, Wolf PA, *et al.* The preclinical phase of Alzheimer disease: a 22-year prospective study of the Framingham Cohort. *Arch Neurol.* 2000;**57**:808–13.

29. Hogervorst E, Lehmann DJ, Warden DR, McBroom J, Smith AD. Apolipoprotein E epsilon4 and testosterone interact in the risk of Alzheimer's disease in men. *Int J Geriatr Psychiatry.* 2002;**17**:938–40.

30. Yaffe K, Haan M, Byers A, Tangen C, Kuller L. Estrogen use, APOE, and cognitive decline: evidence of gene-environment interaction. *Neurology.* 2000; **54**:1949–54.

31. Breteler MM. Vascular risk factors for Alzheimer's disease: an epidemiologic perspective. *Neurobiol Aging.* 2000;**21**:153–60.

32. Luchsinger JA, Mayeux R. Cardiovascular risk factors and Alzheimer's disease. *Curr Atheroscler Rep.* 2004;**6**:261–6.

33. Sudhir K, Komesaroff PA. Clinical review 110: Cardiovascular actions of estrogens in men. *J Clin Endocrinol Metab.* 1999;**84**:3411–15.

34. Arnlov J, Pencina MJ, Amin S, *et al.* Endogenous sex hormones and cardiovascular disease incidence in men. *Ann Intern Med.* 2006;**145**:176–84.

35. Muller M, den Tonkelaar I, Thijssen JHH, Grobbee DE, van der Schouw YT. Endogenous sex hormones in men aged 40–80 years. *Eur J Endocrinol.* 2003;**149**:583–9.

36. Muller M, Grobbee DE, den Tonkelaar I, Lamberts SW, van der Schouw YT. Endogenous sex hormones and metabolic syndrome in aging men. *J Clin Endocrinol Metab.* 2005;**90**:2618–23.

37. Phillips GB, Jing T, Heymsfield SB. Relationships in men of sex hormones, insulin, adiposity, and risk

factors for myocardial infarction. *Metabolism.* 2003;**52**:784–90.

38. Nakhai Pour HR, Grobbee DE, Muller M, van der Schouw YT. Association of endogenous sex hormone with C-reactive protein levels in middle-aged and elderly men. *Clin Endocrinol (Oxf).* 2007;**66**:394–8.

39. Tivesten A, Mellstrom D, Jutberger H, *et al.* Low serum testosterone and high serum estradiol associate with lower extremity peripheral arterial disease in elderly men. The MrOS Study in Sweden. *J Am Coll Cardiol.* 2007;**50**:1070–6.

40. Phillips GB, Pinkernell BH, Jing TY. The association of hyperestrogenemia with coronary thrombosis in men. *Arterioscler Thromb Vasc Biol.* 1996;**16**:1383–7.

41. Muller M, van den Beld AW, Bots ML, *et al.* Endogenous sex hormones and progression of carotid atherosclerosis in elderly men. *Circulation.* 2004;**109**:2074–9.

42. Tivesten A, Hulthe J, Wallenfeldt K, *et al.* Circulating estradiol is an independent predictor of progression of carotid artery intima-media thickness in middle-aged men. *J Clin Endocrinol Metab.* 2006;**91**:4433–7.

43. Abbott RD, Launer LJ, Rodriguez BL, *et al.* Serum estradiol and risk of stroke in elderly men. *Neurology.* 2007;**68**:563–8.

44. de Ronde W, van der Schouw YT, Muller M, *et al.* Associations of sex-hormone-binding globulin (SHBG) with non-SHBG-bound levels of testosterone and estradiol in independently living men. *J Clin Endocrinol Metab.* 2005;**90**:157–62.

45. Hammond GL. Potential functions of plasma steroid-binding proteins. *Trends Endocrinol Metab.* 1995;**6**:298–304.

46. Caldwell JD, Suleman F, Chou SH, *et al.* Emerging roles of steroid-binding globulins. *Horm Metab Res.* 2006;**38**:206–18.

47. Herbert Z, Gothe S, Caldwell JD, *et al.* Identification of sex hormone-binding globulin in the human hypothalamus. *Neuroendocrinology.* 2005;**81**:287–93.

48. Hogervorst E, Bandelow S, Combrinck M, Smith AD. Low free testosterone is an independent risk factor for Alzheimer's disease. *Exp Gerontol.* 2004;**39**:1633–9.

49. Hoskin EK, Tang MX, Manly JJ, Mayeux R. Elevated sex-hormone-binding globulin in elderly women with Alzheimer's disease. *Neurobiol Aging.* 2004;**25**:141–7.

50. Muller M, Schupf N, Manly JJ, Mayeux R, Luchsinger JA. Sex hormone-binding globulin and incident Alzheimer's disease in elderly men and women. *Neurobiol Aging.* 2008. [Epub ahead of print].

51. Garcia-Segura LM, Veiga S, Sierra A, Melcangi RC, Azcoitia I. Aromatase: a neuroprotective enzyme. *Prog Neurobiol.* 2003;**71**:31–41.

52. Longcope C, Billiar RB, Takaoka Y, *et al.* Tissue sites of aromatization in the female rhesus monkey. *Endocrinology.* 1983;**113**:1679–82.

53. Lambert JC, Harris JM, Mann D, *et al.* Are the estrogen receptors involved in Alzheimer's disease? *Neurosci Lett.* 2001;**306**:193–7.

Chapter 25

Testosterone regulates Alzheimer's disease pathogenesis

Christian J. Pike and Emily R. Rosario

Editors' introduction

As aging is associated with decreased estradiol production in women, so is aging associated with decreased testosterone production in men. In this chapter, Pike and Rosario review novel and compelling data indicating testosterone regulation of β-amyloid production in the brain, as well as significant associations between low testosterone levels and risk for Alzheimer's-related dementia in men. Based on these data and on the various mechanisms by which testosterone can exert neuroprotective effects in brain, the authors conclude that low testosterone is a likely risk factor for Alzheimer's-related dementia in men. Their analysis points out the need for research focusing on the development of brain-selective androgen receptor modulators (SARMs) for use in the prevention of Alzheimer's disease (AD) in men.

Introduction

Although the most significant risk factor for AD is advancing age, the age changes that contribute to this risk are not well understood. One consequence of normal aging that is increasingly linked to risk of AD is depletion of sex steroid hormones. An extensive scientific literature of basic and clinical research has established that the loss of estrogen in women at menopause acts as a significant modulator of AD risk. More controversial, as discussed in several chapters in this book, is to what extent and under what circumstances hormone therapy (HT) may reduce AD risk in women. More recently, a much smaller but rapidly growing literature has been asking whether a parallel relationship applies to men: does age-related testosterone loss in men contribute to the development

of AD and, if so, might hormone therapies for men mitigate this risk?

A normal senescent change in aging men with significant clinical consequences is testosterone depletion. Although men do not usually experience complete cessation of reproductive ability akin to menopause, men do experience a somewhat similar process termed andropause. Also called partial androgen deficiency in aging males, andropause refers to normal, age-related depletion of testosterone and the corresponding constellation of symptoms that reflect dysfunction and vulnerability to disease in androgen-responsive tissues including the brain (for a review see [1, 2]). Unlike menopause, aging men do not uniformly experience similar levels of andropause. That is, although nearly all men exhibit significant age-related testosterone loss typically beginning in the third decade of life, men vary in the extent of testosterone loss and the corresponding severity of clinical manifestations. It is estimated that 30% to 70% of men aged 70 and older are hypogonadal, resulting in at least five million aging men in the USA suffering the consequences of andropause and only a small minority of those receive HT [1]. Andropause is associated with increased risk of sarcopenia, osteoporosis, falls, frailty, and all cause mortality [1, 2]. In this chapter, we discuss recent evidence linking andropause with increased risk of AD, the mechanisms that underlie androgen regulation of AD pathogenesis, and therapeutic implications.

Age-related testosterone loss and the risk of Alzheimer's disease

In the past several years, age-related testosterone loss in men has been evaluated as a potential risk factor

---

for the development of AD. Because testosterone and other androgens induce several beneficial actions in the brain, the loss of androgens with age logically would be expected to impair neural function and perhaps elevate vulnerability to neurodegenerative disease. In support of this possibility, an increased risk for the development of AD has been linked to this loss of androgens in men (for a review see [3, 4]). Initial studies examining the relationship between AD and androgens, specifically testosterone, found significantly lower levels of circulating testosterone in men with a clinical diagnosis of AD in comparison to age-matched, cognitively normal men [5, 6]. While several studies support this relationship, there are a few studies that do not find any significant differences in testosterone levels between AD and control subjects [7].

While these initial studies revealed an association in men between low testosterone levels and AD, they were not able to conclude whether testosterone depletion contributed to or resulted from the disease process. Importantly, two complementary studies were able to address this issue and demonstrated that low testosterone is a precursor rather than a consequence of AD pathogenesis. Using samples from the Baltimore Longitudinal Study on Aging, Moffat and colleagues found not only that non-demented men had significantly higher testosterone levels than men with AD, but also that this difference was apparent ten years prior to the clinical diagnosis of dementia [8]. Relying on neuropathological rather than clinical criteria and brain rather than blood levels of testosterone, our research group made similar findings. Using neuropathologically characterized human postmortem brain tissue, we found that brain levels of testosterone but not estradiol exhibit age-related depletion in men lacking neuropathology, an observation that is consistent with numerous prior studies of hormone levels in blood [9]. Also in parallel to prior work on circulating levels of hormones, we found that brain levels of testosterone but not estradiol were significantly lower in male cases with a neuropathological diagnosis of AD [9]. Importantly, we also examined brain levels of testosterone in cases that exhibited mild neuropathological changes consistent with early development of AD (Braak stage 2–3) and found that these cases also had significantly lower levels of testosterone [9]. Together, these two studies indicate that testosterone levels, both circulating levels in blood and tissue levels in brain, are reduced in men prior to the clinical and neuropathological diagnoses of

AD and therefore represent a risk factor for the development of AD.

Testosterone can protect the brain from Alzheimer-related pathologies

Testosterone induces many effects in the brain that improve function, contribute to cognition, and likely increase resistance to AD and related diseases. Besides its established roles in neurodevelopment, aggression, and sexual behaviors, testosterone is involved in a wide range of neural actions, which is consistent with the broad distribution of androgen receptors in brain. Notably, androgens affect neural plasticity by a variety of mechanisms, including regulation of neuronal differentiation, spine density [10], and neurogenesis [11]. Of particular relevance to neurodegenerative diseases including AD is that testosterone is an endogenous neuroprotective factor [12]. For example, androgen depletion resulting from orchidectomy in adult male rats significantly increases hippocampal vulnerability to kainate lesion, an effect that is prevented by androgen replacement [13]. Neuron cell culture studies demonstrate that androgens utilize androgen-receptor dependent mechanisms to protect against a range of insults relevant to AD, including apoptosis induced by β-amyloid protein [12]. Also, relevant to a protective role against AD neuropathology is the androgen action of inhibiting hyperphosphorylation of tau protein [14], an event that left unchecked results in the formation of a neurofibrillary tangles, a significant type of neuropathology common to AD and related disorders.

A particularly important neural action of androgens that likely has a direct role in the development of AD is regulation of β-amyloid (Aβ) accumulation. Although Aβ is a normal protein present as a small soluble peptide in bodily fluids, an extensive body of research implicates abnormal accumulation of Aβ and its adoption of altered conformations in both the initiation and progression of AD [15]. Thus, factors that regulate production, catabolism, and/or clearance of Aβ will affect its accumulation and, by extension, the risk of developing AD. The identification of testosterone as an endogenous regulator of Aβ strongly suggests that this property contributes to its role as a risk factor for AD.

Research findings over the past several years from human tissues, animal models, and cell culture demonstrate that androgens negatively regulate Aβ accumulation [4]. In aged men treated for prostate cancer with anti-androgen therapy (so-called chemical castration that includes both an androgen receptor antagonist and leuprolide acetate, which indirectly reduces testosterone production), several weeks of treatment resulted not only in the desired reduction in plasma levels of testosterone and estradiol but also in elevated plasma levels of Aβ [16, 17]. In aging men with memory loss, plasma levels of testosterone and Aβ are inversely correlated, another observation that links low testosterone with elevated Aβ [18]. Recently, we have found a similar relationship in brain tissue from non-demented men: low testosterone levels were significantly associated with high soluble Aβ (E.R.R. and C.J.P., unpublished observations). Together, these studies establish a relationship between testosterone and Aβ that presumably contributes to the risk of AD associated with low testosterone.

Studies in experimental paradigms confirm a regulatory relationship between testosterone and Aβ. In our laboratory, we found that orchiectomy of adult male Sprague-Dawley rats reduced brain and plasma levels of testosterone while also significantly increasing soluble levels of Aβ in the brain [19]. Restoration of androgen levels in castrated rats with the potent testosterone metabolite dihydrotestosterone (DHT) returned Aβ to levels observed in gonadally intact rats [19]. We recently repeated these observations in the brown Norway rat, a model of reproductive aging in men, showing that natural age-related testosterone depletion in male rats was associated with a robust increase in brain levels of Aβ [51]. Further, in the 3xTg-AD transgenic mouse model of AD we have found that androgen depletion caused by orchiectomy resulted in increased accumulation of Aβ in hippocampus, subiculum, and amygdala as well as impairment in hippocampal-dependent working memory [20]. We also found that treatment of orchiectomized 3xTg-AD male mice with DHT prevented both the increase in Aβ accumulation and the associated deficit in hippocampal behavioral function [20]. Studies performed in cultured neurons and neural cell lines also demonstrated that testosterone and DHT reduce Aβ levels [21, 22]. In summary, findings from several paradigms clearly demonstrate that androgens are associated with regulation of Aβ, a critical event in AD pathogenesis that surely contributes to the relationship between low testosterone and risk of AD. However, because testosterone regulates and is regulated by other hormones and because testosterone

can function directly and indirectly through various pathways, understanding precisely how testosterone regulates Aβ may be complicated but undoubtedly important.

Testosterone protects the brain by multiple mechanisms

In order to pursue clinical interventions that will reduce the risk of AD associated with low testosterone, it is important to understand not only how testosterone acts to regulate AD pathogenesis but also the cellular mechanisms underlying these actions. To begin to investigate the mechanisms through which testosterone regulates Aβ pathology and the risk for development of AD it is important to note that testosterone is a prohormone that is converted in tissues by 5α-reductase to DHT, its active androgen metabolite, and by aromatase to the estrogen 17β-estradiol. The brain contains both 5α-reductase and aromatase, allowing testosterone to act neurally through both androgen- and estrogen-dependent pathways.

Many beneficial neural effects of testosterone are mediated at least in part via estrogen pathways following testosterone conversion to estradiol. During neural development, much of the masculinization due to testosterone is in fact mediated by estradiol. Similarly, testosterone neuroprotection against excitotoxic insult in male rats can involve aromatase action and subsequent activation of estrogen signaling [23] although estrogen-independent pathways also plays a significant role [13]. In the case of testosterone regulation of Aβ, the precise contributions of estrogen versus androgen pathways remain to be fully determined. It is well established that estrogen signaling reduces Aβ accumulation in both cell culture models and in female rodents (for a review see [24]). Although the mechanisms underlying this action have not been fully elucidated, one important pathway is the estrogen-mediated regulation of Aβ production via effects on the trafficking and/or processing of amyloid precursor protein [24]. Testosterone similarly regulates amyloid precursor protein processing by a pathway dependent on aromatase action [25], suggesting that estrogen pathways may contribute to testosterone regulation of Aβ. However, androgen pathways are also important as evidenced by our observation in orchiectomized male rats that DHT but not estradiol significantly reduced levels of soluble

Aβ [19]. By contrast, our recent results in male 3xTg-AD mice suggest that estradiol may reduce Aβ deposition induced by orchiectomy (E.R.R. and C.J.P., unpublished observations). Together, these data suggest the possibility that both estrogen and androgen pathways may contribute to testosterone regulation of Aβ.

In addition to estrogen pathways, there is also a possibility that gonadotropins play a role in the relationships between testosterone, Aβ accumulation, and AD risk in men. Androgens regulate gonadotropin levels through negative feedback of the hypothalamic-pituitary-gonadal axis. Thus, normal aging in men is associated not only with decreases in testosterone but also increases in the gonadotropin luteinizing hormone (LH), although the latter typically increases to significant levels comparatively late in life [2]. Thus, some have argued that the most relevant and perhaps clinically significant age change in the male hypothalamic-pituitary-gonadal axis is not low testosterone but rather elevated LH [26, 27]. In fact, men with AD are reported to exhibit significantly higher levels of LH than non-demented controls [5, 26], although this association between LH and AD appears to be most apparent in men over age 80 [5]. Like estrogen and androgen pathways, there is evidence to suggest that LH may affect AD risk by regulating Aβ. Cell culture studies show that LH increases secreted Aβ levels and reduces non-amyloidogenic processing of amyloid precursor protein suggesting that LH may affect Aβ levels by increasing its production [28]. Reducing LH with leuprolide acetate, a gonadotropin releasing hormone agonist often used as part of androgen suppression therapy in the treatment of prostate cancer, has been observed to decrease soluble Aβ in intact female rats [28] and to reduce Aβ deposition in a transgenic mouse model of AD [27]. These observations suggest that in addition to estrogen pathways, testosterone may indirectly regulate Aβ accumulation and influence AD risk by altering LH levels.

Despite this evidence suggesting involvement of LH in the development of AD, the potential role of gonadotropins as a significant, direct modulator of AD risk is controversial. In our experimental paradigms, we have found that sex steroids rather than gonadotropins appear to be the primary mediators through which testosterone regulates Aβ. In male rodents, it is known that orchiectomy results in both testosterone depletion and a compensatory increase

in LH levels, an effect that is reversed with either DHT or estrogen replacement [29]. Interestingly, we observed that although estrogen treatment of orchiectomized male rats restored LH to normal levels, it did not reduce Aβ levels, a finding that illustrates a disconnection between levels of LH and Aβ ([19], and unpublished data). We found similar results using a rodent model of male reproductive aging, the brown Norway rat. In this model, aging is characterized by gradual depletion of testosterone levels but no significant elevation in plasma LH levels. We find a significant age-related increase in Aβ in male brown Norway rats that correlates with the decrease in testosterone levels; however, we observe no correlation between LH and Aβ in these animals (E.R.R. and C.J.P., unpublished data). In summary, there is an inconsistent literature concerning the role of gonadotropins in Aβ regulation and AD risk, which likely will be clarified by future research.

Although estrogen and LH may contribute to regulation of Aβ, these hormones do not appear to be the primary way through which testosterone regulates Aβ and modulates the development of AD. Rather, our data are most consistent with direct androgen signaling involving activation of androgen receptors. First, the increase in Aβ levels resulting from orchiectomy in both adult male rats [19] and in adult male 3xTg-AD mice [20] is prevented by treatment with DHT, an androgen that is a potent agonist for androgen receptor and is not metabolized to estradiol. As discussed above, our observations in these animal models are also inconsistent with a primary role of LH. Second, we have recently elucidated a novel mechanism of testosterone Aβ regulation. Specifically, we found in the male rodent brain, primary hippocampal neurons, and androgen receptor transfected neural cell lines that testosterone and DHT increase the expression of neprilysin by a classic genomic, androgen receptor dependent pathway [22]. Neprilysin is an Aβ-catabolizing enzyme that degrades Aβ and largely determines the steady state levels of Aβ in the brain [30]. Further, testosterone and DHT reduce Aβ levels in cultured neural cells by a mechanism that is dependent upon both androgen receptors and neprilysin [22]. While these data do not exclude a role for estrogen or gonadotropins in Aβ regulation, they do provide compelling evidence for an androgen-dependent mechanism in the regulation of Aβ and thus development of AD pathology.

Future directions: testosterone-related therapies to prevent Alzheimer's disease

Similar to the use of estrogen-based HTs to prevent and treat AD in women, the parallel use of androgen-based therapies in men will likely be fraught with challenges. In order to minimize such difficulties and maximize the opportunities to deliver effective therapies, it is hoped that basic and clinical researchers will cooperatively pursue interventions, proceed with caution, and be guided on the basis of solid experimental evidence. Based on the currently available research findings, it is logical to conclude that low testosterone in aging men is a risk factor for the development of AD. Further, although testosterone induces many protective actions potentially relevant to AD, the ability of androgens to reduce Aβ accumulation is most likely the primary means by which testosterone regulates AD pathogenesis. Because Aβ accumulation is thought to be the key initiating event in the disease process and because this is thought to occur years prior to the onset of clinical symptoms, testosterone-related interventions are predicted to be most effective in preventing and or delaying disease onset. Further, such interventions would most likely need to begin in middle age, at a time when age-related testosterone loss becomes significant in some men and prior to the development of neural Aβ accumulation. Conversely, once the disease manifests in the form of dementia, significant Aβ accumulation and other neuropathology will exist and the therapeutic efficacy of testosterone-related therapies is predicted to be limited. Thus, a reasonable interpretation of available evidence suggests that testosterone-related therapies may be most useful in the prevention rather than treatment of AD and should be initiated in hypogonadal men in middle age.

In the past few years, there have been several clinical investigations of testosterone in cognitively normal and demented men that have yielded mixed findings (for a review see [31]). In some studies, testosterone use in aged, cognitively normal men was associated with improvement in spatial, visual, verbal, and working memory [32–34]. However, other studies have produced either no evidence of significant increases in cognition [35, 36] or even worsened performance [37]. Similarly, in men with mild cognitive impairment and early AD, testosterone therapy also proved variable, showing improvement only in some studies [38–40]. Because these studies were relatively short term in comparison to the lengthy duration of AD development and progression, it seems likely that the observed testosterone effects reflect testosterone actions on processes associated with cognition (e.g., synaptic plasticity) rather than AD pathology such as Aβ accumulation. Thus, the existing literature suggests that androgens likely benefit select aspects of cognition in hypogonadal men, which may yield modest therapeutic benefit. However, the extent to which testosterone therapy may prevent AD or delay its onset is not known.

An alternative treatment approach for AD that also addresses the age-related depletion of testosterone and associated increase in gonadotropins involves the use of leuprolide acetate. This approach is based upon the hypothesis (discussed above) that elevated levels of the gonadotropin LH may be a key regulator of AD risk. With continued use, leuprolide acetate results in decreased levels of LH and, as a consequence of hypothalamic-pituitary-gonadal function, depletion of endogenous testosterone. One potentially significant caveat of leuprolide acetate treatment is the associated down-regulation of gonadal hormones, which would be expected to have a range of deleterious effects. For example, androgen suppression treatments involving leuprolide acetate for prostate cancer patients have largely been associated with impairments rather than improvements in cognition [16, 32, 41, 42]. Recent findings now discourage the use of such treatments for early-stage prostate cancer due to poor quality of life, an increase in all-cause mortality, and an absence of significant therapeutic benefit [43]. Both men and women with mild to moderate AD have been treated with leuprolide acetate in clinical trials, the results of which have yet to be published. In comparison to the leuprolide acetate approach, testosterone therapy in aged men will not only increase testosterone levels (possibly yielding beneficial effects on cognition) but also decrease LH levels [36], thus providing an intervention that can act via two pathways: restoring androgen signaling and reducing gonadotropins.

Yet another testosterone-related therapy that is currently being developed and evaluated for a variety of andropause-related conditions is a group of compounds collectively called selective androgen receptor modulators (SARMs). The development of SARMs has occurred in response to concerns that testosterone therapy may have undesirable and potentially life-threatening side effects. In particular, there is evidence that testosterone may increase the risk and/or progression of prostate cancer, although this issue is controversial (for a review see [1]). Prostate cancer, which is the second leading cancer among aging men in terms of both prevalence and cause of death [44], is androgen dependent and often treated by androgen suppression therapy. Selective androgen receptor modulators are designed through a variety of strategies to exert androgenic effects in a tissue-selective manner, lacking significant androgen action in prostate but inducing agonist effects in target androgen-responsive tissues of interest, including brain, muscle, and bone.

One class of SARMs that have shown good tissue specificity is novel steroidal compounds that are not substrates for 5α-reductase, the enzyme that converts testosterone to DHT. Prostate growth depends largely on the actions of DHT rather than testosterone because DHT exhibits ∼ten-fold greater net potency, which reflects both a higher binding affinity for AR and a slower dissociation rate from AR [45]. Selective androgen receptor modulators that are not 5α-reductase substrates and thus do not form DHT or DHT-like derivatives have relatively low androgen action in the prostate [46–48]. At this time, the most promising SARM in this category is 7α-methyl-19-nortestosterone, commonly called MENT [47, 48]. MENT, which was developed by the Population Council and is currently in clinical trials as an androgen therapy for hypogonadal men [49], shows low androgen activity in the prostate but is more potent than testosterone in other peripheral androgen-responsive tissues including bone and muscle [47, 48]. Although not a substrate for 5α-reductase, MENT is a substrate for aromatase and thus, like testosterone, generates some estradiol. Because many cellular effects of testosterone result from aromatization to estradiol and subsequent activation of estrogen signaling, there is potentially strong benefit in a SARM that exhibits both androgen and estrogen functions. In addition to MENT, there are numerous recently identified and developed SARMs that show strong initial promise [46, 50]. In the near future, the development of a brain specific SARM is expected with the hope of efficacy in preventing AD while lacking possible deleterious effects on the prostate.

In conclusion, a rapidly growing research literature has established normal age-related loss of testosterone in men with increased risk for AD. Testosterone induces many protective effects in brain relevant to AD, perhaps most importantly it functions as an endogenous negative regulator of Aβ accumulation. However, clinical use of testosterone therapy to prevent and/or treat AD in aging hypogonadal men will likely be as complicated as the ongoing, controversial use of HTs in postmenopausal women. Important considerations include not only when and how to deliver testosterone-related therapies but also what type of therapy. That is, because testosterone activates not only androgen signaling but also affects estrogen and gonadotropin pathways, there are several possible mechanisms that may individually or cooperatively act to regulate AD pathogenesis. As additional research clarifies these issues, we anticipate that one or more emerging testosterone-related therapies will prove useful in maintaining and improving neural health in the aging male.

Acknowledgment

This work was supported by NIH grant AG23739.

References

1. Kaufman JM, Vermeulen A. The decline of androgen levels in elderly men and its clinical and therapeutic implications. *Endocr Rev.* 2005;**26**(6):833–76.

2. Morley JE. Androgens and aging. *Maturitas.* 2001; **38**(1):61–71; discussion 3.

3. Pike CJ, Rosario ER, Nguyen TV. Androgens, aging, and Alzheimer's disease. *Endocrine.* 2006;**29**(2): 233–41.

4. Rosario ER, Pike CJ. Androgen regulation of beta-amyloid protein and the risk of Alzheimer's disease. *Brain Res Rev.* 2008;**57**(2):444–53.

5. Hogervorst E, Combrinck M, Smith AD. Testosterone and gonadotropin levels in men with dementia. *Neuroendocrinol Lett.* 2003;**24**(3/4):203–8.

6. Hogervorst E, Williams J, Budge M, *et al.* Serum total testosterone is lower in men with Alzheimer's disease. *Neuroendocrinol Lett.* 2001;**22**(3):163–8.

7. Pennanen C, Laakso MP, Kivipelto M, Ramberg J, Soininen H. Serum testosterone levels in males with Alzheimer's disease. *J Neuroendocrinol.* 2004; **16**(2):95–8.

8. Moffat SD, Zonderman AB, Metter EJ, *et al.* Free testosterone and risk for Alzheimer disease in older men. *Neurology.* 2004;**62**(2):188–93.

9. Rosario ER, Chang L, Stanczyk FZ, Pike CJ. Age-related testosterone depletion and the development of Alzheimer disease. *JAMA.* 2004;**292**(12):1431–2.

10. MacLusky NJ, Hajszan T, Prange-Kiel J, Leranth C. Androgen modulation of hippocampal synaptic plasticity. *Neuroscience.* 2006;**138**(3):957–65.

11. Galea LA. Gonadal hormone modulation of neurogenesis in the dentate gyrus of adult male and female rodents. *Brain Res Rev.* 2008;**57**(2):332–41.

12. Pike CJ, Nguyen TV, Ramsden M, *et al.* Androgen cell signaling pathways involved in neuroprotective actions. *Horm Behav.* 2008;**53**(5):693–705.

13. Ramsden M, Shin TM, Pike CJ. Androgens modulate neuronal vulnerability to kainate lesion. *Neuroscience.* 2003;**122**(3):573–8.

14. Papasozomenos SC, Papasozomenos T. Androgens prevent the heat shock-induced hyperphosphorylation but not dephosphorylation of tau in female rats. Implications for Alzheimer's disease. *J Alzheimers Dis.* 1999;**1**(3):147–53.

15. Hardy J. Alzheimer's disease: the amyloid cascade hypothesis: an update and reappraisal. *J Alzheimers Dis.* 2006;**9**(3 Suppl):151–3.

16. Almeida OP, Flicker L. Testosterone and dementia: too much ado about too little data. *J Br Menopause Soc.* 2003;**9**(3):107–10.

17. Gandy S, Almeida OP, Fonte J, *et al.* Chemical andropause and amyloid-beta peptide. *JAMA.* 2001;**285**(17):2195–6.

18. Gillett MJ, Martins RN, Clarnette RM, *et al.* Relationship between testosterone, sex hormone binding globulin and plasma amyloid beta peptide 40 in older men with subjective memory loss or dementia. *J Alzheimers Dis.* 2003;**5**(4):267–9.

19. Ramsden M, Nyborg AC, Murphy MP, *et al.* Androgens modulate beta-amyloid levels in male rat brain. *J Neurochem.* 2003;**87**(4):1052–5.

20. Rosario ER, Carroll JC, Oddo S, LaFerla FM, Pike CJ. Androgens regulate the development of neuropathology in a triple transgenic mouse model of Alzheimer's disease. *J Neurosci.* 2006;**26**(51):13384–9.

21. Gouras GK, Xu H, Gross RS, *et al.* Testosterone reduces neuronal secretion of Alzheimer's beta-amyloid peptides. *Proc Natl Acad Sci USA.* 2000;**97**(3):1202–5.

22. Yao M, Nguyen TV, Rosario ER, Ramsden M, Pike CJ. Androgens regulate neprilysin expression: role in reducing beta-amyloid levels. *J Neurochem* 2008.

23. Azcoitia I, Sierra A, Veiga S, Garcia-Segura LM. Aromatase expression by reactive astroglia is neuroprotective. *Ann N Y Acad Sci.* 2003;**1007**:298–305.

24. Xu H, Wang R, Zhang YW, Zhang X. Estrogen, beta-amyloid metabolism/trafficking, and Alzheimer's disease. *Ann N Y Acad Sci.* 2006;**1089**:324–42.

25. Goodenough S, Engert S, Behl C. Testosterone stimulates rapid secretory amyloid precursor protein release from rat hypothalamic cells via the activation of the mitogen-activated protein kinase pathway. *Neurosci Lett.* 2000;**296**(1):49–52.

26. Bowen RL, Isley JP, Atkinson RL. An association of elevated serum gonadotropin concentrations and Alzheimer disease? *J Neuroendocrinol.* 2000;**12**(4):351–4.

27. Casadesus G, Webber KM, Atwood CS, *et al.* Luteinizing hormone modulates cognition and amyloid-beta deposition in Alzheimer APP transgenic mice. *Biochim Biophys Acta.* 2006;**1762**(4):447–52.

28. Bowen RL, Verdile G, Liu T, *et al.* Luteinizing hormone, a reproductive regulator that modulates the processing of amyloid-beta precursor protein and amyloid-beta deposition. *J Biol Chem.* 2004;**279**(19):20539–45.

29. Gharib SD, Wierman ME, Shupnik MA, Chin WW. Molecular biology of the pituitary gonadotropins. *Endocr Rev.* 1990;**11**(1):177–99.

30. Hersh LB, Rodgers DW. Neprilysin and amyloid beta peptide degradation. *Curr Alzheimer Res.* 2008;**5**(2):225–31.

31. Janowsky JS. The role of androgens in cognition and brain aging in men. *Neuroscience.* 2006;**138**(3):1015–20.

32. Cherrier MM, Craft S, Matsumoto AH. Cognitive changes associated with supplementation of testosterone or dihydrotestosterone in mildly hypogonadal men: a preliminary report. *J Androl.* 2003;**24**(4):568–76.

33. Janowsky JS, Oviatt SK, Orwoll ES. Testosterone influences spatial cognition in older men. *Behav Neurosci.* 1994;**108**(2):325–32.

34. Moffat SD, Zonderman AB, Metter EJ, *et al.* Longitudinal assessment of serum free testosterone concentration predicts memory performance and cognitive status in elderly men. *J Clin Endocrinol Metab.* 2002;**87**(11):5001–7.

35. Emmelot-Vonk MH, Verhaar HJ, Nakhai Pour HR, *et al.* Effect of testosterone supplementation on functional mobility, cognition, and other parameters in older men: a randomized controlled trial. *JAMA.* 2008;**299**(1):39–52.

36. Haren MT, Wittert GA, Chapman IM, Coates P, Morley JE. Effect of oral testosterone undecanoate on visuospatial cognition, mood and quality of life in elderly men with low-normal gonadal status. *Maturitas.* 2005;**50**(2):124–33.

37. Maki PM, Ernst M, London ED, *et al.* Intramuscular testosterone treatment in elderly men: evidence of

memory decline and altered brain function. *J Clin Endocrinol Metab.* 2007;**92**(11):4107–14.

38. Cherrier MM, Matsumoto AM, Amory JK, *et al.* Testosterone improves spatial memory in men with Alzheimer disease and mild cognitive impairment. *Neurology.* 2005;**64**(12):2063–8.

39. Tan RS, Culberson JW. An integrative review on current evidence of testosterone replacement therapy for the andropause. *Maturitas.* 2003;**45**(1):15–27.

40. Lu PH, Masterman DA, Mulnard R, *et al.* Effects of testosterone on cognition and mood in male patients with mild Alzheimer disease and healthy elderly men. *Arch Neurol.* 2006;**63**(2):177–85.

41. Green HJ. Altered cognitive function in men treated for prostate cancer with luteinizing hormone-releasing analogues and cyproterone acetate: a randomized controlled trial. *BJU International.* 2002; **90**(4):427–32.

42. Salminen EK, Portin RI, Koskinen A, Helenius H, Nurmi M. Associations between serum testosterone fall and cognitive function in prostate cancer patients. *Clin Cancer Res.* 2004;**10**(22):7575–82.

43. Lu-Yao GL, Albertsen PC, Moore DF, *et al.* Survival following primary androgen deprivation therapy among men with localized prostate cancer. *JAMA.* 2008;**300**(2):173–81.

44. Fleshner N, Zlotta AR. Prostate cancer prevention: past, present, and future. *Cancer.* 2007;**110**(9): 1889–99.

45. Wilson EM, French FS. Binding properties of androgen receptors. Evidence for identical receptors in rat testis, epididymis, and prostate. *J Biol Chem.* 1976;**251**(18):5620–9.

46. Ostrowski J, Kuhns JE, Lupisella JA, *et al.* Pharmacological and x-ray structural characterization of a novel selective androgen receptor modulator: potent hyperanabolic stimulation of skeletal muscle with hypostimulation of prostate in rats. *Endocrinology.* 2007;**148**(1):4–12.

47. Shao TC, Li HL, Kasper S, *et al.* Comparison of the growth-promoting effects of testosterone and 7-alpha-methyl-19-nor-testosterone (MENT) on the prostate and levator ani muscle of LPB-tag transgenic mice. *Prostate.* 2006;**66**(4):369–76.

48. Venken K, Boonen S, Van Herck E, *et al.* Bone and muscle protective potential of the prostate-sparing synthetic androgen 7alpha-methyl-19-nortestosterone: evidence from the aged orchidectomized male rat model. *Bone.* 2005;**36**(4):663–70.

49. von Eckardstein S, Noe G, Brache V, *et al.* A clinical trial of 7 alpha-methyl-19-nortestosterone implants for possible use as a long-acting contraceptive for men. *J Clin Endocrinol Metab.* 2003;**88**(11): 5232–9.

50. Gao W, Reiser PJ, Coss CC, *et al.* Selective androgen receptor modulator treatment improves muscle strength and body composition and prevents bone loss in orchidectomized rats. *Endocrinology.* 2005; **146**(11):4887–97.

51. Rosario ER, Chang L, Head EH, Stanczyk FZ, Pike CJ. Brain levels of sex steroid hormones in men and women during normal aging and in Alzheimer's disease. *Neurobiol Aging,* 2009 May 8 [Epub ahead of print].

Involvement of gonadotropins in cognitive function: implications for Alzheimer's disease

Gemma Casadesus, Kathryn J. Bryan, George Perry, and Mark A. Smith

Editors' introduction

Casadesus and colleagues make a case that hormonal changes associated with the dysregulation of the hypothalamic-pituitary-gonadal (HPG) axis following menopause/andropause are implicated in the pathogenesis of Alzheimer's disease (AD). Experimental support for this postulate has come from studies demonstrating an increase in amyloid-β (Aβ) deposition following ovariectomy/castration. Because sex steroids and gonadotropins are both part of the HPG feedback loop, decrements in sex steroids result in a proportionate increase in gonadotropins. They provide a review of the basic science relevant to luteinizing hormone (LH) and its receptor as a background for considering LH regulation of cognitive behaviors and AD pathology. Results of their analyses suggest that marked increases in serum LH following menopause/andropause is a physiologically relevant signal that could increase Aβ secretion and deposition in the aging brain. Suppression of the age-related increase in serum gonadotropins using anti-gonadotropin agents, such as leuprolide, is proposed as a novel therapeutic strategy for AD.

Etiology of Alzheimer's disease

Alzheimer's disease is characterized by progressive memory loss, impairments in language and visual-spatial skills, episodes of psychosis, aggressiveness, agitation, and ultimately death. Pathological markers of this condition involve a cerebral cortex thinner than normal, senile plaques, and neurofibrillary tangles (NFTs) [1]. As the most prevalent neurodegenerative disease, AD affects approximately five million people in the USA and 15 million people worldwide, and given current population demographic predictions, it is estimated that by 2050, 50 million people will be diagnosed if no successful treatments are found [2].

Despite its discovery 100 years ago, the mechanisms involved in this disease remain to be elucidated. However, the biochemical characterization of senile plaques led to the identification of amyloid-β (Aβ) peptide, the central component of this pathological entity, and a product of the amyloid-β protein precursor (APP). The significance of Aβ/APP in AD became evident by the fact that genetic mutations in the APP gene cause the early onset familial form of the disease. These findings led to the foundation for the Amyloid Cascade Hypothesis [3], which states that mutations in APP (or other genes) lead to an increase in Aβ, which then leads to disease. While the original hypothesis posited Aβ fibrils as the major mediator of the disease, a more recent incarnation of the hypothesis [3] proposes smaller oligomeric forms of Aβ as key. In both cases, Aβ is viewed as being important in mediating the neuronal and synaptic toxicity that leads to the deterioration of cognition [4] suggesting that Aβ may not be the major pathogenic factor [5–8]. In addition, a steady influx of research has begun to elucidate the role of NFTs and their principal protein component, phosphorylated tau, in the brain and how these pathological entities relate to the symptomatology of AD. However, the pathological significance of Aβ and NFT in disease and their interaction is still under much discussion, and other theories of AD, unrelated to NFT and Aβ deposits, are also being actively pursued (for a review see [9–12]). Unfortunately, to date, only palliative treatments of the symptoms are available and it is widely accepted that a better understanding of the etiology and disease pathogenesis is crucial for the

---

Hormones, Cognition and Dementia: State of the Art and Emergent Therapeutic Strategies, ed. Eef Hogervorst, Victor W. Henderson, Robert B. Gibbs, and Roberta Diaz Brinton. Published by Cambridge University Press.
© Cambridge University Press 2009.

development of new drugs capable of forestalling the progression of the disease [13].

Because of the pathogenic plurality of this disease, the lack of successful treatments based on the current hypotheses, and the fact that postmenopausal women are 1.6 to 3 times more likely to develop AD than men, many have turned to the sex steroids for answers [14]. Hormonal influences in AD were initially overlooked due to the assumption that AD incidence in women was higher simply because they lived longer than men. However, findings indicating that women also showed increased AD pathology compared to men led many to a focus on the role of sex steroids on neuronal function and cognition in both men and women [15].

Menopausal changes in hormones: relevance to cognition

Hormones of the hypothalamic-pituitary-gonadal (HPG)-axis include gonadotropin-releasing hormone (GnRH), luteinizing hormone (LH), follicle-stimulating hormone (FSH), 17β-estradiol, progesterone, testosterone, activin, inhibin, and follistatin. Each of these hormones is involved in regulating reproductive function by participating in a complex feedback loop that is initiated by the hypothalamic secretion of GnRH and its stimulation of the anterior pituitary to secrete the gonadotropins, LH and FSH. These gonadotropins, once released into the bloodstream, bind to receptors on the gonads and stimulate oogenesis/spermatogenesis as well as the production of the sex steroids. Sex steroids complete the negative feedback loop by decreasing gonadotropin secretion though the regulation of GnRH in the hypothalamus and directly at the anterior pituitary gland.

The onset of menopause, which occurs around the age of 50, can last for one third of a woman's life and is associated with a disruption of the HPG axis [16]. While the hallmark of menopause is the decreased production of 17β-estradiol and rising levels of gonadotropins, several theories have been proposed to explain this inescapable event in the lives of women. Some theories are ovarian driven, based on the hypothesis that women are born with a finite amount of oocytes and when these are depleted menopause occurs. Others are brain driven, based on evidence associated with perimenopausal declines in inhibins and rising levels of FSH, which can lead to desynchronization of GnRH signals and accelerated follicular loss [17].

Many adverse effects occur during the period surrounding menopause. Some include mood changes, sleep disturbances, urinary incontinence, somatic complaints, sexual dysfunction, hot flashes, and, of direct relevance to this article, cognitive disturbances. Importantly, the majority of women turn to estrogen replacement to alleviate these symptoms [18]. The relevance of estrogen therapy has been extensively studied in relation to cognitive decline because of its link to AD. Early clinical studies determined that low-dose estrogen therapy slightly improved cognition and mood in women diagnosed with AD [19]. Around the same time, another clinical study conducted by Sherwin [20] determined that treatment with estrogen alone, androgen alone, or a combination of the two in premenopausal women who had their uterus and ovaries surgically removed maintained their performance on verbal memory tests. These earlier studies were followed by two decades of research examining estrogen and cognition in both clinical and preclinical studies. As such, behavioral, cognitive, and cellular changes have been under intense investigation and often find that estrogen improves cognition and increases cell survival, synaptic plasticity, and dendritic sprouting [21]. In this regard, ovariectomy reduces synaptic remodeling evidenced by a reduction in spine density in the CA1 region, and this effect is rescued by 17β-estradiol replacement in rodents [22] and in primates [23]. Furthermore, synaptic remodeling has been shown to occur in coordination with the phasic nature of 17β-estradiol as well as after local administration of 17β-estradiol in various brain regions; this is evidenced by dramatic increases in the density of CA1 area spine synapses [23]. Likewise, various synaptic markers are up-regulated after systemic estrogen application, both in vivo [24] and in vitro [25]; namely, synaptophysin, a member of the transmitter vesicle membrane localized in presynaptic boutons [26] and synaptophilin, a cytoskeleton-associated protein, found in postsynaptic spines [27], among others. Furthermore, the ability of 17β-estradiol to change excitability of neurons in the hypothalamus, amygdala, striatum, cerebellum, and hippocampus has also been described [28].

Of direct relevance to AD pathogenesis, estrogen receptors interact with apolipoprotein E (APOE), polymorphisms of which are identified as a major risk factor for AD. APOE is produced by astrocytes and microglia and is important in membrane repair, synaptic plasticity, and reduces the clearance of Aβ. Estrogens can promote the effects of APOE on Aβ clearance, thus reducing Aβ [29]. Additionally, estrogens are well known to interact with the cholinergic system [30]. Since there is decreased expression of choline acetyltransferase activity in AD that correlates well with cognitive dysfunction [31] and 17β-estradiol up-regulates the expression of this enzyme, it was hypothesized that the seemingly positive effects of estrogen therapy on prolonging the onset of AD were likely due to the effects of estrogens on cholinergic dynamics.

Based on these studies, estrogen therapy was extensively investigated for its impact on cognitive dysfunction and AD in women. However, many researchers have been critical of earlier estrogen studies either due to low sample sizes, short-term effects of estrogen treatment, or the timing of the cognitive tests. As such, a study of aging and health in New York City found that hormone therapy (HT) in postmenopausal women decreased the risk of AD and increased performance on some memory tests; however, this finding did not carry over to women who already had mild to moderate AD [14]. Recently, the Women's Health Initiative Memory Study (WHIMS) conducted a large clinical study which included over 4,000 women who received a combination of estrogens and progesterone. Results from the WHIMS produced an upset in the research community; not only did they find that HT did not delay the onset of AD, but that it might actually increase the rate of dementia in a subgroup of women [32, 33]. Many hypotheses have been postulated to explain the perplexing results of the WHIMS (reviewed in [34]) including the form (estradiol versus conjugated equine estrogens), the route of administration (oral versus transdermal) of estrogens, the choice of progestin (natural versus synthetic progestins), the high doses administered, and the type of treatment regimen (continuous versus cyclic). In addition, alternative theories to account for the higher incidence of disease in women [35] include the role of free testosterone and high sex hormone binding globulin (SHBG) levels in AD [36, 37]. A fact of increasing relevance is that women in the WHIMS were 65+ years of age at the onset of the study. Therefore, aspects such as timing of HT onset after menopause and the capacity of HT to modulate other hormones of the HPG-axis must also be taken into account. Here we propose that it is only when the role of the other hormones of the HPG-axis and the

timing of HT are taken into account that cognitive decline and susceptibility, onset, and progression of AD can be more accurately characterized.

Epidemiology of gonadotropin action in Alzheimer's disease

Epidemiological data support a role of gonadotropins in AD, particularly LH. In this regard, and paralleling the female predominance for developing AD [38], LH levels are significantly higher in females as compared to males [39]. Furthermore, while some studies do not show increased serum levels in AD patients [40, 41], other studies indicate significant increases in gonadotropins in patients with this disease [42]. These contradictions are likely related to free hormone levels, different stages of AD and ages of the patients in the different studies, intra-assay variability, assay sensitivity, or to other non-specified factors. Also important is the fact that in Down's syndrome, where the prevalence of AD-like etiology is higher in males than in females (i.e., a reversal to what is observed in the normal population), males have higher serum LH levels compared to females [43]. Therefore, LH levels provide a potential explanation for the reversing of the classical gender-predisposition in AD versus Down's syndrome [44].

Gonadotropins in the brain: are they there and are they functional?

Compared to the abundance of information on the mechanisms of estrogens, there is little research on GnRH and LH in cognition; however, increasing evidence links LH to behavioral endpoints [45] as well as plasticity associated mechanisms such as neurogenesis [46]. One lingering question is whether large molecules such as gonadotropins can cross the blood–brain barrier and thus activate the receptors localized in the brain and whether they are functional once they get there. With regard to the ability of this hormone to reach the brain, LH's "sister" hormone, human chorionic gonadotropin (hCG), which is 80% homologous to LH, shares a common receptor and is slightly larger in size than LH, crosses the blood–brain barrier [47]. Regardless of the origin of the ligand (LH), a mounting body of evidence implicates the functionality of hippocampal LH receptors consistent with a role in modulating cognition. In this regard, LH receptors are highly expressed in the

253

cornu ammonis region of the dentate gyrus of the hippocampus [48], a key region for cognition and devastated in AD. Furthermore, LH protein is clearly observed in hippocampal tissue of individuals with AD but is absent in controls [49]. Also of significance is the fact that in a recent study, two 5'-flanking sequences (approximately 2 kb and 4 kb) of the rat LH receptor (LHR) gene were shown to directly express the lacZ reporter central nervous system (CNS) structures associated with sensory, memory, reproductive behavior, and autonomic functions. Importantly, the transgene activity was confined to neurons and co-localized with the cytochrome P450 side chain cleavage enzyme [50].

The LHR is coupled to the production of cyclic AMP (cAMP), which is an intracellular messenger involved in controlling neuronal excitability in the hippocampus [51]. Under normal conditions, stimulation of LH receptors leads to stimulation of the Gs protein, which then activates the membrane-associated adenylyl cyclase, which increases cAMP [52] and activation of extracellular signal-regulated protein kinases (ERK); both of which are tightly associated with cognition. Luteinizing hormone receptor activation leads to the increased expression of steroidogenic acute regulatory protein (StAR) and facilitates the movement of cholesterol from the outer to the inner mitochondrial membrane for the synthesis of pregnenolone and downstream progesterone synthesis [53], which is also associated with memory function. Importantly, studies demonstrate that StAR is increased in neurons in AD and that expression of this protein co-localizes with the LHR [54]. Furthermore, in vitro studies support these findings such that treatment of differentiated rat primary hippocampal neurons with LH (0, 10 and 100 mIU/mL) induced a rapid (within 30 minutes) increase in the expression of StAR, and a dose-dependent decrease in LH receptor expression. Importantly, suppression of serum LH in young rats treated with leuprolide acetate for four months down-regulated StAR expression and increased LH receptor expression in the brain [55]. Paralleling this, treatment of human neuroblastoma cells with GnRH leads to increases in LH mRNA and protein expression and LH levels are increased in differentiating embryonic rat primary cortical neurons. Furthermore, LH receptors are modulated by 17β-estradiol and are highly expressed after treatments of 0.1 nM of 17β-estradiol in human neurons. With increasing concentrations of 17β-estradiol,

expression of the immature LH receptor decreases, but the mature LH variants increase [56]. These data indicate that estrogen can also modulate the LH receptor and, as such, may directly regulate LH associated events. Collectively, these in vivo and in vitro studies suggest that LHR is functional in the brain.

Targeting LH levels to modulate cognitive function

Various studies report a role of gonadotropins, particularly LH, on cognition. In this regard, an earlier report indicated that intra-cerebral and intra-peritoneal administration of hCG in rats led to deficits in the T-maze test [57]. A more recent report examined cognitive function using the Y-maze in a transgenic mouse that over-expresses LH and found it to be impaired when compared to controls. Interestingly, the LH receptor knockout (LHKO) mouse, which shows equivalent high levels of LH but has no receptor [58], did not show impairment. It is important to note that cognitive impairment in the over-expressor mouse model was evident despite high levels of 17β-estradiol and no cognitive declines were observed in the LHKO mice despite low levels of estrogen. This suggests that changes in 17β-estradiol level were unlikely to be responsible for the cognitive decline; however, because these animals also exhibited deregulated hypothalamus-pituitary-adrenal (HPA) function, further studies are needed to clearly dissect the role of LH from that of HPA deregulation.

More conclusive support for a role of LH on cognition and AD has been gathered from studies using leuprolide acetate to modulate gonadotropins through the GnRH receptor. In this regard, treatment of aged Tg2576, an AD transgenic mouse model, with this selective GnRH agonist, which ablates the levels of both gonadotropins and sex steroids, stabilized cognitive decline in this line and was also effective at reducing Aβ accumulation [59]. Furthermore, a related study showed that leuprolide acetate produced a 1.5- to 3.5-fold reduction in total $A\beta_{1-42}$ and $A\beta_{1-40}$ in C57Bl/6J mice and treatment of cells with LH drove APP processing towards the amyloidogenic, AD-related pathway [60].

Treatments for AD are few and the ones currently available in the clinic are only mildly effective at slowing the development of AD. Based on results from the studies mentioned above, it seems that a therapeutic target that could abolish LH would help increase cognition and decrease Aβ pathology in the AD brain. Leuprolide acetate is a strong candidate for this therapeutic action. Leuprolide acetate is widely used as the treatment for sex steroid-dependent cancers, to shut down sex steroid production and slow down the progression of testosterone-dependent conditions such as prostate cancer. Coincidently, when leuprolide acetate was given to prostate cancer patients who were also suffering from AD, these patients showed a diminution of neurological symptoms associated with the disease [61]. Of note is the fact that premenopausal women treated with leuprolide acetate for estrogen-dependent cancers showed adverse reactions such as depression and cognitive decline. These findings indicate that estrogen has a clear role on cognitive function prior to menopause [62]. However, AD symptoms become evident in the vast majority of the cases after menopause onset, where, as described above, HT may not be playing as prominent a role as once was thought and may even be detrimental.

Importantly, a clinical trial investigating the safety and effectiveness of leuprolide acetate to improve the cognitive function and slow the progression of AD was carried out in 2006. The study included treatment of AD patients 65 years and older with mild to moderate AD. The objective was to evaluate the safety and efficacy of two different doses of leuprolide to improve the cognitive function and slow the progression of AD, as measured by the Alzheimer's Disease Assessment Scale–cognitive subscale ADAS-COG and the Clinical Global Impression (CGI). Measures of behavioral disturbances and quality of life of the care-giver were also carried out. The study design was a randomized, double blind, placebo-controlled, parallel group design with a 2:1 randomization of drug to placebo. Sample size included 90 participants from multiple test sites. The outcome of this clinical trial indicated that treatment of leuprolide acetate at high, but not low, doses sustained cognitive function as measured by ADAS-COG and CGI in women but not in men (http://clinicaltrials.gov/ct/show/nct 00076440?orden=6).

Potential mechanisms

Subjects tested in the WHIMS were 65 years or older, hence hormone replacement therapy (HRT) was begun approximately 15 years earlier, after the onset of menopause in those women. The timing of HRT is becoming the focus with recent clinical studies indicating that only HRT started shortly after menopause is beneficial to cognition, but that it may be detrimental when started a long period after the onset of this process [63] or does not produce improvement [64]. However, little is known with regards to why this dichotomy occurs. Some timing hypotheses focus on the direct effects of 17β-estradiol on the brain, its local production, and how these dynamics change in the aged brain [64]. An alternative hypothesis that is recently emerging is based on evidence indicating that the HPG-axis becomes dysfunctional after chronic lack of negative feedback of 17β-estradiol on GnRH neurons. As such, it is possible that HRT started during perimenopause or early menopause, when the HPG-axis feedback loop system is functional, leads to the equilibration of hormonal function (i.e., reduction of GnRH, LH, FSH, and others). However, when HRT is started in older women, while it may bring the sex steroid levels to premenopausal levels, it is not as effective at regulating these other hormones. As such, some support for a role of HPG-axis function involvement derives from the fact that 17β-estradiol feedback on LH secretion and GnRH gene expression decreases during aging and 17β-estradiol also becomes increasingly less effective at modulating LH expression and biosynthesis the later that HT is started after ovariectomy (OVX) [65]. These latter findings parallel the decline in cognition observed in animals models, such that HRT, begun following a long interval after OVX, fails to rescue cognitive/neuronal function, whereas short delays before the onset of HT are effective [64] and would provide an explanation for the results of the WHIMS and REMEMBER studies [33, 63]. This point is somewhat contested because some studies indicate that the ability of the pituitary to respond to 17β-estradiol and release LH is not impaired in aged animals [66] and a few studies with a very modest amount of subjects indicate that this may not be the case in women. However, more recent and larger studies in women show this may not be the case [67]. Importantly, studies also indicate that the dynamics of LH release by, for example, norepinephrine (NE), are different depending on whether OVX was carried out short or long term. Specifically, in short-term OVX-steroids-primed rats, NE did not alter LH levels in the peripheral plasma but in long-term OVX-steroids-primed rats NE gradually decreased plasma LH concentrations. Furthermore, intraventricular injection of GnRH was differentially efficient at activating LH release such that a brief release of LH was evident in short-term OVX-steroids-primed rats and a prolonged release of LH was evident in long-term OVX-steroids-primed rats.

In summary, the potentially negative impact of increased serum LH on cognition together with dysfunction of the HPG axis may provide, at least partially, an explanation for the conflicting findings in the HRT literature with regards to cognitive function protection.

Acknowledgments

Work in the authors' laboratories is supported by the National Institutes of Health (R01 A6032325) and the Alzheimer's Association. MAS and GP own equity options in, and were previously consultants to, Voyager Pharmaceutical Corporation that is pursuing leuprolide acetate as a potential treatment of Alzheimer's disease.

References

1. Smith MA. Alzheimer disease. *Int Rev Neurobiol.* 1998;**42**:1–54.

2. Hebert LE, Scherr PA, Bienias JL, Bennett DA, Evans DA. Alzheimer disease in the US population: prevalence estimates using the 2000 census. *Arch Neurol.* 2003;**60**:1119–22.

3. Hardy J, Selkoe DJ. The amyloid hypothesis of Alzheimer's disease: progress and problems on the road to therapeutics. *Science.* 2002;**297**:353–6.

4. Walsh DM, Selkoe DJ. Oligomers on the brain: the emerging role of soluble protein aggregates in neurodegeneration. *Protein Pept Lett.* 2004;**11**:213–28.

5. Smith MA, Casadesus G, Joseph JA, Perry G. Amyloid-beta and tau serve antioxidant functions in the aging and Alzheimer brain. *Free Radic Biol Med.* 2002; **33**:1194–9.

6. Lee HG, Zhu X, Nunomura A, Perry G, Smith MA. Amyloid-beta vaccination: testing the amyloid hypothesis? Heads we win, tails you lose! *Am J Pathol.* 2006;**169**:738–9.

7. Joseph J, Shukitt-Hale B, Denisova NA, *et al.* Copernicus revisited: amyloid beta in Alzheimer's disease. *Neurobiol Aging.* 2001;**22**:131–46.

8. Rottkamp CA, Atwood CS, Joseph JA, *et al.* The state versus amyloid-beta: the trial of the most wanted criminal in Alzheimer disease. *Peptides.* 2002;**23**:1333–41.

9. Smith MA, Rottkamp CA, Nunomura A, Raina AK, Perry G. Oxidative stress in Alzheimer's disease. *Biochim Biophys Acta.* 2000;**1502**:139–44.

10. Raina AK, Zhu X, Smith MA. Alzheimer's disease and the cell cycle. *Acta Neurobiol Exp (Wars).* 2004;**64**:107–12.

11. Zhu X, Raina AK, Perry G, Smith MA. Alzheimer's disease: the two-hit hypothesis. *Lancet Neurol.* 2004; **3**:219–26.

12. Casadesus G, Atwood CS, Zhu X, *et al.* Evidence for the role of gonadotropin hormones in the development of Alzheimer disease. *Cell Mol Life Sci.* 2005;**62**:293–8.

13. Marlatt MW, Webber KM, Moreira PI, *et al.* Therapeutic opportunities in Alzheimer disease: one for all or all for one? *Curr Med Chem.* 2005;**12**:1137–47.

14. Tang MX, Jacobs D, Stern Y, *et al.* Effect of oestrogen during menopause on risk and age at onset of Alzheimer's disease. *Lancet.* 1996;**348**:429–32.

15. Barnes LL, Wilson RS, Bienias JL, *et al.* Sex differences in the clinical manifestations of Alzheimer disease pathology. *Arch Gen Psychiatry.* 2005;**62**:685–91.

16. Wu JM, Zelinski MB, Ingram DK, Ottinger MA. Ovarian aging and menopause: current theories, hypotheses, and research models. *Exp Biol Med (Maywood).* 2005;**230**:818–28.

17. Meredith S, Dudenhoeffer G, Butcher RL, Lerner SP, Walls T. Unilateral ovariectomy increases loss of primordial follicles and is associated with increased metestrous concentration of follicle-stimulating hormone in old rats. *Biol Reprod.* 1992;**47**:162–8.

18. Nelson HD. Menopause. *Lancet.* 2008;**371**:760–70.

19. Fillit H, Weinreb H, Cholst I, *et al.* Observations in a preliminary open trial of estradiol therapy for senile dementia-Alzheimer's type. *Psychoneuroendocrinology.* 1986;**11**:337–45.

20. Sherwin BB. Estrogen and/or androgen replacement therapy and cognitive functioning in surgically menopausal women. *Psychoneuroendocrinology.* 1988;**13**:345–57.

21. Garcia-Segura LM, Azcoitia I, DonCarlos LL. Neuroprotection by estradiol. *Prog Neurobiol.* 2001;**63**:29–60.

22. Woolley CS, McEwen BS. Roles of estradiol and progesterone in regulation of hippocampal dendritic spine density during the estrous cycle in the rat. *J Comp Neurol.* 1993;**336**:293–306.

23. Hao J, Janssen WG, Tang Y, et al. Estrogen increases the number of spinophilin-immunoreactive spines in the hippocampus of young and aged female rhesus monkeys. *J Comp Neurol.* 2003;**465**:540–50.

24. Choi JM, Romeo RD, Brake WG, *et al.* Estradiol increases pre- and post-synaptic proteins in the CA1 region of the hippocampus in female rhesus macaques (*Macaca mulatta*). *Endocrinology.* 2003;**144**:4734–8.

25. Kretz O, Fester L, Wehrenberg U, *et al.* Hippocampal synapses depend on hippocampal estrogen synthesis. *J Neurosci.* 2004;**24**:5913–21.

26. Sudhof TC, Jahn R. Proteins of synaptic vesicles involved in exocytosis and membrane recycling. *Neuron.* 1991;**6**:665–77.

27. Feng J, Yan Z, Ferreira A, *et al.* Spinophilin regulates the formation and function of dendritic spines. *Proc Natl Acad Sci USA.* 2000;**97**:9287–92.

28. Qiu J, Bosch MA, Tobias SC, *et al.* Rapid signaling of estrogen in hypothalamic neurons involves a novel G-protein-coupled estrogen receptor that activates protein kinase C. *J Neurosci.* 2003;**23**:9529–40.

29. Bales KR, Verina T, Cummins DJ, *et al.* Apolipoprotein E is essential for amyloid deposition in the APP(V717F) transgenic mouse model of Alzheimer's disease. *Proc Natl Acad Sci USA.* 1999;**96**:15233–8.

30. Gibbs RB, Aggarwal P. Estrogen and basal forebrain cholinergic neurons: implications for brain aging and Alzheimer's disease-related cognitive decline. *Horm Behav.* 1998;**34**:98–111.

31. Luine VN, Khylchevskaya RI, McEwen BS. Effect of gonadal steroids on activities of monoamine oxidase and choline acetylase in rat brain. *Brain Res.* 1975; **86**:293–306.

32. Shumaker SA, Legault C, Rapp SR, *et al.* Estrogen plus progestin and the incidence of dementia and mild cognitive impairment in postmenopausal women: the Women's Health Initiative Memory Study: a randomized controlled trial. *JAMA.* 2003;**289**:2651–62.

33. Rapp SR, Espeland MA, Shumaker SA, *et al.* Effect of estrogen plus progestin on global cognitive function in postmenopausal women: the Women's Health Initiative Memory Study: a randomized controlled trial. *JAMA.* 2003;**289**:2663–72.

34. Baum LW. Sex, hormones, and Alzheimer's disease. *J Gerontol A Biol Sci Med Sci.* 2005;**60**:736–43.

35. Henderson VW. Hormone therapy and Alzheimer's disease: benefit or harm? *Expert Opin Pharmacother.* 2004;**5**:389–406.

36. Hoskin EK, Tang MX, Manly JJ, Mayeux R. Elevated sex-hormone binding globulin in elderly women with Alzheimer's disease. *Neurobiol Aging.* 2004;**25**:141–7.

37. Hogervorst E, Bandelow S, Combrinck M, Smith AD. Low free testosterone is an independent risk factor for Alzheimer's disease. *Exp Gerontol.* 2004;**39**:1633–9.

38. Rocca WA, Hofman A, Brayne C, *et al.* Frequency and distribution of Alzheimer's disease in Europe: a collaborative study of 1980–1990 prevalence findings. The EURODEM-Prevalence Research Group. *Ann Neurol.* 1991;**30**:381–90.

39. Zandi PP, Carlson MC, Plassman BL, *et al.* Hormone replacement therapy and incidence of Alzheimer disease in older women: the Cache County Study. *JAMA.* 2002;**288**:2123–9.

40. Hogervorst E, Williams J, Combrinck M, David Smith A. Measuring serum oestradiol in women with Alzheimer's disease: the importance of the sensitivity of the assay method. *Eur J Endocrinol.* 2003;**148**:67–72.

41. Tsolaki M, Grammaticos P, Karanasou C, *et al.* Serum estradiol, progesterone, testosterone, FSH and LH levels in postmenopausal women with Alzheimer's dementia. *Hell J Nucl Med.* 2005;**8**:39–42.

42. Short RA, Bowen RL, O'Brien PC, Graff-Radford NR. Elevated gonadotropin levels in patients with Alzheimer disease. *Mayo Clin Proc.* 2001;**76**:906–9.

43. Neaves WB, Johnson L, Porter JC, Parker CR, Jr., Petty CS. Leydig cell numbers, daily sperm production, and serum gonadotropin levels in aging men. *J Clin Endocrinol Metab.* 1984;**59**:756–63.

44. Schupf N, Kapell D, Nightingale B, *et al.* Earlier onset of Alzheimer's disease in men with Down syndrome. *Neurology.* 1998;**50**:991–5.

45. Yang EJ, Nasipak BT, Kelley DB. Direct action of gonadotropin in brain integrates behavioral and reproductive functions. *Proc Natl Acad Sci USA.* 2007;**104**:2477–82.

46. Mak GK, Enwere EK, Gregg C, *et al.* Male pheromone-stimulated neurogenesis in the adult female brain: possible role in mating behavior. *Nat Neurosci.* 2007;**10**:1003–11.

47. Lukacs H. Rat as model for studying behavior effects of hCG. *Semin Reprod Med.* 2001;**19**:111–19.

48. Lei ZM, Rao CV, Kornyei JL, Licht P, Hiatt ES. Novel expression of human chorionic gonadotropin/ luteinizing hormone receptor gene in brain. *Endocrinology.* 1993;**132**:2262–70.

49. Bowen RL, Smith MA, Harris PL, *et al.* Elevated luteinizing hormone expression colocalizes with neurons vulnerable to Alzheimer's disease pathology. *J Neurosci Res.* 2002;**70**:514–18.

50. Apaja PM, Harju KT, Aatsinki JT, Petaja-Repo UE, Rajaniemi HJ. Identification and structural characterization of the neuronal luteinizing hormone receptor associated with sensory systems. *J Biol Chem.* 2004;**279**:1899–906.

51. Ji I, Ji TH. Asp383 in the second transmembrane domain of the lutropin receptor is important for high affinity hormone binding and cAMP production. *J Biol Chem.* 1991;**266**:14953–7.

52. Cooke BA. Signal transduction involving cyclic AMP-dependent and cyclic AMP-independent mechanisms

in the control of steroidogenesis. *Mol Cell Endocrinol.* 1999;**151**:25–35.

53. Seger R, Hanoch T, Rosenberg R, *et al.* The ERK signaling cascade inhibits gonadotropin-stimulated steroidogenesis. *J Biol Chem.* 2001;**276**:13957–64.

54. Webber KM, Stocco DM, Casadesus G, *et al.* Steroidogenic acute regulatory protein (StAR): evidence of gonadotropin-induced steroidogenesis in Alzheimer disease. *Mol Neurodegener.* 2006;**1**:14.

55. Liu Q, Merkler KA, Zhang X, McLean MP. Prostaglandin F2alpha suppresses rat steroidogenic acute regulatory protein expression via induction of Yin Yang 1 protein and recruitment of histone deacetylase 1 protein. *Endocrinology.* 2007;**148**:5209–19.

56. Bowen RL, Verdile G, Liu T. Luteinizing hormone, a reproductive regulator that modulates the processing of amyloid-beta precursor protein and amyloid-beta deposition. *J Biol Chem.* 2004;**279**:20539–45.

57. Lukacs H, Hiatt ES, Lei ZM, Rao CV. Peripheral and intracerebroventricular administration of human chorionic gonadotropin alters several hippocampus-associated behaviors in cycling female rats. *Horm Behav.* 1995;**29**:42–58.

58. Casadesus G, Milliken EL, Webber KM, *et al.* Increases in luteinizing hormone are associated with declines in cognitive performance. *Mol Cell Endocrinol.* 2007; **269**:107–11.

59. Casadesus G, Puig ER, Webber KM, *et al.* Targeting gonadotropins: an alternative option for Alzheimer disease treatment. *J Biomed Biotechnol.* 2006; **2006**(3):39508.

60. Bowen RL, Atwood CS, Perry G, Smith MA. Mechanisms involved in gender differences in

Alzheimer's disease: the role of leuteinizing and follicle stimulating hormones. In Legato ML, ed. *Principles of Gender Specific Medicine.* San Diego CA: Academic Press, 2004, pp. 1234–7.

61. Bowen RL. Sex hormones, amyloid protein, and Alzheimer disease. *JAMA.* 2001;**286**:790–1.

62. Varney NR, Syrop C, Kubu CS, *et al.* Neuropsychologic dysfunction in women following leuprolide acetate induction of hypoestrogenism. *J Assist Reprod Genet.* 1993;**10**:53–7.

63. MacLennan AH, Henderson VW, Paine BJ, *et al.* Hormone therapy, timing of initiation, and cognition in women aged older than 60 years: the REMEMBER pilot study. *Menopause.* 2006;**13**:28–36.

64. Daniel JM, Hulst JL, Berbling JL. Estradiol replacement enhances working memory in middle-aged rats when initiated immediately after ovariectomy but not after a long-term period of ovarian hormone deprivation. *Endocrinology.* 2006;**147**:607–14.

65. King JC, Anthony EL, Damassa DA, Elkind-Hirsch KE. Morphological evidence that luteinizing hormone-releasing hormone neurons participate in the suppression by estradiol of pituitary luteinizing hormone secretion in ovariectomized rats. *Neuroendocrinology.* 1987;**45**:1–13.

66. Joshi D, Lekhtman I, Billiar RB, Miller MM. Gonadotropin hormone-releasing hormone induced luteinizing hormone responses in young and old female C57BL/6J mice. *Proc Soc Exp Biol Med.* 1993;**204**:191–4.

67. Weiss G, Skurnick JH, Goldsmith LT, Santoro NF, Park SJ. Menopause and hypothalamic-pituitary sensitivity to estrogen. *JAMA.* 2004;**292**:2991–6.

The role of gonadotropins and testosterone in the regulation of beta-amyloid metabolism

Giuseppe Verdile and Ralph N. Martins

Editors' introduction

Verdile and Martins review the relationship between dysfunction of the hypothalamic-pituitary-gonadal (HPG) axis, reduced levels of testosterone in men, cognitive decline, and risk of Alzheimer's disease (AD). Regulation of testosterone and luteinizing hormone (LH) are tightly linked, and following reproductive senescence declines in sex hormones are coupled with elevated gonadotropin levels. Several studies have reported that compared to controls, men with AD and other dementias have lower serum testosterone levels. Testosterone has been shown to have a number of neuroprotective effects, including reducing oxidative stress and inflammatory processes, which are key events in the AD brain. While animal and in vitro analyses have provided support for the therapeutic potential of testosterone, definitive benefits of testosterone therapy remain to be determined. The APOE ε4 allele appears to be a determining factor in the association between testosterone and the risk of developing dementia in men. It appears that both testosterone and LH can impact beta-amyloid accumulation and AD pathogenesis, although the relative contributions of each hormone remain undefined. Verdile and Martins propose that combinational hormone therapy (HT) may prove to be more efficacious in the prevention of AD.

Introduction

Hormonal changes associated with aging have been implicated in the increased risk of developing dementia and in the pathogenesis of AD. Although age and the possession of the apolipoprotein ε4 allele (*APOE ε4*) are major risk factors for AD the actual trigger(s) of disease onset remain to be established. Sex hormones

are considered likely candidates. Low serum levels of estrogen in postmenopausal women and testosterone in andropausal men have been shown to be associated with AD. These hormones also play important roles in modulating beta-amyloid (Aβ) levels, the accumulation of which has a critical role in the cascade of pathogenic events that lead to neuronal degeneration in AD.

It is also now becoming apparent that elevated levels of gonadotropins (particularly luteinizing hormone, LH) are also associated with increased risk of developing AD and have a role in the metabolism and accumulation of Aβ. The complete mechanisms that underlie the effects of the sex steroids and gonadotropins on AD pathogenesis and whether one is secondary to the other or whether both have a role to play remains to be elucidated. This review focuses specifically on the sex hormone, testosterone, and the gonadotropin, luteinizing hormone (LH). It outlines the role of these hormones in regulating Aβ metabolism and amyloid precursor protein (APP) processing and discusses their potential as targets for developing effective therapeutic agents for AD.

Beta-amyloid: a key molecule in AD pathogenesis

One of the key histopathological elements of AD is the abnormal deposition of amyloid plaques. The major protein component of these plaques is a small peptide termed beta-amyloid (Aβ). In the human brain, there are two main forms of Aβ, a 40 amino acid peptide, $A\beta_{1-40}$, and the longer, more toxic peptide comprising 42 amino acids, $A\beta_{1-42}$. Under physiological conditions, the predominant Aβ species is 40 amino acids long ($A\beta_{1-40}$). $A\beta_{1-42}$ is thought to be the more toxic species since it aggregates much

Hormones, Cognition and Dementia: State of the Art and Emergent Therapeutic Strategies, ed. Eef Hogervorst, Victor W. Henderson, Robert B. Gibbs, and Roberta Diaz Brinton. Published by Cambridge University Press.
© Cambridge University Press 2009.

(A)   Non-amyloidogenic pathway   (B)   Amyloidogenic pathway

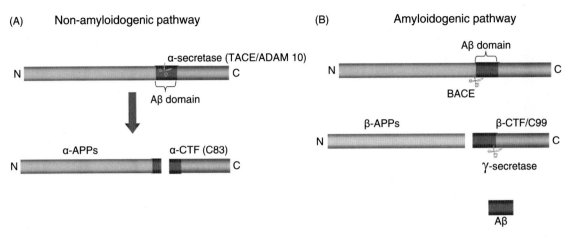

Fig. 27.1 The non-amyloidogenic and amyloidogenic pathways of APP processing. A schematic representation of the two competing APP processing pathways. (A) In the non-amyloidogenic pathway APP is cleaved by α-secretase, within the Aβ domain, precluding the formation of Aβ. (B) The sequential cleavage of APP by first the β-APP cleaving enzyme (BACE) and then by γ-secretase in the amyloidogenic pathway results in Aβ production.

more rapidly than $A\beta_{1-40}$ and is demonstrated to be more neurotoxic in numerous in vitro studies. This Aβ species is central to the "amyloid hypothesis." In this hypothesis $A\beta_{1-42}$ acts as the seed for further Aβ deposition and induces a cascade of events that include the generation of free radicals, oxidative damage, and inflammatory processes. The primary event that results in the abnormal accumulation of Aβ is thought to be the dysregulated proteolytic processing of its parent molecule, the amyloid precursor protein (APP) (reviewed in [1]).

The APP molecule is a transmembrane glycoprotein that is proteolytically processed by two competing pathways, the non-amyloidogenic and amyloidogenic (Aβ forming) pathways (Fig. 27.1). How these pathways are regulated remains unclear. However, there are many factors including diet, hormonal status, and genetic mutations that influence the processing of APP to generate Aβ (reviewed in [1]). Three major secretases are postulated to be involved in the proteolytic cleavage of APP. These include α-secretase (of which the metalloproteases ADAM 17/TACE and ADAM 10 are likely candidates), beta APP cleaving enzyme (BACE, formally known as β-secretase), and the γ-secretase. The α-secretase enzyme cleaves within the Aβ domain of APP thus precluding the formation Aβ and generating non-amyloidogenic fragments and a secreted form of APP (α-APPs). In the amyloidogenic pathway, BACE cleaves near the N-terminus of the Aβ domain on the APP molecule, liberating another soluble form of APP, β-APPs, and a C-terminal fragment (C99)

containing the whole Aβ domain. The final step in the amyloidogenic pathway is the intramembranous cleavage of the C99 fragment by γ-secretase, to liberate the Aβ peptide (reviewed in [1]). This enzyme is a multisubunit enzyme complex consisting of four proteins (presenilins, nicastrin, APH-1, and PEN-2) of which the presenilins are thought to be the catalytic subunit (reviewed in [2]). Recently, other components of the complex have been identified that appear to function in regulating/modulating Aβ production (reviewed in [3]).

Numerous studies have shown that Aβ is neurotoxic and can inhibit synapse formation as evident by long-term potentiation studies (reviewed in [4]). Although toxicity has been demonstrated with fibrillar Aβ, the current focus is on the non-fibrillar, soluble, aggregates as the toxic species of Aβ. These include Aβ derived diffusible ligands (ADDLs) "$A\beta_{1-42}$ globulamers" and Aβstar56* (reviewed in [5]). These Aβ oligomers have been shown to be neurotoxic, impair memory in vivo, inhibit synapse formation, and correlate well with the severity of neurodegeneration in AD [6, 7]. The mechanism(s) by which Aβ induces neurotoxicity is unclear; however, metal-induced generation of reactive oxygen species has a critical role (reviewed in [4]).

The role of testosterone in AD risk and pathogenesis

The major biologically active androgen in men is testosterone, and its action is mediated via binding to the androgen receptor (AR), either directly or after 5α-reduction to the more active dihydroxytestosterone (DHT). In contrast to estrogen in postmenopausal women, age-related reductions in testosterone are very gradual. Levels of bioavailable testosterone decline in men by approximately 1% every year from the third to fourth decade of life, and the gradual decline in androgen levels that occurs, combined with other factors that increase resistance to androgen action, such as rising sex hormone binding globulin (SHBG) levels with age, causes androgen deficiency symptoms often referred to as andropause [8].

Reduced levels of testosterone in men have been associated with cognitive decline and AD. Several studies have reported that compared to controls, men with AD and other dementias have lower serum testosterone levels [9, 10, 11, 12]. One study of subjects with mild neuropathology consistent with initial AD found that the brain testosterone levels in these subjects were similar to those found in more advanced AD cases, yet significantly lower than age-matched control levels [13]. Further, longitudinal studies have shown that lower free testosterone levels can be detected five to ten years prior to the diagnosis of AD [14]. In addition, we have recently reported an association between serum testosterone concentrations and cognitive performance in healthy elderly men [15]. From this evidence it is clear that low testosterone levels are associated with an increased risk of developing AD. Evidence has also been presented for a key role of testosterone in the pathogenesis of AD.

Testosterone has been shown to have a number of neuroprotective effects, including reducing oxidative stress and inflammatory processes, which are key events in the AD brain. Testosterone has been shown to exhibit neuroprotective effects in cerebellar granule cells against oxidative insults mediated by reactive oxygen species, hydrogen peroxide, and nitric oxide [16]. Testosterone does not have antioxidant properties due to the lack of a phenol that is present in estradiol [17]. Therefore, it was suggested that these neuroprotective effects of testosterone were through its aromatization to estrogen [18]. However, the antioxidant properties of testosterone can be attenuated by flutamide, an androgen receptor antagonist [16]. It is now thought that testosterone mediates its antioxidant effects by the up-regulation of the antioxidant enzymes superoxide dismutase and catalase through the androgen receptor (AR), rather than via conversion

to estrogen or via direct scavenging activity [16]. Testosterone has also been implicated in the regulation of the free radical scavenger glutathione, with increased levels reported in rat brain homogenate following testosterone supplementation [19]. Testosterone and dehydroepiandrosterone (DHEA), along with estradiol and progesterone, have been shown to reduce reactive gliosis in ovariectomized/castrated rats following brain injury [20]. Evidence also exists that brain injury up-regulates *de novo* synthesis of estrogen from testosterone in astrocytes [20].

Cell culture studies provided the initial evidence that testosterone regulates Aβ levels and APP processing. Treatment of neuronal cells in culture resulted in an increase in the secretion of the soluble, neuroprotective, α-APPs molecule and a reduction in Aβ production [21, 22] suggesting activation of the α-secretase pathway in the processing of APP. Indeed Goodenough and colleagues [22] showed that testosterone activates the MAP-kinase signaling pathway, which has previously been shown to induce APP through the non-amyloidogenic pathway favoring α-APP production and thus precluding Aβ formation [23]. It has also been suggested that testosterone or other androgens may mediate their effects through the AR. Evidence for androgen activation of the MAP-kinase signaling pathway has come from one study showing that DHT increased phosphorylation of MAP-kinase signaling molecules (ERK-1 and ERK-2) in cells over-expressing the AR, but not in wild-type cells or cells expressing the empty vector [24]. Further, DHT attenuated Aβ-induced toxicity in neuronal cells expressing the AR. However, as yet, no direct evidence has been provided to suggest that testosterone-mediated secretion of α-APPs is AR dependent.

The aromatization of testosterone to estrogen has also been shown to be involved in the testosterone-induced secretion of APP, as inhibition of aromatase in the presence of testosterone results in a reduction in α-APPs [22]. Estrogen itself can activate the MAP-kinase pathway [25] and has also been shown to induce α-APP secretion through the MAP-kinase pathway [26]. Thus it is also plausible that testosterone could be altering APP metabolism through estrogen-dependent pathways. There is no evidence to date that other androgens such as the non-aromatizable DHT, can mediate the non-amyloidogenic processing of APP to generate α-APPs. In fact, in vivo data indicate that DHT has no effect on α-APP levels but reduces Aβ levels in rat brain ([27]; see below).

This suggests that although both testosterone and DHT have neuroprotective effects (that are possibly AR dependent), they have independent effects on APP processing, with testosterone effects mediated by the aromatization of testosterone to estrogen.

In vivo studies have confirmed that androgens can influence Aβ levels. Our studies showed that a reduction in testosterone level is associated with increased plasma Aβ levels in dementia cases and in men that have undergone chemical castration [28, 29, 30] providing the first clinical evidence that testosterone can regulate Aβ levels in vivo. A recent study in the triple transgenic mouse model of AD (3xTg-AD mouse) showed similar results [31]. In this study depletion of androgens (by gonadectomy) led to an acceleration in Aβ accumulation in the brains of the transgenic mice without altering the levels of the APP C-terminal fragment, suggesting that the effect was independent of the processing of APP. In addition, impairments in hippocampal-dependent behavioral performance were observed in androgen-depleted animals. Further, mice administered DHT (which doesn't undergo aromatization to estrogen) exhibited reduced cerebral Aβ levels and improved hippocampal behavior [31]. This effect of DHT suggests that the effects of androgens on Aβ metabolism are estrogen independent. Similar results were shown in a previous study where supplementation of DHT to rats reduced brain Aβ levels [27]. This study also showed that, unlike in cell culture studies, supplementation of DHT to the rats did not alter α-APP brain levels suggesting that androgens may alter Aβ through mechanisms independent of APP processing, though this latter finding needs verification in independent studies.

Interestingly, the study by Ramsden and colleagues [27] showed no effect of DHT on plasma Aβ levels and also showed that androgen depletion did not alter plasma Aβ levels. Recent data from our laboratory has shown that androgen depletion in guinea pigs results in a significant increase in both cerobrospinal fluid (CSF) and plasma Aβ levels (Fig. 27.2). However, at high doses while CSF Aβ levels decreased further, plasma levels actually increased at this dose of testosterone. These results indicate tissue-specific action of testosterone, but could also suggest enhanced clearance of Aβ from the CSF into the periphery. This process may be modulated by testosterone as this hormone can also enter the CSF [32, 33].

Animal and cell culture studies have provided support for testosterone in having potential therapeutic benefits. However, clear benefits of testosterone replacement therapy have not been forthcoming. Only a few studies have assessed the effects of testosterone supplementation on cognition in AD. Results from these studies have been inconclusive with some showing benefits of testosterone replacement on selective cognitive functions including spatial memory and constructive ability of AD patients, while others have shown minimal effect on cognition but an improvement in quality of life (reviewed in [34]). However, these studies assessed the effects of testosterone in a small number of subjects (range 18–32) and had relatively short time periods of treatment (i.e., six weeks). In addition these studies have not controlled for the presence of the major genetic risk factor for AD, APOE ε4. It is likely, though, that testosterone may play a more effective role in prevention rather than treatment.

The APOE genotype has been shown to strongly determine the outcome of estrogen replacement therapy in women. Studies where the APOE genotype was assessed showed a benefit to APOE ε4 carriers, though cognition was enhanced in non-carriers [35, 36]. The APOE ε4 allele also appears to modulate the association between testosterone and the risk of developing dementia in men. We have recently reported an association between serum testosterone concentrations and cognitive performance in healthy elderly men [15]. This study showed that higher levels of free, bioavailable testosterone were associated with better cognitive function only in men who did not possess the APOE ε4 genotype. However, in animal studies the therapeutic benefit of testosterone therapy was present even in the presence of the ε4 allele. One study showed that inhibiting the effects of testosterone by blocking the androgen receptor (AR) in male mice expressing APOE ε4 results in the development of prominent deficits in spatial learning and memory [37]. Interestingly, female APOE ε4 mice, when compared to female APOE ε3 mice, exhibit such deficits in learning and memory without AR blockade, yet treatment with either testosterone or DHT attenuates the deficits [37]. These animal studies provide a precedence to assess testosterone as a substitute for estrogen in assessing the efficacy of these sex steroids at improving cognition in women.

It is clear from the studies above that large-scale randomized, placebo-controlled intervention studies that assess cognitive, biochemical, and brain imaging parameters are required to determine if testosterone

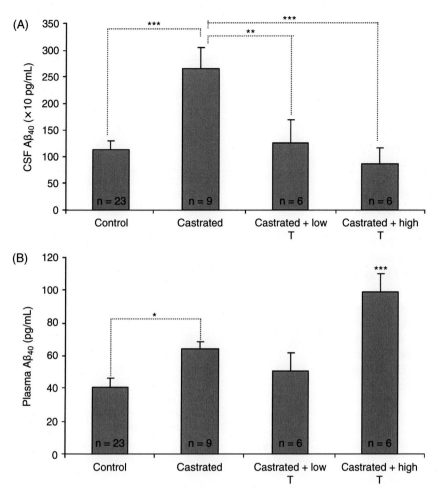

Fig. 27.2 The effect of testosterone (T) on CSF and plasma $A\beta_{40}$ levels in castrated guinea pigs. Castration results in a reduction in testosterone levels (not shown) and an increase in (A) levels of CSF $A\beta_{40}$ and (B) plasma $A\beta_{40}$ compared to controls. This effect is altered significantly by supplementation with testosterone. All data are shown as mean $\pm$ SEM (* $p < 0.05$; ** $p < 0.01$; *** $p < 0.001$).

has benefits for AD. In addition, considering the importance of the *APOE* gene in so many aspects of AD and in the outcome of potential therapeutics for the disease, this gene will require consideration when assessing the benefits of testosterone therapy.

We are currently undertaking a study in which testosterone was administered to a group of hypogonadal men to assess the potential therapeutic benefit in reducing $A\beta$ levels and improving memory. The results thus far ($N = 21$) show a reduction in plasma $A\beta$ levels after four months' treatment. This reduction was associated with a decrease in serum LH levels. These results suggest testosterone reduces plasma $A\beta$ levels indirectly, through altering the feedback loops of the HPG axis resulting in lower LH levels. High LH levels are associated with both increased risk and

pathogenesis of AD (see below). Cognitive assessment showed that testosterone therapy showed a slight improvement in verbal recall (as assessed by the California Verbal Learning Test, CVLT). We are continuing to recruit a larger number of participants to improve the statistical power of the study.

Gonadotropins

Sex steroid production is under the control of complex feedback loops within the hypothalamic-pituitary-ovary/gonadal axis that regulate the levels of the pituitary gonadotropins, follicle stimulating hormone (FSH), and luteinizing hormone (LH), in turn controlling estrogen and testosterone levels. Therefore, when understanding the mechanisms of sex hormones in AD pathogenesis it is important to consider gonadotropins and their role in the etiology and pathology of the disease.

The release of the gonadotropins from the pituitary gland is under the control of a small peptide called gonadotropin-releasing hormone (GnRH), which is produced and secreted from the hypothalamus to act on the anterior pituitary. In menopause/andropause the loss of negative feedback by estrogen or testosterone results in increases in serum levels of gonadotropins.

Sex steroid hormones are derived from a common sterol precursor, cholesterol. The conversion of cholesterol to pregnenolone marks the first step in the formation of these hormones and is the rate limiting step [38]. The steroid biosynthesis pathway is initiated by the binding of ligands such as LH to receptors initiating downstream cascade responses including the 1,4,5-triphosphate (IP3) and diacylglycerol (DAG) pathway to release Ca^{2+} and activate protein kinase C or to modulate the activity of adenyl cyclase to generate cAMP, both pathways are involved in the conversion of cholesterol esters to cholesterol, which is subsequently converted to pregnenolone.

The role of gonadotropins in Alzheimer's disease

The gonadotropins have been implicated in the pathogenesis of AD. Previous reports have shown in a small cohort that the serum levels of gonadotropins are higher in AD patients compared to age-matched controls [9, 39]. We have unpublished data to show that age-related increases in LH serum levels are associated with a reduction in cognition in a large cohort of elderly women without dementia (n = 450, Fig. 27.3A). Interestingly, in contrast to an increase in LH levels, high serum levels of FSH were associated with improved cognition in the same cohort of women (Fig. 27.3B). The significance of this contrasting effect with FSH requires further investigation and suggests that increases in FSH levels with age are a protective effect against cognitive decline. The role of FSH in cognition and memory has been largely unexplored and further in vitro and in vivo work should determine whether this gonadotropin has neuroprotective properties or attenuates Aβ accumulation.

Evidence for a role of LH in the disease process has been provided by a number of studies. The first

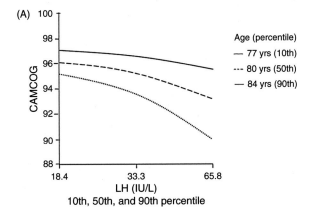

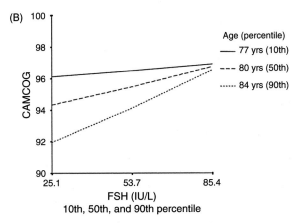

Fig. 27.3 Diagrammatic presentation of the direction of influence and the interactive nature of the FSH, LH, and age on the Cambridge Cognitive Test (CAMCOG) for the non-*APOE* ε4 subsample group. Low, average, and high values of LH, FSH, and age represent the 10th, 50th, and 90th percentiles. (A) CAMCOG scores decreased with age and increasing LH levels. (B) CAMCOG scores increased with age and increasing FSH levels.

showed that LH accumulates intracellularly in the pyramidal neurons of AD compared with age-matched control brains [40]. More recently, we investigated the role of gonadotropins in promoting amyloidogenesis where neuronal cells were treated with LH. Intracellular levels of APP [41] were not altered; however, the proteolytic processing of APP was, as evidenced by increased secretion and insolubility of Aβ [41]. This report was the first to show that LH could modulate Aβ levels. Recently, we investigated whether serum LH levels were positively correlated with plasma Aβ levels in a small group of elderly men (r = 0.5, p = 0.038, unpublished data). The results showed that the serum levels of LH were positively correlated with plasma Aβ levels in this group of elderly men.

No association was shown between free, bioavailable levels of testosterone and plasma Aβ levels. However, this is a relatively small study ($n = 40$) and it could not be ruled out that this effect may be due to androgen insensitivity or as a response to changes in the HPG feedback system. It is highly likely that increases in LH may actually be a marker of decreased testosterone activity akin to high thyroxine stimulating hormone as a marker for low thyroxine. Large cross-sectional human studies and appropriate animal studies are required to determine whether availability or response to circulating testosterone have additional important roles.

The mechanisms by which LH modulates Aβ metabolism remain to be determined. It is not clear whether LH in the periphery can have effects in the CNS. Some evidence has been provided to show that LH is synthesized in the brain [40, 42]. However, the effects of *de novo* synthesis of LH on normal brain function and in AD pathogenesis remain unknown. Evidence for a role of LH in the CNS has been presented by investigating the LH receptor. Although a high density of the gonadotropin receptors are found in steroidogenic cells such as Leydig, luteal, and granulosa cells, they are also found in the brain indicating that the CNS may be one of the target tissues for LH (reviewed in [43]). Investigation of the distribution of the LH receptors in the adult rat brain has shown that the highest levels are found in the hippocampus [43] an area of the brain that is involved in memory and is severely affected in AD containing large amounts of amyloid deposits, which characterize the disease. Strong LH immunoreactivity is observed within neurons in the AD brain but not in control brain, consistent with higher LH levels in AD and suggestive of their uptake by LH receptors [40].

The LH receptor (LHR) is a member of the seven transmembrane receptor family and once activated (through ligand binding) induces adenyl cyclase to produce cAMP and phospholipase C, which in turn catalyzes the production of inositol phosphates and diacylglycerol [44] ultimately activating the rate limiting step, which is the conversion of cholesterol to pregnenolone. A protein that is critical for this conversion is the steroidogenic acute regulatory (StAR) protein. This protein transports cholesterol to the inner mitochondrial membrane where the conversion of cholesterol to pregnenolone occurs. Currently, only one study has provided evidence that the StAR protein is present in hippocampal neurons and is up-regulated in the AD brain [45]. Furthermore, this study showed that StAR co-localized with the LH receptor within the neurons. Although this study suggests that StAR may have a role in AD pathogenesis, further evidence is required to conclusively show that LH may modulate APP processing through the activation of cAMP signaling pathways and up-regulation of the StAR protein. However, this notion cannot be ruled out as inhibition or activation of cAMP dependent pathways has been shown to alter APP metabolism and Aβ generation [46, 47].

Although blood levels of LH are associated with cognitive decline and AD, whether peripheral levels can mediate its effects in the CNS remains unclear. It has classically been thought that gonadotropins do not cross the blood–brain barrier as they are lipid-soluble molecules. Early studies have demonstrated the presence of gonadotropins in the CSF and synchrony between serum and CSF gonadotropin levels in both primates and humans [33, 48]. Subsequent studies in rodents have demonstrated that a small percentage of LH and its more potent analog, hCG, but not FSH, can cross the blood–brain barrier [49]. These studies indicate that transport of LH across the blood–brain barrier into the CNS can occur. However, more recently there is some evidence that LH can be synthesized within neurons.

Evidence has been provided to show that the gonadotropin releasing hormone (GnRH) can stimulate neurons to generate LH [42]. The authors found evidence that a receptor for GnRH (GnRHR I) was present in the cell bodies and dendrites of neurons in the human hippocampus, entorhinal cortex, and occipitotemporal gyrus. No difference in expression was observed between AD and aged-matched control brain samples. However, reductions in a GnRHR I variant in an AD brain sample was observed particularly in a high molecular weight variant of the receptor, which is thought to be a receptor complex/post-translational modified active protein. Further they showed that treatment of neuronal cells with GnRH I led to increased LH expression and down-regulation of the GnRH I receptor. These results suggest that LH synthesis occurs in neurons and is regulated by GnRH. Coupled together with previous findings that LH is present in pyramidal neurons of the AD brain [40], it could be argued that its presence reflects increased *de novo* synthesis of LH thereby promoting Aβ production and accumulation in the

AD brain. Further in vivo studies are required to determine the relative contributions of peripheral and CNS LH to APP processing and Aβ metabolism within the brain.

Although the mechanism(s) of action of gonadotropins in AD are still unknown, they are a target for developing appropriate therapeutic agents for AD. One such agent, leuprolide, showed promise and entered human clinical trials. Leuprolide is a GnRH agonist that initially stimulates the production of LH, but continuous administration results in a down-regulation and desensitizing of the HPG axis and a decline in LH levels. Mainly used for the treatment of hormone-responsive cancers such as prostate and breast cancer, it was shown to have potential as a therapeutic agent for AD. Initial studies in transgenic and non-transgenic mice showed that leuprolide could reduce brain Aβ accumulation and levels of $Aβ_{40}$ and $Aβ_{42}$ [41, 50]. A 48-week Phase II human clinical trial administering leuprolide acetate to women over 65 years with mild to moderate AD has recently been completed by Voyager Pharmaceuticals, with promising results. The results showed memory and cognition (assessed by ADAS-cog) and ability to perform activities of daily living (assessed by Alzheimer's Disease Cooperative Study-Activities of Daily Living inventory, ADCS-ADL) improved in a group of women with AD (n = 109) receiving acetyl-choline esterase inhibitor (AChEI) and a high dose of leuprolide acetate, compared to those women receiving placebo and AChEI. A Phase III clinical trial commenced early last year, but unfortunately was prematurely halted due to funding constraints. While the early clinical trial to lower LH as an effective treatment for mild to moderate AD was encouraging, a Phase III clinical trial is required to obtain a definitive answer.

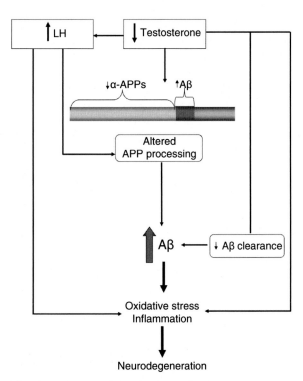

Fig. 27.4 Schematic of the role of LH and testosterone in promoting Aβ accumulation. High LH levels and low testosterone levels can promote Aβ accumulation by a number of pathways, leading to a cascade of pathogenic events such as oxidative stress and inflammation, resulting in neurodegeneration. Low levels of testosterone could alter APP processing such that the amyloidogenic pathway (Aβ production) is favored over the non-amyloidogenic pathway (α-APP production). The overproduction of Aβ would lead to accumulation of this protein. Testosterone could also influence Aβ clearance, where impaired clearance would lead to an accumulation of this protein in the CNS. Increases in LH can also stimulate the amyloidogenic pathway of APP processing leading to the overproduction and accumulation of Aβ. Changes in the levels of LH and/or testosterone could also directly influence oxidative stress and inflammatory pathways leading to neurodegeneration. It is also conceivable that combined effects of low testosterone and high LH levels would also contribute to Aβ accumulation and neurodegeneration in AD.

Concluding remarks

Regulation of testosterone and LH is tightly linked, and following reproductive senescence, sex hormone reductions are coupled with elevated gonadotropin levels. It appears that both hormones have roles in Aβ accumulation and AD pathogenesis (Fig. 27.4). Although mechanism(s) are yet to be determined, hormone-induced receptor mediated signaling pathways appear to have an important role in modulating APP processing and Aβ metabolism. The relative contributions of LH and testosterone to AD remain a challenge to be overcome by further experimentation. Indeed, it is conceivable that the combined effects of testosterone and gonadotropins can influence not only Aβ accumulation but also other features of neurodegeneration such as oxidative stress and inflammation (Fig. 27.4). Given the diverse actions of the reproductive hormones, combinational hormone therapy may prove to be more efficacious in the prevention of AD. However, this notion requires further validation in appropriate in vivo animal studies followed by clinical trials.

References

1. Verdile G, Fuller S, Atwood CS, *et al.* The role of beta amyloid in Alzheimer's disease: still a cause of everything or the only one who got caught? *Pharmacol Res.* 2004;**50**(4):397–409.

2. Verdile G, Gandy SE, Martins RN. The role of presenilin and its interacting proteins in the biogenesis of Alzheimer's beta amyloid. *Neurochem Res.* 2007;**32**(4/5):609–23.

3. Zhou S, Zhou H, Walian PJ, Jap BK. Regulation of gamma-secretase activity in Alzheimer's disease. *Biochemistry.* 2007;**46**(10):2553–63.

4. Cappai R, Barnham KJ. Delineating the mechanism of Alzheimer's disease abeta peptide neurotoxicity. *Neurochem Res.* 2008;**33**(3):526–32.

5. Walsh DM, Selkoe DJ. A beta oligomers – a decade of discovery. *J Neurochem.* 2007;**101**(5):1172–84.

6. McLean CA, Cherny RA, Fraser FW, *et al.* Soluble pool of Abeta amyloid as a determinant of severity of neurodegeneration in Alzheimer's disease. *Ann Neurol.* 1999;**46**(6):860–6.

7. Fonte J, Miklossy J, Atwood C, Martins R. The severity of cortical Alzheimer's type changes is positively correlated with increased amyloid-beta levels: resolubilization of amyloid-beta with transition metal ion chelators. *J Alzheimers Dis.* 2001;**3**(2):209–19.

8. Pike CJ, Rosario ER, Nguyen TV. Androgens, aging, and Alzheimer's disease. *Endocrine* 2006;**29**(2):233–41.

9. Bowen RL, Isley JP, Atkinson RL. An association of elevated serum gonadotropin concentrations and Alzheimer disease? *J Neuroendocrinol.* 2000;**12**(4):351–4.

10. Hogervorst E, Williams J, Budge M, *et al.* Serum total testosterone is lower in men with Alzheimer's disease. *Neuro Endocrinol Lett.* 2001;**22**(3):163–8.

11. Hogervorst E, Combrinck M, Smith AD. Testosterone and gonadotropin levels in men with dementia. *Neuro Endocrinol Lett.* 2003;**24**(3/4):203–8.

12. Hogervorst E, Bandelow S, Combrinck M, Smith AD. Low free testosterone is an independent risk factor for Alzheimer's disease. *Exp Gerontol.* 2004;**39**(11/12):1633–9.

13. Rosario ER, Chang L, Stanczyk FZ, Pike CJ. Age-related testosterone depletion and the development of Alzheimer disease. *JAMA.* 2004;**292**(12):1431–2.

14. Moffat SD, Zonderman AB, Metter EJ, *et al.* Free testosterone and risk for Alzheimer disease in older men. *Neurology.* 2004;**62**(2):188–93.

15. Burkhardt MS, Foster JK, Clarnette RM, *et al.* Interaction between testosterone and apolipoprotein E epsilon4 status on cognition in healthy older men. *J Clin Endocrinol Metab.* 2006;**91**(3):1168–72.

16. Ahlbom E, Prins GS, Ceccatelli S. Testosterone protects cerebellar granule cells from oxidative stress-induced cell death through a receptor mediated mechanism. *Brain Res.* 2001;**892**(2):255–62.

17. Behl C, Skutella T, Lezoualch F, *et al.* Neuroprotection against oxidative stress by estrogens: structure-activity relationship. *Mol Pharmacol.* 1997;**51**(4):535–41.

18. Azcoitia I, Sierra A, Veiga S, *et al.* Brain aromatase is neuroprotective. *J Neurobiol.* 2001;**47**(4):318–29.

19. Atroshi F, Paulin L, Paalanen T, Westermarck T. Glutathione level in mice brain after testosterone administration. *Adv Exp Med Biol.* 1990;**264**:199–202.

20. Garcia-Estrada J, Luquin S, Fernandez AM, Garcia-Segura LM. Dehydroepiandrosterone, pregnenolone and sex steroids down-regulate reactive astroglia in the male rat brain after a penetrating brain injury. *Int J Dev Neurosci.* 1999;**17**(2):145–51.

21. Gouras GK, Xu H, Gross RS, *et al.* Testosterone reduces neuronal secretion of Alzheimer's beta-amyloid peptides. *Proc Natl Acad Sci USA.* 2000;**97**(3):1202–5.

22. Goodenough S, Engert S, Behl C. Testosterone stimulates rapid secretory amyloid precursor protein release from rat hypothalamic cells via the activation of the mitogen-activated protein kinase pathway. *Neurosci Lett.* 2000;**296**(1):49–52.

23. Desdouits-Magnen J, Desdouits F, Takeda S, *et al.* Regulation of secretion of Alzheimer amyloid precursor protein by the mitogen-activated protein kinase cascade. *J Neurochem.* 1998;**70**(2):524–30.

24. Nguyen TV, Yao M, Pike CJ. Androgens activate mitogen-activated protein kinase signaling: role in neuroprotection. *J Neurochem.* 2005;**94**(6):1639–51.

25. Bi R, Broutman G, Foy MR, Thompson RF, Baudry M. The tyrosine kinase and mitogen-activated protein kinase pathways mediate multiple effects of estrogen in hippocampus. *Proc Natl Acad Sci USA.* 2000;**97**(7):3602–7.

26. Manthey D, Heck S, Engert S, Behl C. Estrogen induces a rapid secretion of amyloid beta precursor protein via the mitogen-activated protein kinase pathway. *Eur J Biochem.* 2001;**268**(15):4285–91.

27. Ramsden M, Nyborg AC, Murphy MP, *et al.* Androgens modulate beta-amyloid levels in male rat brain. *J Neurochem.* 2003;**87**(4):1052–5.

28. Gandy S, Almeida OP, Fonte J, *et al.* Chemical andropause and amyloid-beta peptide. *JAMA.* 2001;**285**(17):2195–6.

29. Gillett MJ, Martins RN, Clarnette RM, *et al.* Relationship between testosterone, sex hormone binding globulin and plasma amyloid beta peptide

40 in older men with subjective memory loss or dementia. *J Alzheimers Dis.* 2003;**5**(4):267–9.

30. Almeida OP, Waterreus A, Spry N, Flicker L, Martins RN. One year follow-up study of the association between chemical castration, sex hormones, beta-amyloid, memory and depression in men. *Psychoneuroendocrinology.* 2004;**29**(8):1071–81.

31. Rosario ER, Carroll JC, Oddo S, LaFerla FM, Pike CJ. Androgens regulate the development of neuropathology in a triple transgenic mouse model of Alzheimer's disease. *J Neurosci.* 2006;**26**(51):13384–9.

32. Hobbs CJ, Jones RE, Plymate SR. The effects of sex hormone binding globulin (SHBG) on testosterone transport into the cerebrospinal fluid. *J Steroid Biochem Mol Biol.* 1992;**42**(6):629–35.

33. Dubey AK, Herbert J, Abbott DH, Martensz ND. Serum and CSF concentrations of testosterone and LH related to negative feedback in male rhesus monkeys. *Neuroendocrinology.* 1984;**39**(2):176–85.

34. Moffat SD. Does testosterone mediate cognitive decline in elderly men? *J Gerontol A Biol Sci Med Sci.* 2006;**61**(5):521.

35. Yaffe K, Haan M, Byers A, Tangen C, Kuller L. Estrogen use, APOE, and cognitive decline: evidence of gene-environment interaction. *Neurology.* 2000;**54**(10):1949–54.

36. Burkhardt MS, Foster JK, Laws SM, *et al.* Oestrogen replacement therapy may improve memory functioning in the absence of APOE epsilon4. *J Alzheimers Dis.* 2004;**6**(3):221–8.

37. Raber J, Bongers G, LeFevour A, Buttini M, Mucke L. Androgens protect against apolipoprotein E4-induced cognitive deficits. *J Neurosci.* 2002;**22**(12):5204–9.

38. Johnson MEBJ. *Essential Reproduction.* London: Blackwell Science, 2000.

39. Short RA, Bowen RL, O'Brien PC, Graff-Radford NR. Elevated gonadotropin levels in patients with Alzheimer disease. *Mayo Clin Proc.* 2001;**76**(9):906–9.

40. Bowen RL, Smith MA, Harris PL, *et al.* Elevated luteinizing hormone expression colocalizes with neurons vulnerable to Alzheimer's disease pathology. *J Neurosci Res.* 2002;**70**(3):514–18.

41. Bowen RL, Verdile G, Liu T, *et al.* Luteinizing hormone, a reproductive regulator that modulates the processing of amyloid-beta precursor protein and amyloid-beta deposition. *J Biol Chem.* 2004;**279**(19): 20539–45.

42. Wilson AC, Salamat MS, Haasl RJ, *et al.* Human neurons express type I GnRH receptor and respond to GnRH I by increasing luteinizing hormone expression. *J Endocrinol.* 2006;**191**(3):651–63.

43. Lei ZM, Rao CV. Neural actions of luteinizing hormone and human chorionic gonadotropin. *Semin Reprod Med.* 2001;**19**(1):103–9.

44. Wood JR, Strauss JF, 3rd. Multiple signal transduction pathways regulate ovarian steroidogenesis. *Rev Endocr Metab Disord.* 2002;**3**(1):33–46.

45. Webber KM, Stocco DM, Casadesus G, *et al.* Steroidogenic acute regulatory protein (StAR): evidence of gonadotropin-induced steroidogenesis in Alzheimer disease. *Mol Neurodegener.* 2006;**1**:14.

46. Marambaud P, Chevallier N, Ancolio K, Checler F. Post-transcriptional contribution of a cAMP-dependent pathway to the formation of alpha- and beta/gamma-secretases-derived products of beta APP maturation in human cells expressing wild-type and Swedish mutated beta APP. *Mol Med.* 1998;**4**(11):715–23.

47. Su Y, Ryder J, Ni B. Inhibition of Abeta production and APP maturation by a specific PKA inhibitor. *FEBS Lett.* 2003;**546**(2/3):407–10.

48. Bagshawe KD, Orr AH, Rushworth AG. Relationship between concentrations of human chorionic gonadotrophin in plasma and cerebrospinal fluid. *Nature.* 1968;**217**(5132):950–1.

49. Lukacs H, Hiatt ES, Lei ZM, Rao CV. Peripheral and intracerebroventricular administration of human chorionic gonadotropin alters several hippocampus-associated behaviors in cycling female rats. *Horm Behav.* 1995;**29**(1):42–58.

50. Casadesus G, Webber KM, Atwood CS, *et al.* Luteinizing hormone modulates cognition and amyloid-beta deposition in Alzheimer APP transgenic mice. *Biochim Biophys Acta.* 2006;**1762**(4): 447–52.

Chapter 28

Epilogue

Wulf H. Utian

Surveys of women transiting menopause at the usual age of 45 to 55 years overwhelmingly confirm that their greatest fear regarding hormone therapy (HT) is that of breast cancer. Survey women a decade older or more, and you learn that their greatest concern has now become memory loss and Alzheimer's disease (AD). As recently as a decade ago there was increasing optimism that replacement of the female sex steroids – estrogens and progesterone – as well as testosterone for women beyond menopause could be the key to maintenance or recovery of memory. Then came studies like the Women's Health Initiative Memory Study (WHIMS) to dampen expectations and sow confusion. The preceding chapters demonstrate that the entire subject of memory and cognition, and the pathological aspects thereof, is far more complex, and it cannot be explained away by one simple mechanism.

Recently, a committee of experts was convened by the North American Menopause Society (NAMS) to attempt to digest the existing literature into a set of clinical recommendations [1]. They commenced by defining the term "cognition" as a group of mental processes by which knowledge is acquired or used, encompassing such mental skills as concentration, learning and memory, language, spatial abilities, judgment, and reasoning. They recognized that cognitive abilities change throughout life, and that with advancing age performance tends to decline on many, but not all, cognitive tests.

The expert panel concluded that although memory complaints are common in midlife, findings from well characterized cohorts suggest that natural menopause has little effect on memory performance or other areas of cognitive function. They further concluded that limited, short-term clinical trial data among younger postmenopausal women suggest that estrogen–progestogen HT does not have a substantial impact on cognition after natural menopause. As inferred from very small, short-term clinical trials, estrogen therapy initiated promptly after bilateral oophorectomy may improve verbal memory. Several observational studies report no association between age at menopause and AD. However, a case-control study found that bilateral oophorectomy before menopause was associated with an elevated risk of cognitive impairment or dementia, and this risk increased with younger age at oophorectomy. All this information has been expanded on in depth in the pages of this book.

For postmenopausal women over the age of 60, the NAMS panel noted that findings from several large, well designed clinical trials indicate that HT does not improve memory or other cognitive abilities. One trial within the Women's Health Initiative – WHIMS – of women aged 65 to 79 reported an increase in dementia incidence with estrogen therapy and estrogen–progestogen therapy. The estimate of dementia cases attributed to HT was 12 per 10,000 persons per year of use of conjugated estrogens, and 23 per 10,000 persons per year of use of conjugated estrogens and medroxyprogesterone acetate.

By way of contrast, a number of observational studies have reported associations between HT use and reduced risk of developing AD. Hormone therapy exposure in observational studies is more likely to involve use by younger women closer to the age of menopause than women eligible for the WHIMS trial. Speculatively, this difference implies an early window during which HT use might reduce AD risk.

Hormones, Cognition and Dementia: State of the Art and Emergent Therapeutic Strategies, ed. Eef Hogervorst, Victor W. Henderson, Robert B. Gibbs, and Roberta Diaz Brinton. Published by Cambridge University Press.
© Cambridge University Press 2009.

However, recall bias and the healthy-user bias may account for protective associations in the observational studies, many of which are difficult to interpret because of fairly small numbers of study participants. The window of opportunity perspective is supported by limited evidence, but no clinical trial data address long-term cognitive consequences of HT exposures during the menopause transition and early postmenopause. For women with AD, limited clinical results suggest that therapy with an estrogen has no substantial effect on dementia symptoms or progression.

Based on these considerations, the NAMS expert panel concluded that HT cannot be recommended at any age for the sole or primary indication of preventing cognitive aging or dementia. Hormone therapy seems to increase the incidence of dementia when initiated in women age 65 and older. Similarly, HT should not be used to enhance cognitive function in younger postmenopausal women with intact ovaries, although very small clinical trials support the use of estrogens initiated immediately after menopause induced by bilateral oophorectomy. Available data do not adequately address whether HT used soon after menopause increases or decreases later dementia risk. Limited data do not support the use of HT as treatment of AD.

Clearly the existing data, despite demonstrating the limitations of current knowledge, open ideas and offer possibilities for further research into the relationships between hormones and cognition. Where that research is at present is well described in the previous chapters, covering the basics of cell culture, the use of artificial neural networks, study of animal biology and behavior, other hormone systems like insulin pathways and gonadotropins, protein metabolism, and eventually translating this basic scientific endeavor into clinical research studies. Epidemiological observations help to direct some lines of research, although in themselves they cannot directly link cause and effect. This raises the necessity for testing multiple steroidal drugs in varying doses, combinations, and routes of delivery. The transnasal approach, as described in one of the chapters, is just one intriguing approach. Beyond that will be the testing of earlier generation estrogen agonist–antagonist molecules, and as an area of rapid drug development in a relatively early stage, the potential of testing new and ever better designed molecules. As basic mechanisms of brain cell metabolism and neural pathways are revealed, the possibility exists for specific ligand receptor products to be developed with planned and precisely targeted activity.

The contents of this book reveal the exciting frontier of the new science of brain and memory research, and should act as a stimulus to basic science and clinical researchers going forward. We are just scratching the surface of the science and the potential for defeating what is one of the most devastating problems facing humanity, namely the loss of memory and its impact on the individual and the family.

Reference

1. Utian WH, Archer DF, Bachmann GA, *et al.* Estrogen and progestogen use in postmenopausal women: July 2008 position statement of the North American Menopause Society. *Menopause.* 2008;**15**:584–602.

Chapter 29

Concluding remarks

Eef Hogervorst, Victor W. Henderson, Robert B. Gibbs, and Roberta Diaz Brinton

The Women's Health Initiative Memory Study (WHIMS), an ancillary study of the Women's Health Initiative, comprised two large parallel randomized placebo-controlled clinical trials, one of women with a uterus and one of women who had undergone hysterectomy. The largest study of its kind, the WHIMS had been set up to further investigate the promising protective effects of estrogen treatment on the aging brain. The primary outcomes were specified as all-cause dementia or Alzheimer's disease, but other cognitive outcomes were explored as well. The WHIMS reported a completely unexpected increased risk of dementia with combined conjugated equine estrogens (CEE) and medroxy-progesterone acetate (MPA) treatment in women of 65 years of age and older and a trend for increased risk with CEE alone. The number of incident cases was too small to consider Alzheimer's disease as a separate outcome. Secondary ancillary analyses also showed negative effects on verbal memory functions after an average of three years of treatment. This was particularly surprising, as verbal memory functions were thought to be more likely to benefit from estrogens treatment and are usually the earliest affected cognitive functions in dementia due to Alzheimer's disease.

Many researchers argued that there may have been subgroups for whom hormone treatment (HT) would have been successful. Perhaps women from the WHIMS might not have been representative because they were too often obese or had too many other risk factors for dementia. In Chapter 2 authors presented novel statistical techniques to analyze data using artificial neural networks to identify treatment responders. The models derived from subsets of data using artificial neural network analyses with cross-validation techniques showed good predictive value for the simplest models. These would be comparable to logistic regression models limited to only main effects (not including interactions). More complex models that included non-linear interactions could fit the training data with 100% accuracy, but did not achieve better predictive accuracy on novel data. The results of Chapters 1 and 2 thus suggested that there were no particular subgroups of older women for whom estrogen treatment would be indicated to reduce dementia risk or improve aspects of cognition tested in the WHIMS. This finding, however, does not explain why positive results of estrogens on cognition were reported in observational studies or in some earlier smaller treatment trials.

The WHIMS had included women of 65 years and older for whom HT for vasomotor menopausal complaints would ordinarily not be considered. Most observational studies on dementia risk had included estrogens used by younger, relatively recent menopausal women for whom treatment would perhaps be more often considered. This difference, backed up by evidence from animal and observational human studies, led to the "window of opportunity," or "critical window," theory. The "window of opportunity" theory is introduced from both the animal (Chapter 5) and human perspective (Chapter 4). This theory suggests that estrogens may be effective and may have positive effects on brain function when given close to the age of menopause; however, this would not explain the negative effects of estrogens on dementia risk in women over the age of 65.

The "healthy cell bias" hypothesis (Chapter 6) attempts to explain these negative findings using convincing evidence from cell culture studies. This theory suggests that estrogens would not have beneficial effects on neurons that are undergoing pathological changes such as those observed in dementia. This chapter also discusses the possibility of optimal estrogens dosage for beneficial effects on the brain, and the evidence for interactions of estrogens treatment with the APOE genotype. This genotype is associated with an increased risk of dementia and is thought to modify the effect of HT. This intriguing possibility is further discussed in Section 4 in more detail, which suggests that genetic screening would be a future possibility in the assessment of risks and benefits.

Observational data presented in Chapter 3 from a cohort of women over 90 years of age also suggest an increased risk of dementia with HT, which further substantiate the "healthy cell bias" hypothesis. On the other hand, mortality was lowered with hormone use in this study, similar to other cohorts investigating this association. The data presented suggested a significantly increased risk of hormone use only between 5 to 9 years duration. It is possible that survival effects and power issues may have affected these analyses, and more data from older women who used HT for a prolonged period of time need to be analyzed.

In the second section of the book scientists discuss alternative reasons for the negative results found in the WHIMS and the possibility of using alternative treatment strategies. For instance, some authors suggested that the type of estrogens given could be responsible for the negative effects found in the WHIMS. Transdermal estradiol might be a safer form of HT than oral forms of estrogens. The positive effects of transdermal estradiol in healthy women and women with dementia were discussed in Chapters 7 and 8. A large currently ongoing trial using estradiol is also described in Chapter 7, which, it is to be hoped, will provide answers to the many questions raised by the WHIMS.

Another theory is that continuous treatment with estrogens has negative effects on the brain. The use of a more natural form of estradiol treatment for menopausal complaints is discussed in Chapter 9. Administration of estradiol using a nasal spray allows pulsatile fluctuations of estradiol levels, which may mimic the natural rhythmic secretion of estradiol in premenopausal women more closely and may therefore have a safer and more effective profile than continuous oral administration. Selective estrogen receptor modulators

have traditionally been described for estrogen-sensitive cancers. The effect of these forms of HT on cognitive function is discussed in Chapter 10. In the chapters of Section 2, both risks and benefits are discussed for alternative treatments, which, it is to be hoped, enables the clinician to make a better judgment about the use of these potential alternatives for menopausal complaints.

In the third section of this book, possible modifiers of the effect of estrogens on the brain are described. These modifiers could perhaps explain some of the discrepancies found among studies. For instance, many scientists have suggested that the addition of a progestogen was detrimental to the effect of estrogens. This evidence is discussed in more detail in Chapter 11. In particular medroxy-progesterone acetate does not seem to be the first progestogen of choice for treatment of menopausal complaints. Its negative effects on the vascular system were already described in the 1980s.

Chronic cortisol elevations produced during stress appear to have a negative impact on the aging brain. Estradiol could have protective effects in this context either by reducing hypothalamic-pituitary-adrenal activity or by preventing glucocorticoid-induced adverse effects on neuronal integrity. However, other short-term data suggested that elevated cortisol can counteract the positive effects of estrogens on the brain. This might explain why women who are in certain (stressful, anxious, etc.) psychophysiological or perhaps ill states would not benefit from estrogen treatment. These hypotheses are discussed in more detail in Chapter 14.

There are many other potential interactions of sex steroids with other hormones that are not discussed in this section, simply because of lack of time and space, such as the interaction with growth hormone, thyroid function, and insulin, for instance. Work presented by Craft [1] suggested that, like many of the other hormones mentioned, insulin can act as a neuromodulator and has been found to be involved in neuronal maintenance, energy metabolism, neurogenesis, and neurotransmitter regulation, as well as neuronal firing and long-term potentiation involved in memory and other cognitive activity. Data suggest that postmenopausal women experience an increased risk of developing type 2 diabetes mellitus, but that estrogen treatment increases insulin sensitivity. Craft found that women with

AD had lower rates of insulin-mediated glucose disposal, and thus have lower insulin sensitivity. Diabetes mellitus has also been found to be a risk factor for dementia. However, studies by Craft [1] showed that women with AD who received HT had a three-fold increase in their insulin-mediated glucose disposal rates and lower insulin levels in the hyperinsulinemic condition compared with AD subjects not receiving HT. The authors suggested that improvements in insulin sensitivity may mediate potential beneficial effects on estrogens on memory and attention.

Others have suggested that it is the modification of estrogens on mood and sleep during the menopausal transition that mediates the positive effect on memory. This possibility is discussed in Chapter 12 and would explain why the largest effect sizes of treatment studies have been seen in women with severe menopausal complaints. As selective serotonin reuptake inhibitors (SSRI) also treat flashes and may affect sleep, these may be considered as an alternative treatment for women with severe menopausal complaints. Future studies should investigate the efficacy of SSRI versus HTs in improving cognitive function in women with severe mood and sleep disorders resulting from hormonal fluctuations in the perimenopause.

Lastly, data from Oxford showed that folate could counteract the negative effects of estrogens in older women. Data from phytoestrogens (plant estrogens abundant in soy products), with and without folate, and their association with cognitive functions and possible dementia were discussed in Chapter 13. Intriguingly, these data also showed increased risks for memory impairment and dementia with high levels and high intake of these estrogen-like compounds in women and men over 68 years of age. However, optimal phytoestrogen levels for optimal cognitive functions (curvilinear associations) were seen in those who were young-old (52–68 years of age). This suggests modification of estrogen-like compounds on cognition by both age and dosage.

These data of Section 2 combined could thus suggest that other morbidity such as insulin resistance, anxiety, depression, and sleep disorders, but also low folate levels, could significantly interact with the efficacy obtained from estrogen treatment. Investigating these modifiers using higher order interactions requires large datasets. In addition, the biochemistry

assays to assess these compounds are costly, and funding for hormone studies has been more difficult to obtain after the WHIMS data were published. Section 4 discussed the possibility that genetics further modify the risk for dementia with use of estrogens and testosterone. This could suggest that genetic screening may be an option when deciding on risks and benefits associated with HT in the future. The potentially relevant genetic polymorphisms have been discussed, but these need to be further substantiated in future studies. The current development of cheaper and faster ways of large-scale genetic screening will hopefully enable researchers to do so.

In Section 5 the effects of testosterone in men and women were discussed from various angles. There were observational data, including novel brain scan data from the Baltimore Longitudinal Study on Aging, and treatment results for both men and women. Some of the observational data suggested negative effects of high levels of estrogens on cognitive function, not only for older women but also for older men, which would be in line with the "healthy cell bias" theory. The role of sex hormone binding globulin in age-related decline and dementia was highlighted. Lowering levels of this globulin using Danazol® and thereby increasing bioavailable estrogens and testosterone levels may be a novel treatment strategy worth investigating in the future. Section 6 discussed the possibility of another treatment angle for dementia. Animal, cell culture, and small treatment studies suggest that research should focus on lowering gonadotropins, which are very neurotoxic, rather than on increasing levels of estrogens or testosterone. Evidence for and against the use of leuprolide acetate in older men versus use of testosterone which also lowers gonadotropin levels, was discussed from the perspective of animal cell culture and human studies.

In summary, this book brings together basic scientists and clinical investigators using a variety of experimental and observational approaches to attempt to find an answer to apparent discrepancies between the negative effects of estrogens found in the WHIMS and conflicting data showing the protective effects of estrogens on the aging brain. As with many risk factors for dementia, a consensus seems to be growing that midlife is a crucial time to intervene to reduce the risk for late-life dementia. Lowering blood pressure, cholesterol, and body weight in midlife is mentioned as important to reduce the risk for dementia and cardiovascular disease in later life. Whether HT has a role in this approach, or whether hormone use was only part of a "healthy lifestyle" adopted by women who were at a general lower risk for dementia remains to be further investigated.

Reference

1. Craft S. Insulin resistance and Alzheimer's disease pathogenesis: potential mechanisms and implications for treatment. *Curr Alzheimer Res.* 2007;4(2):147–52.

Index

275

Printed in the United States
by Baker & Taylor Publisher Services